Perspectives on →

Occupational Therapy Education

Past, Present, and Future

Perspectives on ⟶

Occupational Therapy Education

Past, Present, and Future

Steven D. Taff, PhD, OTR/L, FNAP, FAOTA
Director, Division of Professional Education
Associate Professor of Occupational Therapy and Medicine
Program in Occupational Therapy
Washington University School of Medicine
St. Louis, Missouri

Lenin C. Grajo, PhD, EdM, OTR/L
Director, Post-Professional Doctor of Occupational Therapy Program
Assistant Professor, Programs in Occupational Therapy
Department of Rehabilitation and Regenerative Medicine
Vagelos College of Physicians and Surgeons
Columbia University
New York City, New York

Barbara R. Hooper, PhD, OTR/L, FAOTA
Program Director and Division Chief
Occupational Therapy Doctorate Division
Duke University
Durham, North Carolina

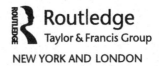

Routledge
Taylor & Francis Group

NEW YORK AND LONDON

Perspectives on Occupational Therapy Education: Past, Present, and Future includes ancillary materials specifically available for faculty use. Included are PowerPoint Slides. Please visit https://www.routledge.com/9781630915476 to obtain access.

First published in 2020 by SLACK Incorporated

Published 2024 by Routledge
605 Third Avenue, New York, NY 10017

and by Routledge
4 Park Square, Milton Park, Abingdon, Oxon OX14 4RN

Routledge is an imprint of the Taylor & Francis Group, an informa business

© 2020 Taylor & Francis Group

Cover Artist: Anita Santiago

Library of Congress Cataloging-in-Publication Data

Names: Taff, Steven D., author. | Grajo, Lenin C., author. | Hooper,
  Barbara, Ph. D., author.
Title: Perspectives in occupational therapy education : past, present, and
  future / Steven D. Taff, Lenin C. Grajo, Barbara R. Hooper.
Description: Thorofare, NJ : SLACK Incorporated, 2019. | Includes
  bibliographical references and index.
Identifiers: LCCN 2019034967 | ISBN 9781630915476 (paperback)
Subjects: MESH: Occupational Therapy--education | United States
Classification: LCC RM735.42 | NLM WB 18 | DDC 615.8/515071--dc23
LC record available at https://lccn.loc.gov/2019034967

ISBN: 9781630915476 (pbk)
ISBN: 9781003525615 (ebk)

DOI: 10.4324/9781003525615

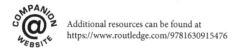

Additional resources can be found at
https://www.routledge.com/9781630915476

DEDICATION

This book is dedicated to all occupational therapy educators—past, present, and future. These occupational therapy educators are visionary leaders who have and continue to form communities of learners, enhance the student experience, and influence the continual growth of the occupational therapy profession by inspiring future practitioners.

CONTENTS

Section III: Future

ACKNOWLEDGMENTS

We would like to thank our contributing authors who have shared with us our vision for this first comprehensive text on occupational therapy education. These authors are accomplished educators who have made and continue to make outstanding contributions in occupational therapy education in the United States and all over the world.

We also thank our colleagues and friends at SLACK Incorporated: Brien Cummings, our Acquisitions Editor; Allegra Tiver, our Managing Editor; and Joe Lowery, our Project Editor. Thank you for advocating for this project and moving it forward.

From Dr. Steven D. Taff

Thank you to all my teachers and mentors over the years. I am especially grateful to those in my doctoral program who helped transform my thoughts about teaching and learning: Scot Danforth, Phil Ferguson, Virginia Navarro, Marvin Berkowitz, and Matt Keefer. I am so thankful to have worked with a stellar team of scholars in occupational therapy education including Andrea Bilics, Barb Hooper, Sheama Krishnagiri, Maralynne Mitcham, and Pollie Price. A special nod to Andrea Bilics for her mentorship and support as I navigated the complexities of academia. Finally, thanks to my colleagues in education in our profession and the faculty at Washington University School of Medicine, particularly the Program in Occupational Therapy; I learn from each of you every day.

Thanks also to the talented and dedicated teachers and support staff with whom I worked as a clinician in the school setting. A sincere thank you to all the students with whom I've learned since entering academia. Creating communities of learning with you has been a highlight of my career.

Last, but certainly not least, I want to thank my family and friends, particularly my wife Helen and our boys Aidan and Ryan; you provide the foundation for everything I do.

From Dr. Lenin C. Grajo

Thank you to all my teachers and educators who have mentored me, inspired me to become an effective educator, and challenged the way I learned and taught. Most especially, thank you to Prof. Maria Concepcion Cabatan, Dr. Cathy Candler, and Dr. Sally Schultz.

Thank you to three outstanding centers that continue to advance excellence in teaching and learning, prepare and advance skills of educators, and have made significant contributions to my professional development as an educator: The National Teacher Training Center for the Health Professions of the University of the Philippines Manila, the Reinert Center for Transformative Teaching and Learning at Saint Louis University, and the Center for Teaching and Learning at Columbia University. Thank you to my ever-supportive colleagues in the Programs in Occupational Therapy at Columbia University, and most especially to Dr. Janet Falk-Kessler and Dr. Glen Gillen who took a chance on me as a young educator and welcomed me to this great family.

Thank you to my Aunt Elnora who has always, and sometimes ambivalently, supported my passion and dream to become an educator; and to my sister Marijo who inspires me in all that I do.

Lastly, I want to thank all my former and current students at the bachelor's, master's, and doctoral levels. Every small and big teaching-learning moment and encounter with each of you have made me the educator I am today.

From Dr. Barbara R. Hooper

What a privilege it is to get to design learning experiences through which students connect—mind, body, and spirit—with the profession of occupational therapy. For all those educators and mentors who led me through that threshold and fueled my passion for learning, teaching, and occupation; for all who showed me the craft of designing learning experiences; and for the students who have been courageous enough to go on the journey with me and teach me, I am immensely grateful. And I thank my spouse, Dr. Wendy Wood, my co- in everything.

ABOUT THE EDITORS

Steven D. Taff, PhD, OTR/L, FNAP, FAOTA is the Director of the Division of Professional Education and Associate Professor in the Occupational Therapy and Department of Medicine Program, and Director of the Teaching Scholars Program at Washington University School of Medicine in St. Louis, Missouri. He is also co-founder of the Cross-Campus Educational Research Group, a multidisciplinary community of educational scholars and innovators at Washington University in St. Louis. Dr. Taff served as the Chair of the Commission on Education of the American Occupational Therapy Association (AOTA) from 2016 to 2019 and is also a member of the leadership group of the AOTA Scholarship of Teaching and Learning Program. He was a recipient of the Emerson Excellence in Teaching Award in 2017.

Lenin C. Grajo, PhD, EdM, OTR/L is the Director of the Post-Professional Doctor of Occupational Therapy Program and Assistant Professor in the Programs in Occupational Therapy, Department of Rehabilitation and Regenerative Medicine in the Vagelos College of Physicians and Surgeons at Columbia University Irving Medical Center in New York, NY.

Dr. Grajo was elected Chairperson of the Academic Education Special Interest Section (AESIS) of the AOTA and a member of the Commission on Education of AOTA from 2016 to 2019. Through AESIS, he has co-developed mentoring programs for new occupational therapy and occupational therapy assistant educators and fieldwork coordinators. He is a multi-awarded educator who has taught in the Philippines and the United States.

Barbara R. Hooper, PhD, OTR/L, FAOTA is the occupational therapy doctorate Program Director and Division Chief at Duke University. Dr. Hooper is the director of the Center for Occupational Therapy Education (COTE), an education research and professional development center for occupational therapy educators and programs. Barb has been involved in several national-level occupational therapy education initiatives, including the American Occupational Therapy Foundation (AOTF) Curriculum Mentors project, AOTA Future of Education Task Force, founding committee for the AOTF (now AOTA) Scholarship of Teaching and Learning Program, co-author of the original AOTA Educational Research Agenda, and co-author of the previous AOTA Educational Philosophy Statement. She served as the principal investigator on a national study of occupational therapy education co-sponsored by the Society for the Study of Occupation—USA and the AOTF. She has received teaching awards at the University of New Mexico and Colorado State University.

Contributing Authors

Rebecca M. Aldrich, PhD, OTR/L
(Chapter 11)
Associate Professor of Clinical
Occupational Therapy
University of Southern California
Los Angeles, California

Sue Baptiste, OTDip, MHSc, FCAOT
(Chapter 14)
Professor Emerita
Faculty of Health Sciences
McMaster University
Hamilton, Canada

Andrea R. Bilics, PhD, OTR/L, FAOTA
(Foreword)
Professor Emeritus
Worcester State University
Worcester, Massachusetts

Maria Concepcion Cabatan, MHPEd,
OTRP, OTR, FPAOT (Chapter 12)
Professor
Department of Occupational Therapy
College of Allied Medical Professions
University of the Philippines—Manila
Manila, Philippines

Catherine Candler, PhD, OTR, BCP
(Chapter 4)
Professor
Department of Occupational Therapy
Abilene Christian University
Abilene, Texas

Nancy E. Carson, PhD, OTR/L, FAOTA
(Chapter 20)
Associate Professor
Division of Occupational Therapy
Medical University of South Carolina
Charleston, South Carolina

Susan M. Cleghorn, DrOT, OTR/L, TRS,
CAPS, FNAP (Chapter 6)
Associate Professor of Occupational
Science and Therapy
Grand Valley State University
Grand Rapids, Michigan

Susan Coppola, OTD, OT/L, FAOTA
(Chapter 19)
Professor
Division of Occupational Science and
Occupational Therapy
University of North Carolina at Chapel Hill
Chapel Hill, North Carolina

Tina DeAngelis, EdD, OTR/L (Chapter 3)
Director, Doctorate Program in
Occupational Therapy
Jefferson College of
Rehabilitation Sciences
Thomas Jefferson University
Philadelphia, Pennsylvania

R. Lyle Duque, MSc, OTRP, FPAOT
(Chapter 12)
Program Director and Founder
Life Skills Therapy Center
Chairperson
Continuing Professional Development
Council for Occupational Therapy
Member
Professional Regulatory Board for Physical
Therapy and Occupational Therapy
Manila, Philippines

Amy R. Early, OTD, OTR/L (Chapter 9)
Behavioral Health Occupational Therapist
UI Health
University of Illinois at Chicago
and MemoryCare Corporation
Chicago, Illinois

Maria Luísa Guillaumon Emmel, OT, PhD
(Chapter 13)
Senior Professor
Occupational Therapy Postgraduate Program
Federal University of São Carlos
São Paulo, Brazil

Mirela de Oliveira Figueiredo, OT, PhD
(Chapter 13)
Professor
Occupational Therapy Postgraduate Program
Federal University of São Carlos
São Paulo, Brazil

Roshan Galvaan, PhD, MSc (OccTher),
BSc (OccTher) (Chapter 17)
Professor
Department of Health and
Rehabilitation Sciences
Division of Occupational Therapy
University of Cape Town
Cape Town, South Africa

Amanda K. Giles, OTD, OTR/L
(Chapter 18)
Assistant Professor
Division of Occupational Therapy
Medical University of South Carolina
Charleston, South Carolina

Sharon A. Gutman, PhD, OTR, FAOTA
(Chapter 7)
Professor
Programs in Occupational Therapy
Department of Rehabilitation and
Regenerative Medicine
Columbia University
New York, New York

Neil Harvison, PhD, OTR, FNAP, FAOTA
(Chapter 21)
Chief Officer
Knowledge
American Occupational Therapy Association
Bethesda, Maryland

Susan M. Higgins, OTD, OTR/L
(Chapter 19)
Academic Fieldwork Coordinator/Lecturer
Boston School of Occupational Therapy
Tufts University
Middlesex County, Massachusetts

William E. Janes, OTD, MSCI, OTR/L
(Chapter 18)
Assistant Professor and
Academic Fieldwork Coordinator
Department of Occupational Therapy
University of Missouri School of
Health Professions
Columbia, Missouri

Sheama Krishnagiri, PhD, OTR/L, FAOTA
(Chapter 10)
Occupational Therapist
Private Practice
Tarzana, California

Giulianne Krug, PhD, OTR, CLA
(Chapter 3)
Founding Program Director and Professor
Occupational Therapy Program
University of Mary Hardin-Baylor
Belton, Texas

Wanda J. Mahoney, PhD, OTR/L
(Chapter 2)
Associate Professor
Program in Occupational Therapy
Washington University School of Medicine
St. Louis, Missouri

Daniel Marinho Cezar da Cruz, PhD, OT
(Chapter 13)
Professor
Occupational Therapy Graduate Program
Universidade Federal de São Carlos
São Paulo, Brazil

Lauren E. Milton, OTD, OTR/L (Chapter 5)
Assistant Professor
Occupational Therapy and Medicine
Program in Occupational Therapy
Washington University School of Medicine
St. Louis, Missouri

Matthew Molineux, BOccThy, MSc,
PhD, MBA (Chapter 16)
Professor and Head
Discipline of Occupational Therapy
School of Allied Health Sciences
Griffith University
Queensland, Australia

Jaime P. Muñoz, PhD, OTR/L, FAOTA
(Chapter 9)
Department Chair and Associate Professor
Duquesne University
Pittsburgh, Pennsylvania

Monica S. Perlmutter, OTD, OTR/L, SCLV,
FAOTA (Chapter 6)
Associate Professor
Program in Occupational Therapy and
Ophthalmology and Visual Sciences
Washington University School of Medicine
St. Louis, Missouri

Liesl Peters, BSc (OccTher), MSc (OccTher)
(Chapter 17)
Senior Lecturer
Division of Occupational Therapy
Department of Health and
Rehabilitation Sciences
Faculty of Health Sciences
University of Cape Town
Cape Town, South Africa

Bridgett Piernik-Yoder, PhD, OTR
(Chapter 3)
Associate Professor and Chair
Department of Occupational Therapy
University of Texas Health Science Center
at San Antonio
San Antonio, Texas

Pollie Price, PhD, OTR/L, FAOTA
(Chapter 10)
Associate Professor
Post-Professional OTD Program Director
Associate Chair
Department of Occupational and
Recreational Therapies
University of Utah
Salt Lake City, Utah

Melanie Roberts, BAppSc (OccThy), MClinRehab
(Chapter 16)
Senior Lecturer
Discipline of Occupational Therapy
School of Allied Health Sciences
Griffith University
Queensland, Australia

Patricia Schaber, PhD, OTR/L, FAOTA
(Chapter 4)
Associate Professor
Program in Occupational Therapy
University of Minnesota
Minneapolis, Minnesota

Stacy Smallfield, DrOT, MSOT, OTR/L,
BCG, FAOTA (Chapter 5)
Assistant Director
Entry-Level Professional Programs
Associate Professor
Occupational Therapy and Medicine
Program in Occupational Therapy
Washington University School of Medicine
St. Louis, Missouri

Yolanda Suarez-Balcazar, PhD (Chapter 9)
Professor and Head
Department of Occupational Therapy
Professor
Department of Disability and
Human Development
Affiliate Faculty
Department of Psychology
University of Illinois
Chicago, Illinois

Hanneke van Bruggen, BSc OT, Hon. Dscie,
FWFOT (Chapter 15)
Director of Facilitation and Participation
of Disadvantaged Groups (FAPADAG)
Apeldoorn, Netherlands
Adjunct Professor
Dalhousie University
Halifax, Canada

Lyn Westcott, MSc, BSc, DipCOT,
MRCOT, HCPC Registered (Chapter 15)
Associate Professor
Deputy Head
School of Health Professions
University of Plymouth
Plymouth, England
Chair of the Royal College of
Occupational Therapists Board:
Learning and Development
London, England

Hirokazu Yoshikawa, PhD (Chapter 8)
Courtney Sale Ross Professor of
Globalization and Education
University Professor
New York University
New York, New York

FOREWORD

Occupational therapy education faces numerous challenges in the 21st century. Pressing challenging issues include which entry-level degree or degrees will be offered, how to attract and educate students who represent the diversity of the population they serve, what skills and knowledge practitioners will need in 5 and 10 years, and what constitutes best practices in occupational therapy education.

The American Occupational Therapy Association (AOTA) Centennial Vision 2017 imagined the profession as "a powerful, widely recognized, science-driven, and evidence-based profession with a globally connected and diverse workforce meeting society's occupational needs" (AOTA, 2007, p. 613). Vision 2025 continues to press toward this vision as represented in its four pillars: Effective (evidence based, science driven), Leaders (powerful, widely recognized), Collaborative (globally connected), and Accessible (diverse workforce) (AOTA, 2018). How will occupational therapy education prepare future practitioners to achieve Vision 2025 and to meet the challenges ahead? How will occupational therapy education prepare future practitioners to serve the occupational needs of people around the globe in culturally relevant ways? How will educators know if their students achieved the intended outcomes of their teaching?

In *Perspectives on Occupational Therapy Education: Past, Present, and Future*, Drs. Taff, Grajo, and Hooper provide valuable information about occupational therapy education. In reading and thinking about the book, I recalled Maralynne Mitcham's 2014 Eleanor Clarke Slagle Lecture, "Education as Engine." I find the framework she presented useful for organizing and further examining the breadth of information in this book. Mitcham's framework consists of three aspects of education: Education as Product, Learning as Process, and Living as Progress.

Mitcham referred to Education as Product as the "stuff" of education, such as the content, pedagogies, and technologies, among other stuff. When I think of Education as Product, I wonder how occupational therapy education came to incorporate so much stuff. I recall how challenging it was as an educator to include and organize required content into the curriculum and specific courses. The multitude of stuff to learn overwhelmed many students. Given the sheer amount of content, were students able to learn at a deep level, such that they could demonstrate occupational therapy's distinct value in meeting the occupational needs of the people and communities? Reading in this text about the history and philosophies of occupational therapy education, I see a pattern of increasing content, experiences, and pedagogies over time. As per Mitcham's encouragement, educators need to examine the products in occupational therapy education for what to keep, what to eliminate, and what to add. Beyond individual content areas, is there a way we can organize the stuff that would best facilitate students' learning the stuff at deep levels?

Mitcham referred to Learning as Process as a focus on the learner—the process where students learn to think like occupational therapists. Shulman writes about profession's signature pedagogies through which "novices are instructed in critical aspects of the three fundamental dimensions of professional work: *to think, to perform, and to act with integrity*" (2005, p. 52). How do occupational therapy educators socialize students into the profession? Do we have one or more signature pedagogies? In this text, Schaber and Candler propose several signature pedagogies including relational learning, affective learning, and highly contextualized active learning. Other chapters of this text inform us about additional pedagogies such as internationalization, interprofessional education, and learning on fieldwork. Hooper, Krishnagiri, and Price offer principles that help center a curriculum and all its content on occupation. Could that approach be another signature pedagogy? Would adopting signature pedagogies facilitate and/or organize learning the large amount of stuff contained in Education as Product? Do signature pedagogies prepare graduates with a solid understanding of occupation and its influence on health and well-being so they can advocate for the profession and its distinct value to societies in ways that are culturally relevant and integrated with other health care services?

If Learning as Process focuses on student learning, we need to determine if students are learning what we want them to learn. In *Occupational Therapy: 2001* (1979), Nedra Gillette wrote about the relationship among practice, education, and research. She stressed the importance of research, aka knowledge, as the link between education and practice. Teaching future practitioners is a practice area; as such, it is important that educators research their teaching and students' learning. It is important to research the effectiveness of the curriculum. What are the learning outcomes for our courses and curricula? How do we measure student learning? Are we measuring what we think is important and central to our distinct value? On a more macro level, how are we preparing future practitioners? Are they prepared to practice in the current environment? In future environments? Grajo and Gutman's chapter on measuring educational outcomes and Yoshikawa's chapter on educational research, along with the AOTA Occupational Therapy Education Research Agenda—Revised (2018a), guide educators to examine teaching and learning and longer-range impact on meeting society's occupational needs.

Mitcham referred to Living as Progress as the transformations that can come from disruptions to the status quo. Is occupational therapy education disrupting students' thinking so they will be better able to meet the needs of the people and communities—the people whose lives have been disrupted and the communities whose fabric is fraying? I find myself using the Person-Environment-Occupation-Performance (PEOP) model when thinking about disruptions that could impact occupational therapy education. Students and faculty are increasingly diverse across a number of domains. Around the world, people are migrating for many reasons. The environment is rapidly changing, be it technology, development, or infrastructure. Climate change is visibly altering the world in which we live. New occupations are being created while others are evolving and disappearing. Health care and higher education systems are rapidly changing in ways that are difficult to predict. In response to the high cost of higher education, institutions are cautious to add additional credits to programs of study. How then will occupational therapy education continue to have all the Education as Product stuff (and possibly add more) to address the unknown societal disruptions in the future? Performance continues to change as new ways of accomplishing the same tasks have created opportunities for previously marginalized persons to more fully participate in society. All of these are responses to disruptions and simultaneously create new disruptions. Who knows what disruptions will occur in our future. In the last chapter of this text, Imagining the Occupational Therapy Educational Landscape in 2050, Harvison and the editors identified contextual pressures that the profession and education will likely face. The road ahead for occupational therapy education will continue to adjust to disrupting contextual changes—some anticipated, some not.

Mitcham challenges educators to carefully and consistently examine occupational therapy education. From the focus of Education as Product, we need to carefully identify what should stay and what could go in order to facilitate the Learning as Process that transforms students into occupational therapy practitioners prepared to contribute occupational therapy's distinct value in disrupted community and health care environments. This book provides a foundation to start that inspection of education at a critical point in the profession's history. I encourage the reader to accept Mitcham's challenge and use this textbook to engage in a critical examination of education to strengthen the profession and move it forward. Enjoy your journey.

—*Andrea R. Bilics, PhD, OTR/L, FAOTA*
Professor Emeritus
Worcester State University
Worcester, Massachusetts

References

American Occupational Therapy Association. (2007). AOTA's Centennial Vision and executive summary. *American Journal of Occupational Therapy, 61*(6), 613–614. Retrieved from http://ajot.aota.org on 02/14/2019

American Occupational Therapy Association. (2018a). Occupational Therapy Education Research Agenda— *Revised. American Journal of Occupational Therapy, 72*(Suppl. 2), 7212420070. https://doi.org/10.5014/ajot.2018.72S218

American Occupational Therapy Association. (2018b). Vision 2025. *OT Practice, 23*(1), 20-21. https://www.aota.org/Publications-News/otp/Archive/2018/Vision-2025.aspx

Gillette, N. (1979). Practice, education and research. In *Occupational Therapy: 2001: Papers Presented at the Special Session of the Representative Assembly, November 1978.* Bethesda, MD: American Occupational Therapy Association.

Mitcham, M. D. (2014). Education as engine (Eleanor Clarke Slagle Lecture). American Journal of Occupational Therapy, 68, 636–648. http://dx.doi.org/10.5014/ajot.2014.686001 11. Available at: https://doi.org/10.15453/2168-6408.1347

Shulman, L. S. (2005). Signature pedagogies in the professions. *Dædalus, 134*(3), 52-59. Retrieved from http://gold.worcester.edu:2096/apps/doc/A135697726/AONE?u=mlin_c_worstate&sid=AONE&xid=7d6c195f. on 2/17 2019.

Introduction: Occupational Therapy Education— Weaving Together the Past, Present, and Future

John Dewey's (1925/2000) concept of growth provides a unifying theme for evolution of the profession of occupational therapy and its associated educational training over the past century. Growth, the constant process of change is, for Dewey, a universal concept, applicable to situations biological, inanimate, and social (Cutchin, 2004; Taff & Danforth, 2016). The growth of any entity or phenomenon is equivalent to the accumulation of experience over time. Therefore, growth, time, history, and place are closely related concepts instructive to our present discussion of occupational therapy education over the past century and into the future. History, broadly configured as a correlate of time and growth, offers important lessons as we reflect upon the continuity of events and experiences that have shaped and will continue to shape professional education.

French philosopher Henri Bergson's concept of duration is also instructive in helping us reframe time as a representation of both history and growth (Bergson, 1910/2014, 1911/1998). In relation to duration, time is a qualitative concept that embodies continuous experiences and subsequent changes (Linstead & Mullarkey, 2003). For Bergson (1910/2014), duration includes past, present, and future as additive experiences that unfold along the same continuum. Therefore, time is indivisible, and the points along the continuum cannot be separated into historical epochs but must instead be viewed as a series of growth events.

Dewey (1939/1988) shares Bergson's conception of time as a series of interconnected events, a "temporal seriality" (Mozur, 1991, p. 322) that defines the essence or identity of a person, object, or in the present case, a profession. From a Deweyan standpoint, the professional essence of occupational therapy is an inherent growth capacity or potential to evolve. This potential is realized only through the profession's interaction with the environment through time. Just as humans experience the process of becoming through contextualized occupational engagement, so too the profession moves towards its potential, guided by key environmental factors at each point along the continuum of time. The trajectory of occupational therapy education has typically paralleled that of the profession at large, each event and consequent change part of a constant pattern of growth. For these reasons, we believe that the publication of this text *Perspectives on Occupational Therapy Education: Past, Present, and Future* is timely. The text, as indicated in its title, has three main sections—past, present, and future—each weaving a unique perspective on the growth of occupational therapy education.

Examining the Past

Section I authors narrate two histories of occupational therapy education. One history told in Chapter 1 examines critical philosophies such as progressivism and essentialism, which prevailed at the time occupational therapy was founded. The chapter traces the influences those philosophies had on the emergence of the profession broadly and education specifically. Chapter 2 narrates a history of occupational therapy in search of its status as a profession. The chapter's premise is that occupational therapy education in the United States grew from tensions between the profession, higher education systems, and health care systems over time.

From these tensions grew new and expanded accreditation standards, new programs offering the entry-level professional degree for occupational therapy, new understandings of desired competencies for practice, and more.

Responding to Present Trends in Health Care and Higher Education

Section II authors address trends in the American health care and higher education systems and illustrate how occupational therapy education is responding to or resisting those trends. The initial chapter analyzes current issues and trends in health care and how occupational therapy education is addressing those to prepare the workforce of the future. The remainder of Section II addresses this series of critical issues in occupational therapy education: an examination of pedagogies that are unique to occupational therapy; a discussion on how to bridge the gap between what is learned in entry-level education and expectations in clinical practice; the use of competency exams to help students develop critical thinking and professional reasoning; measuring outcomes of occupational therapy education; expanding educational research in occupational therapy; promoting diversity and inclusion among faculty and students; and the principles of occupation-centered education mapped to best practices in education.

A Global Lens to View the Future of Occupational Therapy Education

In Section III, authors write about occupational therapy education from around the world, collectively offering a global and international perspective on occupational therapy education—past, present, and future. The The opening chapter describes efforts to internationalize occupational therapy education and enhance the cultural awareness of students. Next, an outstanding group of leaders and scholars discuss the development and the future of occupational therapy education in their home countries and regions of the world. These perspectives come from occupational therapy education in the Philippines (Southeast Asia), Brazil (South America), Canada (North America), the European Union (Europe), Australia, and South Africa (Africa). Subsequent chapters present trends in educational technology, fieldwork competencies and requirements, and interprofessional education. The section concludes, and the book ends, with an imagining of the landscape of occupational therapy education in the next 30 years.

How to Use Perspectives on Occupational Therapy Education

Each chapter in *Perspectives on Occupational Therapy Education* represents one point in a single and endless narrative of becoming, which chronicles the growth of professional education forging ahead to reach its potential. While the sections of the book weave a theoretical dimension of time as temporal seriality, each chapter is a single and unique point on the continuum reflecting the expert lenses of its authors. We purposefully wanted each chapter to represent the unique voices and perspectives of the contributing authors and the creative ways by which they articulated and exemplified their own perspectives on occupational therapy education. So rather than consuming information from one chapter to another, we encourage readers to use individual sections and chapters that are of critical importance to their teaching and scholarship.

This text is an essential resource for educators in occupational therapy programs across a wide range of academic experiences. For new educators who may be transitioning from clinical practice, new graduates of doctoral programs, or educators transitioning to a full-time academic position from adjunct or part-time teaching, this book provides context and practical guidance for your new academic role. The text combines helpful tips for, and important perspectives on, the multi-faceted dimensions of academic education. For seasoned educators, we hope this text offers fresh insights and perspectives on occupational therapy education as well as new tools for teaching and education research. We also hope that you can use this text as an essential reference when teaching doctoral students, preparing them as future occupational therapy educators, or entry-level students interested in exploring a career in academia. Further, the contents of this text can help current and future educators develop teaching and learning philosophies and pedagogies rooted in occupation and the historical perspectives of occupational therapy education.

Occupational therapy education has often borrowed its body of knowledge from higher education, educational psychology, and cognitive psychology to examine and support its scholarship of teaching and learning and to develop theoretical frameworks for best practices in teaching. We hope that this text facilitates the use and development of profession-specific research, pedagogies, and philosophies to guide our teaching moving forward.

Ann Wilcock and Clare Hocking (2015) emphasized the power of occupation to lead the process of becoming. Becoming is a process, an unfolding awareness that allows us to become who we are and who we want to be, a set of potentialities that when actualized brings occupational therapy education into full fruition. We hope that this text can help you become the best occupational therapy educator and educational researcher you can be and help move occupational therapy education toward its potentialities.

> "The best teachers assume that learning has little meaning unless it produces a sustained and substantial influence on the way people think, act, and feel."
> —Ken Bain

REFERENCES

Bain, K. (2004). *What the best college teachers do*. Cambridge, MA: Harvard University Press.

Bergson, H. (1998). *Creative evolution* (A. Mitchell, Trans.). Mineola, NY: Dover Publications, Inc. (Original work published 1911)

Bergson, H. (2014). *Time and free will: An essay on the immediate data of consciousness* (F. L. Pogson, Trans.). New York: Routledge. (Original work published 1910)

Cutchin, M.P. (2004). Using Deweyan philosophy to rename and reframe adaptation-to-environment. *American Journal of Occupational Therapy, 58*, 303-312.

Dewey, J. (1988). Time and individuality. In J. A. Boydston (Ed.), *John Dewey: The later works, 1925–1953, Vol. 14* (pp. 98-114). Carbondale: Southern Illinois University Press. (Original work published 1939)

Dewey, J. (2000). *Experience and nature*. Mineola, NY: Dover Publications, Inc. (Original work published 1925)

Linstead, S., & Mullarkey, J. (2003). Time, creativity and culture: Introducing Bergson. *Culture and Organization, 9* (1), 3-13.

Mozur, G. E. (1991). Dewey on time and individuality. *Transactions of the Charles S. Peirce Society, 27* (3), 321-340.

Taff, S. D. & Danforth, S. (2016). John Dewey and philosophy of disability. In M. A. Peters (Ed.), *Encyclopedia of Educational Philosophy and Theory*. Singapore: Springer.

Wilcock, A., & Hocking, C. (2015). *An occupational perspective of health* (3rd edition). Thorofare, NJ: SLACK Incorporated

Section I

Past

1

Educational Philosophies Influencing the Development of Early Occupational Therapy Curricula

Steven D. Taff, PhD, OTR/L, FNAP, FAOTA

Chapter Objectives

By the end of this chapter, the reader will be able to:

1. Understand the basic concepts, goals, and thinkers associated with essentialism, progressivism, perennialism, and social reconstructionism.
2. Relate the context of early educational philosophies to present-day issues impacting professional training.
3. Recognize traces of the four educational philosophies currently present in his or her teaching or curriculum.
4. Value the influence of social issues, philosophy, and politics in the development of curricula.

INTRODUCTION

Occupational therapy historians have identified the major factors that influenced the origination of the profession, including pragmatist philosophy, the social reform movement, and the need for rehabilitation of soldiers returning from World War I (Andersen & Reed, 2017; Quiroga, 1995). I suggest here that additional forces were at play in terms of influencing all levels of educational systems during the Progressive Era, including scientific management, the growth of clinical psychology, and the rise in influence of educationally focused philosophies that steered curriculum design. The educational landscape of the times, as driven by sociopolitical factors, had as much of an impact on the development of early occupational therapy education (what was taught) as did the forces that shaped the development of the profession (what therapists did in practice). This chapter explores four foundational educational philosophies that were embedded within the historical context from which occupational therapy emerged. These philosophies guided schools and professions at the time in their curricular decisions of *what* to teach and *why*.

Taff, S. D., Grajo, L. C., & Hooper, B. R. (Eds.). *Perspectives on Occupational Therapy Education: Past, Present, and Future* (pp. 3-11).
© 2020 Taylor & Francis Group.

The United States in the Progressive Era (roughly 1890-1930) was represented by a unique mix of historical, social, and political factors that fundamentally altered the face of American society (Taff, 2005). With the abrupt shift from an agrarian to an industrialized society, a new middle class (professionals) emerged, altering society's status hierarchy. Hofstadter (1955) views the Progressive Era as a status revolution catalyzed by a growing middle class eager to make its mark on society. Progressivism was both a "progressive impulse" that exposed and addressed social maladies and an attempt by the new middle class to forge an identity and cultivate that identity into preferred social status (i.e., the progressive impulse was used by new professionals as a way to bolster their public status as valuable social problem solvers). Thus, Hofstadter (1955) defined progressivism as "that broader impulse toward criticism and change that was everywhere so conspicuous after 1900, when the already forceful stream of agrarian discontent was enlarged and redirected by the growing enthusiasm of middle-class people for social and economic reform" (p. 5). Diner (1998) additionally suggested that the progressive impulse was driven by three common goals: economic security, personal autonomy, and social status. Competition for authority over these three goals among different groups of people created the progressive landscape of reform.

The Progressive Era was laden with incongruities, as illustrated by the settlement house and social gospel reform movements occurring simultaneously with institutionalization of people with disabilities, involuntary sterilization, political isolationism, and suspicion and intolerance of immigrants. This complex context created the dynamics surrounding the development of occupational therapy and other new professions. Buenker, Burnham, and Crunden (1977) noted that the "imperialism, the racism, the prohibitionism and the narrow fundamentalism of many legitimate progressive leaders and voters are inseparable from the efforts at conservation, financial reform, tariff reduction, initiative, referendum, and recall that seem so much more attractive" (p. 108).

Rothman (1980) framed the presumably opposing purposes of mitigating social ills and seeking status promotion as "conscience and convenience." This dualistic perspective paved the way for policy enactment and a heightened trend toward segregation and institutionalization, which placed increasing value on classifying, sorting, and improving the efficiency of processes, both industrial and social. Therefore, the Progressive Era saw the rise of business and industry as the best cultural guides for all of society, which led to "America's subsequent saturation with business-industrial values and practices" (Callahan, 1962, p. 2).

Clearly, a common theme in most historical accounts of the Progressive Era is the rise of the middle class and a corresponding development of professions vying for legitimacy (Taff, 2005). Occupational therapy surely was included in this struggle, and it necessitated the development of suitable training to underpin and legitimize the young profession (Andersen & Reed, 2017; Quiroga, 1995).

THE RISE OF EDUCATIONAL PHILOSOPHIES

Given the relatively low status and power of education as a profession, schools responded to criticism by adopting "scientifically" efficient manufacturing methods as part of their administrative and instructional structures (Callahan, 1962). Education was in danger of losing its intended role as a liberal equalizer of democratic citizens informed by knowledge. Instead, schools had to reshape education in terms of process and product. The process of education needed to become much more efficient; waste had to be minimized, and excess paperwork, instructional practices, supplies, and even staff needed to be streamlined. The passive thinker of abstract ideals was less relevant; what America now needed was people of practical action to best support a manufacturing economy. Scientific management as forwarded by theorists such as Frederick Taylor accompanied the rise in industrial manufacturing common in the early 20th century (Haber, 1964). In this paradigm, schools were now expected to turn out socially efficient products, which required reshaping curricula to concentrate on vocational and manual training designed for the masses, not individual learners. In the name of

Table 1-1			
EDUCATIONAL PHILOSOPHIES AND PURPOSES			
EDUCATIONAL PHILOSOPHY	**FOUNDATIONAL PHILOSOPHY**	**FOCUS**	**ROLE IN SOCIETY**
Progressivism	Pragmatism	Experience	Problem solving/ growth
Essentialism	Realism	Science	Specialization/ professionalization
Perennialism	Idealism	Ideas/intellect	Stability
Social reconstructionism	Critical theory	Critique	Social justice/ change

efficiency, schools became "sorters," places where students could be tracked into the course of study most suitable for their abilities (largely determined through intelligence testing) (Callahan, 1962). Although the efficiency movement in education was more aggressively pursued in the elementary and secondary levels, higher education and professional training still felt its presence, and curricula became more focused on pragmatic skills that yielded professionally sustaining results.

Influenced by the context of the Progressive Era, educational leaders struggled with fundamental philosophical questions surrounding the purpose of education and closely related discussions of what to teach in a social landscape newly dominated by concerns for pragmatic and efficient solutions to the modern consequences of industrialization and urbanization (Bowles & Gintis, 1976; Cremin, 1961; Kliebard, 1986). As compulsory school attendance and immigration compelled educational systems to accommodate the sheer number of students, different perspectives of how to best educate this new citizenry also arose (Taff, 2005). In the early 20th century, four distinct (yet overlapping in some ways) foundational educational philosophies (Table 1-1) emerged as intellectual and theoretical touchstones for framing the educational systems of the time: progressivism, essentialism, perennialism, and social reconstructionism (Brameld, 1956a). Although elements of essentialism and perennialism existed well before the Progressive Era, progressivism and particularly social reconstructionism were recent philosophical developments in the grand discussion of the goals of education and how curricula should be designed to achieve those outcomes.

Progressivism

Not surprisingly, the influence of progressive educational philosophies was at its height during the early decades of the 20th century. Progressivism as originally implemented in educational systems was a mix of many factors, including pragmatist philosophy, a reform mindset, and scientific management or social efficiency chief among them. The pragmatist philosopher John Dewey is well known in educational circles and acknowledged as a primary influence on the development of occupational therapy as a profession (Andersen & Reed, 2017). Dewey's thought heavily influenced other contemporary educational progressivists such as William Kilpatrick, Boyd Bode, and Booker T. Washington. Progressivist education strives to stimulate learners to "think with effectiveness … to analyze, to criticize, to select among alternatives … to carry on continuous, intelligent adjustments with the natural and social environment of which everyone is a part" (Brameld, 1956a, pp. 74-75). Schools should foster a sense of democratic living through cooperative problem solving (Dewey, 1916). This communal experiment is supported through individual experience and a focus on growth as evolving learners (Dewey, 1900). Progressivist educators favor a broad curriculum and active learning that is student centered and facilitated by a teacher who is the guide, resource, and creative arranger of experiences (Ozmon & Craver, 1999). Progressivist curricula can be organized by traditional subject areas but not limited within those, allowing for flexibility and exploration. Harold Rugg (1936) proposed an "experience-centered curriculum," which dissolved content area lines and emphasized contextualized units that spanned multiple disciplinary fields. Progressivist educators assist learners to think through experimentation rather than abstract concepts, often in groups centered on a project-based approach (Kilpatrick, 1926). A progressive education considers the whole child, not simply the intellectual elements. Motivation, emotions, habits, and the social and physical environment all impact growth and learning.

Essentialism

Essentialist philosophy favors a conservative, traditional curriculum that is "grounded, first of all, upon the *essentials*, that is, upon the tried and tested heritage of skills, facts, and laws of knowledge that have come down to us through modern civilization" (Brameld, 1956a, p. 74). Essentialist education grew more influential in the Progressive Era because technical knowledge and specialization became increasingly necessary to support the industrial and scientific development of the United States. Major proponents of the essentialist perspective during the Progressive Era included William Bagley, William Harris, and Ross Finney (Brameld, 1956a). Essentialism as educational philosophy draws strongly from the larger philosophical school of realism, which suggests that objective knowledge and value exist independently of the individual consciousness or intellect (Ozmon & Craver, 1999). Science as a discipline is looked to as the only valid source of knowledge. As such, basic truths of the world generated through the scientific method are the basis of any essentialist curriculum. Therefore, knowledge "is not a process of creation, but of disclosure of reality" (Brameld, 1956a, p. 245). Foundational content areas such as reading, writing, mathematics, science, and history are priorities. While sharing with progressivism a fondness for the scientific method, essentialism discourages exploration and places learning in the hands of subject matter experts who transmit their knowledge to students, who are responsible for mastering that content. Character and moral development are also important aspects of an essentialist education. Indeed, the essentialist view of education rests not only on truth but also fundamental goodness. Education should inculcate norms and values because the school "is an agent for preserving the inherited values and adjusting man to society" (Brameld, 1956a, p. 239). In terms of instruction, essentialist educators stress the use of objects, illustrations, and lecture as primary avenues for learning. The role of the teacher is subject matter expert; the responsibility of the learner is to take in the knowledge offered and minimize subjective evaluation. Essentialists support efforts to measure and evaluate learning and individual student capabilities (such as intelligence) and achieve this outcome largely through examinations and standardized tests.

Perennialism

Perennialism is perhaps the least represented in practice of the four educational philosophies. Perennialists hold that education and society itself depend on "restoration of the spirit that governed education in the Middle Ages … the eternal principles of truth, goodness, and beauty" (Brameld, 1956a, p. 75). Perennialism shares with essentialism a premium on truth; however, its means for arriving at those truths rests less on scientific investigation than on "great ideas of great men." The aim of a perennialist education is to train intellectual leaders who rely on ideas rather than the ever-changing world around them (Brameld, 1956a). Perennialist educators may rely on lecture, but even that method of instruction must be accompanied by interpretations and asking students the implications of content. In this way, perennialists agree that "exercising and disciplining the mind is one of the highest obligations of learning" (Brameld, 1956a, p. 322). Unlike progressivism, which views education as a continual process in experimentation, perennialism (particularly with younger students) adopts a more staged approach in which each succeeding level of schooling prepares learners for the next step. Philosophically, perennialism is most closely associated with idealism and favors religion and the classics as foundational curricular content that is relevant to contemporary issues (Ozmon & Craver, 1999). A broad preparation is preferred over narrow specialization, and this is reflected in the curriculum design, which frequently includes reading "great books" (Van Doren, 1943). Likewise, Hutchins (1936) advocated focus on the basics and classics, avoiding social issues or reform-minded discussions.

Social Reconstructionism

Of the four educational philosophies, social reconstructionism was the last to emerge (during the Great Depression) and was represented by such thinkers as George Counts and Theodore Brameld. (Harold Rugg, initially more of a progressivist, later included strands of social reconstructionism in his work.) Although both social reconstructionism and perennialism agree that modern civilization needs clarification and reform, social reconstructionism looks to the future for solutions to reconstruct schools and society. Social reconstructionism advocates for a "world in which the technological potentialities ... are released for the creation of health, abundance, and security for the masses of people of every color, nationality, and creed" (Brameld, 1956a, pp. 75-76). Social reconstructionism, although similar to progressivism, takes a more collective and radical path in which schools and institutions are vehicles for advocacy and social reform (Stanley, 1992). Social reconstructionists believe that social change requires both a "reconstruction of education and the use of education in reconstructing society" (Ozmon & Craver, 1999, p. 176). Contrasting the essentialist view that education adjusts learners to society, social reconstructionism suggests that people should learn the skills and knowledge that allow them to change society for the better.

The leading social reconstructionist theorist during the Progressive Era was George Counts, who argued that education be used to establish new cultural values and promote social equity (Counts, 1932). Theodore Brameld (1956b) held a similar position, although he was more focused on the humane application of technology and an internationally oriented perspective of change. A curriculum influenced by social reconstructionism would feature experiential, collaborative, and community-based learning supplemented by broad topics such as problem solving, activism/advocacy, and alternative narratives (Ozmon & Craver, 1999). Social and world studies, history, languages, and cultural awareness also fit within the social reconstructionist curriculum model. Social reconstructionist educators must keep current on national and world events, facilitate tough conversations, and model social activism. Instruction should be as relevant as possible to real-life situations and offer students the skills to enable active democratic citizenship and critically evaluate the knowledge they encounter.

IMPACT ON PROFESSIONS: THE CLINICAL PSYCHOLOGY EXAMPLE

Clinical psychology experienced a similar developmental arc to occupational therapy in the first decades of the 20th century. Likewise, clinical psychologists sought a social standing and authority sufficient enough to claim social utility and relevance. Brown (1992) suggests that every developing profession requires three basic elements: knowledge, practitioners, and a clientele. Clinical psychology, like occupational therapy, had acquired a knowledge base influenced by the scientific and objective ways of experimental psychology and medicine. The maturing group of clinical psychologists attempted to enhance their image as professional experts through both scientific objectivity and an association with medicine that borrowed physician's healing aptitude and applied it in a novel setting—the schools (Taff, 2005). The twin phenomena of immigration and compulsory schooling essentially guaranteed clinical psychology's acquisition of a clientele (Brown, 1992). Confronted with an unprecedented number of students and a newfound pressure to educate socially and industrially efficient citizens, the schools welcomed the advent of experts who could identify, classify, segregate, and even cure children with learning challenges or language barriers. The increasing adoption of intelligence tests as diagnostic tools further enhanced the stature of clinical psychologists (Fancher, 1985). The rise of clinical psychologists, who focused their work primarily in schools, fundamentally transformed the purpose of education toward an emphasis on identifying learning levels and classifying students as determined in part by standardized assessments.

Clinical psychology provides an informative example for how each of the four educational philosophies permeated the fledgling profession during its initial growth phase. Essentialism was present through a strong foundation in the basic sciences and notions of adjusting learners to society's needs rather than considering the role of the environment on individual thinking. Perennialism, with its high value on individual intellect and the separation of thinkers from their context, also surfaced in more understated ways. The progressivist perspective was represented through empirical measurement and the goals of increased efficiency of educational systems and maximizing future productivity of individuals. Clinical psychology also was viewed as a solution to a high-profile social problem, that of immigrant learners and children with mild disabilities (Taff, 2005). In many respects, social reconstructionism's preference of democratic learning community over hierarchical social segregation was the antithesis of the basic tenets underpinning clinical psychology. However, it did surface in clinical psychology through their common esteem of innovative thinking and use of technological tools.

EARLY OCCUPATIONAL THERAPY CURRICULA: 1924 TO 1943

As was the case with many new professions at the time occupational therapy was established, there was a need to simultaneously develop training programs to prepare practitioners and provide legitimacy as a growing profession. The first formal training requirements were issued in 1924 (American Occupational Therapy Association, 1924) and consisted of a minimum of 12 months of training, 8 months in "theoretical and practical work" and no less than 3 months of "hospital practice." The standard curriculum included anatomy, orthopedics, kinesiology, psychology, sociology, "mental diseases," tuberculosis, and hospital ethics and management as well as training in arts and crafts such as woodworking, weaving, sheet metal, basketry, drawing, and applied design. The first minimum standards did not explicitly include liberal arts or humanities, and the relationship between the basic and applied sciences was not clearly articulated (Presseller, 1984). Similarly, Presseller (1984) noted that, in the history of occupational therapy education, "there has never been consensus on the proper balance of the liberal and technical components of professional education" (p. iv). This has resulted in a theory/practice gap in the profession that is still evident today. By 1935, the length of training had increased to a minimum of 25 months total, 16 months of theoretical/didactic work and 9 months of clinical training (American Medical Association, 1935). The 1935 Essentials saw an increase in basic sciences content, whereas applied science did not display a similar increase in focus (Presseller, 1984). Although the 1924 Essentials could be viewed as subtly including the humanities and liberal arts, the 1935 version included no mention of either. Curricula included anatomy, physiology, neurology, kinesiology, psychology, psychiatry, social sciences, theory of occupational therapy, and clinical topics such as orthopedics, tuberculosis, cardiac diseases, and blindness and deafness. Practical craft work was also required, including design, leather, wood, metal, plastic arts, recreation, and textiles. Perhaps fueled by lobbying for a closer tie to the medical profession, curriculum debates involving more biomechanical treatment techniques such as massage and electrotherapy ensued (Doan, 1934; Presseller, 1984). Shortly thereafter, the 1939 Essentials (American Medical Association, 1939) were issued, demonstrating a slight shift away from a strict medical model curriculum by infusing more social sciences content. Finally, the 1943 Essentials (American Medical Association, 1943) retained the length of training from the 1935 version and required a similar blend of theoretical training (adding "individual readjustment") and fine and applied arts and crafts. The 1943 Essentials also specified that occupational therapists must work under physicians and "not as independent practitioners of occupational therapy" (Presseller, 1984, p. 50).

Throughout the first four iterations of essential training requirements, curricular content was fairly consistent and reflected a strong essentialist (mostly) and progressivist philosophical base. Essentialist notions of the primacy of the basic sciences and specialization were keystones to training practitioners in a newly developing profession. Strong basic sciences content was the clearest way for the young profession to ally its training model with that of physicians. Progressivist thought might have been better reflected in the hospital/field portion of occupational therapy training, where the basic sciences were put into practice through mentored supervision and engaged, in-context learning. Despite not being represented as explicitly as essentialism, progressivism, with its focus on problem solving and adaptation, was a key underpinning for the development of clinical reasoning gained through didactic and field training.

The perennialist and social reconstructionist philosophies were not well represented given the applied and scientifically based nature of the training model. Perennialist views centered on classical literature were not well aligned with the evolutionary ideas of growth and pragmatic decision making in a modern society. The relative lack of humanities content in early occupational therapy curriculum also illustrated the limited presence of a perennialist perspective, though emphasis on the liberal arts would grow and be debated in ensuing years. Meanwhile, social reconstructionism was often future oriented, and the problems facing the new profession were "now" issues. Critical theory, a key influence in social reconstructionist thought, was just starting to arise concurrently with the "ills" of modern society. Additionally, the drive to legitimize the profession through rigorous and rigid curricula (an essentialist view) outweighed opportunities for advocacy and social reform.

INFLUENCES OF EDUCATIONAL PHILOSOPHIES IN CONTEMPORARY CURRICULA

Although all four educational philosophies first rose to prominence in the early 20th century, these same paradigms still exert considerable influence today, even if subtly and not framed as "philosophies" per se. Perennialism seems to surface most in times of social crisis when conservative values are threatened by change. Its presence is still felt in religious education, homeschooling, and learning enhancements such as mindfulness and metacognitive processes. It could also be argued that the movement toward Common Core educational standards in kindergarten through 12th grade settings has elements of perennialist philosophy at its foundation. Likewise, essentialism is present in a wide variety of contexts including standardized testing; the focus on science, technology, engineering, and mathematics education; and the role of cognitive science in informing teaching practices. Progressivist perspectives, in particular, have endured in curricula through more recent developments such as constructivism, student-centered learning, team and project-based learning, community experiences, quality improvement initiatives, and the increased use of simulation and standardized patients. Social reconstructionism also is very apparent in contemporary curricula through critical pedagogy, evidence-based practice, interprofessional education, internationalization, diversity and inclusion initiatives, and the explosion of online learning and instructional technologies.

CONCLUSION

Largely driven by the social issues endemic to the Progressive Era in U.S. history, four distinct yet connected educational philosophies surfaced in educational systems for the first time in an applied fashion. These philosophies provided a fusion of intellectual and practical foundations on which professional curriculum specifications were constructed. Early occupational therapy curricula focused heavily on essentialist and progressivist modes of thought, which aligned closely to the needs of a youthful profession struggling to justify its place in an era rife with competing professionalization. The multilayered blend of professional legitimacy, social issues, scientific advances, and political ideologies has consistently shaped occupational therapy curricula throughout the past century. Aspects of the four philosophies continue to influence curricular content despite the gradual decrease in status of philosophy and a generalized anti-intellectualism in both mainstream and academic arenas. Perhaps occupational therapy's second century will see a return to prominence of the valuable and unique lens offered by philosophy; only time will tell.

Implications for Occupational Therapy Education

- Early occupational therapy curricula were dictated by an urgency to legitimize the profession alongside the rise of educational philosophies.
- Elements of the four educational philosophies exist in contemporary professional education; these (and more recent approaches) impact teaching styles and curricular content.
- The early influences on the development of occupational therapy education were multifaceted, complex, and guided largely by sociopolitical factors. Although contemporary factors are different than in the 1920s or 1930s, the sociopolitical context still drives educational policy and decision making.

Key Reflection Questions

1. Where do you see the four educational philosophies embedded in the content and learning activities in the courses you teach?
2. Consider how the four educational philosophies connect with Pratt's five perspectives on teaching or Fink's taxonomy of significant learning.
3. If the sociopolitical context is a major influence on curriculum and instruction, what roles could occupational therapy educators play to contribute to the ongoing processes that determine "what" is taught?

What led you to become an occupational therapy educator?

I grew up in a "teaching" home where education was highly valued. Both of my parents were teachers, and I often was in schools even when I was not in class! The educational setting has always been comfortable for me, and I came to understand that all experiences in life are educational events. My passion for education was only heightened by a collective of encouraging and energetic mentors in my PhD program. They modeled a mindset of "humane critique," a deep curiosity for learning, and a duty to frame every teaching/ learning encounter as an opportunity to contribute to the greater good of individuals and society. This is a perspective to which I hold as I design learning experiences and teach in the classroom.

Steven D. Taff, PhD, OTR/L, FNAP, FAOTA

REFERENCES

American Medical Association. (1935). Essentials of an acceptable school of occupational therapy. *JAMA: The Journal of the American Medical Association, 108,* 1632-1633.

American Medical Association. (1939). Essentials of an acceptable school of occupational therapy. *JAMA: The Journal of the American Medical Association, 112,* 926-927.

American Medical Association. (1943). Essentials of an acceptable school of occupational therapy. *JAMA: The Journal of the American Medical Association, 115,* 541-542.

American Occupational Therapy Association. (1924). Minimum standards for courses of training in occupational therapy. *Archives of Occupational Therapy, 3*(4), 295-298.

Andersen, L. T., & Reed, K. L. (2017). *The history of occupational therapy: The first century.* Thorofare, NJ: SLACK Incorporated.

Bowles, S., & Gintis, H. (1976). *Schooling in capitalist America: Educational reform and the construction of economic life.* New York, NY: Basic Books.

Brameld, T. (1956a). *Philosophies of education in cultural perspective.* New York, NY: The Dryden Press.

Brameld, T. (1956b). *Toward a reconstructed philosophy of education.* New York, NY: The Dryden Press.

Brown, J. (1992). *The definition of a profession: The authority of metaphor in the history of intelligence testing, 1890-1930.* Princeton, NJ: Princeton University Press.

Buenker, J. D., Burnham, J. C., & Crunden, R. M. (1977). *Progressivism.* Cambridge, MA: Schenkman Publishing Company, Ltd.

Callahan, R. E. (1962). *Education and the cult of efficiency.* Chicago, IL: University of Chicago Press.

Counts, G. (1932). *Dare the schools build a new social order?* Carbondale, IL: Southern Illinois University Press.

Cremin, L. A. (1961). *The transformation of the school: Progressivism in American education, 1876-1957.* New York, NY: Alfred A. Knopf.

Dewey, J. (1900). *The school and society.* Chicago, IL: University of Chicago Press.

Dewey, J. (1916). *Democracy and education: An introduction to the philosophy of education.* New York, NY: Macmillan.

Diner, S. A. (1998). *A very different age: Americans of the progressive era.* New York, NY: Hill and Wang.

Doan, J. C. (1934). Presidential address. *Occupational Therapy and Rehabilitation, 13,* 355-360.

Fancher, R. E. (1985). *The intelligence men: Makers of the IQ controversy.* New York, NY: W.W. Norton & Company.

Haber, S. (1964). *Efficiency and uplift: Scientific management in the progressive era 1890-1920.* Chicago, IL: University of Chicago Press.

Hofstadter, R. (1955). *The age of reform.* New York, NY: Alfred A. Knopf.

Hutchins, R. M. (1936). *No friendly voice.* Chicago, IL: University of Chicago Press.

Kilpatrick, W. H. (1926). *Education for a changing civilization.* New York, NY: Century.

Kliebard, H. M. (1986). *The struggle for the American curriculum, 1893-1958.* Boston, MA: Routledge & Kegan Paul.

Ozmon, H. A., & Craver, S. M. (1999). *Philosophical foundations of education* (6th ed.). Upper Saddle River, NJ: Merrill.

Quiroga, V. A. M. (1995). *Occupational therapy: The first 30 years, 1900-1930.* Bethesda, MD: American Occupational Therapy Association.

Presseller, S. R. (1984). *Occupational therapy education: Yesterday, today, and tomorrow* (Unpublished master's thesis). Boston University School of Education, Boston, MA.

Rothman, D. J. (1980). *Conscience and convenience: The asylum and its alternatives in Progressive America.* Boston, MA: Little, Brown and Company.

Rugg, H. O. (1936). *American life and the school curriculum.* Boston, MA: Ginn & Company.

Stanley, W. B. (1992). *Curriculum for utopia: Social reconstructionism and critical pedagogy in the postmodern era.* Albany, NY: State University of New York Press.

Taff, S. D. (2005). *The phenomenology of the "backward" child: A history of school failure in progressive era America, 1890-1930* (Unpublished doctoral dissertation). University of Missouri-St. Louis, St. Louis, MO.

Van Doren, M. (1943). *Liberal education.* New York, NY: Henry Holt & Company.

2

A Historical Overview of Occupational Therapy Education

Wanda J. Mahoney, PhD, OTR/L

Chapter Objectives

By the end of this chapter, the reader will be able to:

1. Describe major changes in occupational therapy education in the United States from the early 1900s to present.

2. Examine how tensions within the occupational therapy profession, higher education system, and health care systems in the United States influenced changes in occupational therapy education.

3. Evaluate patterns in the history of occupational therapy education to recognize and anticipate possibilities and challenges in the future.

INTRODUCTION

Although the formation of the National Society for the Promotion of Occupational Therapy (NSPOT) in 1917 is celebrated as the birth of occupational therapy in the United States, occupational therapy education began more than 10 years earlier when the first occupational training courses were offered. Susan Tracy is credited with starting the first program in 1906 at the Adams Nervine Hospital in Boston (Dunton, 1947). This was followed soon after in 1908 with courses at the Chicago School of Civics and Philanthropy that transitioned to become the Henry B. Favill School of Occupations, which was headed by Eleanor Clarke Slagle (Dunton, 1947). Most of the founders of NSPOT, renamed the American Occupational Therapy Association (AOTA), had prior involvement with preparing individuals to practice occupational therapy, and educational preparation was an important concern for the early organization (Peters, Martin, & Mahoney, 2017).

The goal of occupational therapy education has always been to prepare competent occupational therapy practitioners, reflecting a reciprocal relationship between occupational therapy education

Taff, S. D., Grajo, L. C., & Hooper, B. R. (Eds.). *Perspectives on Occupational Therapy Education: Past, Present, and Future* (pp. 13-28).
© 2020 Taylor & Francis Group.

and practice. However, the knowledge, skills, and dispositions for competence among occupational therapy practitioners have changed as the profession, health care, and societal systems have changed. Furthermore, while educators prepare graduates for competent practice in the current environment, they also anticipate the competencies that will be needed in the future to help the profession evolve. This chapter refers to the *profession* of occupational therapy to distinguish it from occupational therapy education.

The profession of occupational therapy has been striving to attain professional status since its inception, which has been a driving force behind major changes in occupational therapy education. Thus, occupational therapy education reflects the formation and development of the profession in response to internal and external tensions. Within the profession, tensions include professionalization, the primacy of art or science, philosophical underpinnings, student diversity, and changing visions of what the profession was and desired to become. Occupational therapy practitioners' shifting perceptions of themselves, their work, and who they want to become as professionals have also changed the structure and function of occupational therapy education. Externally, tensions result from competing expectations between occupational therapy, the educational institutions that house them, health care systems where occupational therapy practitioners provide service, and broader societal systems including health care, legislation, funding, and the community. This chapter explores such tensions for how they prompted educational changes.

Descriptions of major changes in occupational therapy education in this chapter were informed by published interpretations of events in occupational therapy education and historical analysis of selected archived or published sources. Although occupational therapy assistant education is briefly mentioned, especially as it began in the 1950s, the focus is on educational preparation for occupational therapists in the United States. Existing historical scholarship focuses on events before the 1990s; therefore, the bulk of this chapter concentrates on occupational therapy education from its inception through the 1990s. Although historians recognize the need for temporal distance from events in order to understand their implications, connections to current issues in occupational therapy education are included. Major changes in education covered in this chapter include the expansion in the number of programs, students' academic preparation, and additional requirements to enter the field. Why these changes occurred is organized into three major sections: factors internal to the profession, educational systems that house academic programs, and health care and societal systems in which occupational therapy practitioners provide services.

MAJOR CHANGES IN OCCUPATIONAL THERAPY EDUCATION

Occupational therapy education program accreditation standards are key sources that reflect major changes in occupational therapy education. AOTA passed the first educational requirements in 1924, with enforcement only through Eleanor Clarke Slagle's informal approval (AOTA, 1924; Colman, 1986). In 1935, AOTA joined with the American Medical Association (AMA) to formally accredit occupational therapy education programs (AOTA, 2016; Peters et al., 2017). This AMA/AOTA relationship continued until 1994 when the new agency, Accreditation Council for Occupational Therapy Education (ACOTE), was established (AOTA, 2016). As the number of programs expanded, the accreditation standards attempted to ensure consistency among the programs as a mechanism to assist the professionalization of occupational therapy.

Expansion of Programs

One of the easiest ways to see change in occupational therapy education in the United States is in the steady increase in the number of accredited entry-level programs (Table 2-1). At the end of World War I when the workforce emergency need for reconstruction aides ended, many of the short courses closed (Dunton, 1947). Five programs continued to offer diplomas in the United

Table 2-1

ACCREDITED OCCUPATIONAL THERAPY PROGRAMS IN THE UNITED STATES: 1940 TO 2018[a]

YEAR	NUMBER OF PROGRAMS (REGISTERED OCCUPATIONAL THERAPIST)	NUMBER OF PROGRAMS (OCCUPATIONAL THERAPY ASSISTANT)	CITATION
1940	5	N/A	Dunton, 1947
1950	24	N/A	AOTA, 1950
1960	29	N/A[b]	AOTA, 1960
1970	36	N/A[b]	AOTA, 1970
1980[c]	55	52	AOTA, 1983b
1990	69	68	AOTA, 1990
2000	138	169	AOTA, 2000
2010	154	150	AOTA, 2010
2018	196	220	AOTA, 2018

Abbreviation: N/A, not applicable.
[a]Developing or inactive programs not included. Additional locations counted separately if listed separately. Each institution with multiple entry-level degrees (i.e., doctorate and master's) counted as one program.
[b]Although AOTA began accrediting occupational therapy assistant programs in 1958, they were not included in the published list of programs until 1976.
[c]Data are from 1983 because of the availability in published records.

States, and they were the first programs to be accredited by AOTA: Boston School of Occupational Therapy, Kalamazoo School of Occupational Therapy, Milwaukee-Downer College, St. Louis School of Occupational Therapy, and Philadelphia School of Occupational Therapy (PSOT) (Dunton, 1947; Peters et al., 2017). The 1940s, 1970s, and 1990s were decades of substantial growth in the number of occupational therapist programs. The emergency need for occupational therapists in World War II was a major factor in the growth in the 1940s. The growth in the 1970s corresponded with an overall surge in the number of people, especially women, seeking college degrees. The growth in the 1990s was likely a result of a substantial increase in health care spending that enhanced the appeal of health care education programs to both potential students and educational institutions. Although individual programs have closed during the past 100 years, including several of the original programs, overall there has been a significant increase in the number of programs offering entry-level occupational therapy degrees, resulting in 416 accredited programs (occupational therapists and occupational therapy assistants) in 2018.

Academic Preparation

The education necessary for entry into occupational therapy practice has undergone numerous changes across the history of occupational therapy and has been a source of debate from the inception of the field through the present. Some of these changes include the academic degree required for entry into the field, educational content of programs, requirements for students and faculty, and additional prerequisites for practice.

Academic Degree

Susan Cox Johnson, NSPOT founder and chair of the first teaching and education committee, felt that a college degree was necessary to practice occupational therapy (Quiroga, 1995). Other founders disagreed, and diploma-granting, independent schools of occupational therapy became the norm in the 1920s and 1930s, with Milwaukee-Downer College as a notable exception. In the years before an academic degree requirement, the standards specified the minimal length of time to be spent in academic preparation. The initial requirement was 12 months of training in 1924, which doubled to 2 years in 1930 (AOTA, 1924, 1930). The accreditation standards developed with the AMA specified that the program had to be at least 25 months or 100 weeks long (AMA, 1935).

Major changes in the occupational therapy education standards often started as recommendations. For example, the 1935 and 1943 standards specified that "affiliation with a college, university or medical school is highly desirable but is not an absolute requirement" (AMA, 1935, p. 683; Council on Medical Education and Hospitals, 1943, p. 541). The World War II crisis that prompted the need for more occupational therapists resulted in temporarily relaxed standards for war emergency courses (Colman, 1990). This workforce emergency during the war was not the time to increase standards to require occupational therapy schools to affiliate with higher education institutions. However, indications of the impending requirement were clear before 1949 when the standards required occupational therapy programs to be part of an approved college or medical school (Council on Medical Education and Hospitals, 1950). This requirement added an additional layer of higher education system accountability for occupational therapy education.

Occupational therapy programs, many of which previously developed formal affiliations with a university, became part of a university system in the late 1940s and early 1950s (Grant, 1991; Peters et al., 2017). Although bachelor's degrees became more common, occupational therapy certificate and diploma programs persisted, especially for students with prior college experience (Grant, 1991; Peters et al., 2017). With this push toward college education for entry-level practice, technical programs primarily based in hospitals also emerged, serving a new level of practitioner, the occupational therapy assistant, beginning in 1958 (Cottrell, 2000; West, 1992). The 1965 standards required occupational therapist programs to award a bachelor's degree for practice in the United States, ending the debate about whether a college degree would be required for occupational therapists (AOTA, 1967).

However, the college degree requirement did not end the debate about the necessary academic preparation and degree for entry-level practice. In addition to a push for postprofessional education, discussion about an entry-level master's degree, which began at least as early as the 1940s, heated up in the 1970s, and 10 programs had developed entry-level master's degrees by the mid-1980s (AOTA, 1983b; Lucci, 1974). Occupational therapy programs responded to the 1991 recommendation for the entry-level degree to move to a master's; the number of new entry-level master's programs grew from 12 in 1990 to 44 in 1998 (AOTA, 1990, 1991, 1998; Fisher, 2000). In 1999, the Representative Assembly followed the tradition of turning a recommendation to increase standards into a mandate and passed Resolution J, which required an entry-level master's degree for occupational therapists (AOTA, 2016; Brown, Crabtree, Mu, & Wells, 2015). By that time, almost half of the occupational therapist programs in the United States (65/138) offered a master's degree (AOTA, 2000).

In the United States, the discussion and debate about the degree required to practice occupational therapy continue to be a current issue (AOTA, 2017). In 2019, after several years of contention, AOTA and ACOTE issued a joint statement that occupational therapists' entry-level degree may be doctoral or master's and occupational therapy assistants' entry-level degree may be bachelor's or associate's level (AOTA & ACOTE, 2019). Although the content of the debate has changed over time as influenced by higher education, health care, and societal policies, the core issue of the academic education necessary to practice occupational therapy has been a source of tension in the profession since its inception.

Student Requirements

Until the 1960s, potential students' education, age, character, and health had specified criteria in the occupational therapy accreditation standards. Before 1943, the occupational therapy standards dictated age requirements for students that included a minimum age at graduation of 20 or 21 (AMA, 1935; AOTA, 1924, 1930). In 1930, there was also a maximum age of 40 specified, and some programs continued to specify age minimum and maximum requirements in their published admission criteria (AOTA, 1930). For example, PSOT specified entrance requirements as age 18 to 35, although exceptions to the maximum age were made on an individual basis (Nimbkar, 1980; PSOT, 1941). "Good character" was a stated admission requirement for occupational therapy students until the 1960s, and even after it was no longer specified in the accreditation standards, it continued to be an expectation without a clear definition (e.g., Council on Medical Education and Hospitals, 1950). Until 1983, the standards also required "good health," defined in 1943 as individuals being free from tuberculosis and with current vaccinations (e.g., Council on Medical Education and Hospitals, 1943). By 1973, the requirement was broader, and applicants had to "submit evidence of good mental and physical health, consistent with the demands of the total educational program" (AOTA, 1975, p. 488). This requirement for good health may have formed a basis for excluding applicants with disabilities, an issue of recent significance to the field. In the 1960s, occupational therapy accreditation standards shifted the responsibility for defining student admission requirements to individual occupational therapy programs. The 1973 standards added stipulations that programs use published criteria, follow the practices of the educational institution, and involve occupational therapy faculty in student selection, but each program determined its own requirements for admission (AOTA, 1975).

Faculty Requirements

The only mention of faculty in the first occupational therapy standards was that "some properly qualified member of the staff" should "interpret" the medical content into the practical work of occupational therapy for the students (AOTA, 1924, p. 298). Once accreditation standards began to specify requirements for faculty starting in 1935, the main areas of concern were registration as an occupational therapist, clinical experience, teaching competence or experience, and, later, the faculty member's academic degree. Additional requirements for program directors became codified in 1943 with the recommendation that the program director have an academic degree (Council on Medical Education and Hospitals, 1943). Following the pattern of other occupational therapy standards, initially, there were recommendations for faculty criteria, which later became requirements, such as the program director's academic preparation. Because programs were required to affiliate with colleges and universities, additional language in the standards ensured that requirements for faculty were consistent with other programs in the educational institution (AOTA, 1967).

Educational Content

Early occupational therapy standards provided specific requirements for the content programs must teach, including the number of hours for each content area. For example, the 1930 standards specified 165 hours total, split between psychology and other mental sciences, physiology and other physical sciences, medical conditions, and occupational therapy principles and history (AOTA, 1930). The bulk of the coursework (1000 hours) consisted of "training in occupations" with a long list of specific crafts that had to be included in entry-level education (AOTA, 1930). The content categories and the amount of time required in each category changed with subsequent standards. In 1965, the number of semester hours devoted to crafts substantially decreased from the previous requirement of 25 semester hours to 9 semester hours (AOTA, 1967; Council on Medical Education and Hospitals, 1950). Rather than lowering standards, this was seen as a way to support students learning how to use crafts therapeutically rather than acquiring a wide range of craft skills (AOTA, 1963, 1967). In 1973, the standards stopped prescribing the curriculum for occupational therapy programs and instead provided resources to serve as a guide for curriculum development for each program to organize their context (AOTA, 1975). The 1965 and 1973 standards incorporated AOTA's curriculum study consensus recommendations to consider the following changes: (a) emphasize function and dysfunction rather than diagnosis-based treatment, (b) increase the emphasis on behavioral sciences to be equal to biological sciences, (c) de-emphasize crafts, (d) change aspects of fieldwork education to increase quality rather than quantity, and (e) integrate fieldwork with academic education (AOTA, 1963). The content that programs needed to address became more detailed with subsequent standards. In 1983, specific outcomes of entry-level education, beyond assuring entry-level competence, were explicitly stated. These outcomes expanded to include additional roles that experienced occupational therapists could hold such as "consultant, educator, researcher, and health planner" (AOTA, 1983a, p. 817). By 1999, the outcomes of occupational therapy education expanded beyond essential requirements for practice to include preparation "to be a lifelong learner" and other characteristics associated with being a professional (AOTA, 1999, p. 575).

Fieldwork and Clinical Education

The earliest occupational therapy training programs included observation and work with hospital patients as part of the curriculum (Quiroga, 1995). The first occupational therapy education standards specified that a minimum of 3 of the 12 months of the program needed to be spent in supervised hospital training (AOTA, 1924). In 1930, this substantially increased to 9 months of the minimum 2-year program and included the additional requirements for "competent supervision" by an occupational therapist and specific settings where the "practice training" needed to occur, including "mental hospitals, tuberculosis hospitals, general hospitals, children's hospitals, and orthopedic hospitals" (AOTA, 1930, p. 2). The requirement for 9 months of clinical education remained in place until the 1965 standards decreased the minimum time to 6 months, a rare example of reducing standards (AOTA, 1967). The setting requirements changed to 3 months in a psychosocial setting, 3 months in a physical dysfunction setting, and, as needed, up to 2 additional months to work with medical and surgical conditions if not addressed in previous settings (AOTA, 1967). The decision to lower the standard related to time is noteworthy because it came after the AOTA "curriculum study" that recommended additional, high-quality clinical training opportunities infused in the curriculum (AOTA, 1963). The 1973 standards implemented that recommendation by instituting and delineating Level I and Level II fieldwork requirements (AOTA, 1975). Subsequent editions of the standards required that Level I fieldwork align with the curriculum design. It was not until 2011 that the standards specified a setting requirement for Level I that at least one fieldwork rotation, whether Level I or II, focus on psychosocial needs (ACOTE, 2012). The other substantial changes to fieldwork came in 1999 when Level II fieldwork increased from 6 months that could include 3 months of part-time work up to 6 months of full-time practice or its equivalent. The 2011 standards included more fieldwork-specific requirements (ACOTE, 2012; AOTA, 1999).

Additional Requirements for Entry Into Practice

The occupational therapy registry was one of the earliest attempts to regulate practice beyond educational programs. AOTA initially developed the registry in 1931 as a way to enforce the minimum standards for occupational therapy education programs (AOTA, 1930). After grandfathering in practicing therapists regardless of their educational preparation, AOTA required graduation from an approved educational program to qualify for registry and use the official designation "OT Reg" (West, 1992). Occupational therapy programs strongly encouraged their graduates to join the registry to promote higher standards for the profession because there was no formal regulation of the profession beyond AOTA (Klinefelter, 1939; Peters et al., 2017).

Because the number of schools offering occupational therapy programs significantly expanded in the 1940s, AOTA created the certification examination in 1947 (Brandt, 1956). The national examination confirmed that graduates met basic standards and that there was a consistent way to ensure entry-level competence (Brandt, 1956). Passing the examination became a requirement for national registration (AOTA, 1967; Brandt, 1956). For a brief time in the 1970s until 1982, criteria for entry into the profession were relaxed, and the certification examination was available as a non–education-based mechanism for occupational therapy assistants to become occupational therapists (Colman, 1992a; Cottrell, 2000).

Occupational therapy licensure is another mechanism beyond education to control entry into the profession and provide consumer protection. Since the 1970s, AOTA has supported state regulation of occupational therapy and a legal definition of occupational therapy, although some continued to argue that educational accreditation and the national certification examination provided sufficient consumer protection (Davy & Peters, 1982; Low, 1992).

In sum, major changes in occupational therapy education included increases in the numbers of educational programs; advances in educational standards that detailed criteria for content, student requirements, and faculty requirements; and additional requirement to enter practice. The following sections explore why these changes occurred.

WHY CHANGES IN OCCUPATIONAL THERAPY EDUCATION OCCURRED

Tensions within occupational therapy and from external forces have prompted changes in occupational therapy education. The common vision of occupational therapy education is to graduate competent occupational therapy practitioners. However, what constituted competence and the ideas about how to create such competence have been sources of debate in occupational therapy education. The following sections discuss historical examples of tensions and their relationship to changes in occupational therapy education.

Occupational Therapy: Who Are We and Who Do We Want to Become?

Occupational therapy leaders, educators, and clinicians hold beliefs about what the profession is and should be, who the practitioner is and should be, and what occupational therapy practitioners do and should do. These beliefs differ across individuals and groups, change over time, and reflect personal and professional values. As occupational therapy historian Wendy Colman (1986) argued, the debates about values guiding occupational therapy education have propelled professional growth and development.

Becoming a Profession

Many of the internal debates in occupational therapy impacting occupational therapy education stemmed from the goal to achieve the status of "profession." Characteristics of professions include having a unique knowledge base and skill set learned through extensive education and using that knowledge to serve society (Brown et al., 2015; Grant, 1986; MacDonald, 1995). As a traditionally women-dominated field, occupational therapy was considered a semiprofession or trade rather than a profession; men-dominated fields were more likely to be granted status as a profession (Linker, 2005; Quiroga, 1995). Becoming recognized as a profession has been a major factor in the debate over entry-level degree requirements. The need for a unique knowledge base fueled the development of occupational science that is now named within the liberal arts and sciences foundation in the occupational therapy education standards (ACOTE, 2012; Yerxa, 1994). Good moral character, a common criterion for entry into a profession, was removed as an admission criterion from occupational therapy accreditation standards, but it continues to be a requirement in half of the states' occupational therapy licensure requirements (AOTA State Affairs Group, 2017; Craddock, 2008). Additionally, licensure for occupational therapists served as an external validation of professional status; thus, advocacy for licensure intensified in the 1970s when the debate included whether occupational therapy qualified as a profession if it was not licensed (Low, 1992).

The early discussion about the primacy of art or science in occupational therapy was another manifestation of the quest for professionalization through occupational therapy education. Although the combination of art and science is a long-standing hallmark of occupational therapy, science was more consistent with the professionalization goal of the field (AOTA, 1972; Quiroga, 1995). The relative dominance of art or science and changing definitions of what constitutes art or science prompted shifts in how crafts, interaction with clients, and medically focused topics were emphasized in occupational therapy standards and across occupational therapy curricula (e.g., Peters et al., 2017). Debates continue about how and to what extent basic sciences and crafts should be included in occupational therapy curricula. However, the importance of both client-centered therapeutic relationships, associated with art, and evidence-based practice, associated with science, is well established in current occupational therapy education.

The philosophies of both pragmatism and structuralism have also coexisted throughout the history of occupational therapy, with changes in the dominance of the ideas informing education and visions of what occupational therapy wants to become (Hooper & Wood, 2002). Related to the nature of humans, pragmatism focuses on human agency and individual experience, whereas structuralism understands humans as a sum of parts and generalizable patterns (Hooper & Wood, 2002). Although occupational therapy currently leans toward a pragmatist view of the human, both ideas continue to infuse occupational therapy and create a tension between what occupational therapists think and what they prioritize with clients. Influences of this tension on education are reflected in how explicitly educators discuss assumptions underlying one's clinical thinking, explore how some of these assumptions may be in conflict with each other, and encourage students to consider how their assumptions play out in therapeutic planning (Hooper & Wood, 2002).

The philosophical conceptualization of knowledge has a huge impact on what and how occupational therapy educators teach, but educators may be less aware of their assumptions about the nature of knowledge unless they are prompted to explore them. Pragmatism considers knowledge as situational such that knowledge changes based on the context, and structuralism posits that knowledge is more objective and universal (Hooper & Wood, 2002). These different views of knowledge impact how educators teach occupational therapy students to develop therapeutic reasoning skills. Early occupational therapy education was designed to ensure sufficient "foundational" knowledge, and although what information was considered important changed over time, the structuralist view of knowledge was clear (Hooper, 2006; Hooper & Wood, 2002). Until the 1990s, educational standards addressed the variety and amount of information students needed to learn more than their process for evaluating information and determining therapeutic actions. Recognizing the need for this shift was one of the major rationales for the mandate for entry-level graduate education. This relatively recent shift to a pragmatist view of knowledge in occupational therapy requires educators to set up situations to enable student learning that avoid perpetuating knowledge as universal, concrete, and static (Hooper, 2006). This current pragmatist view of knowledge is consistent with the type of reasoning needed to meet occupational therapy's goal to be a profession with a distinct knowledge base and skill set that practitioners assemble in each therapeutic encounter.

Student Recruitment and Diversity

Demographics are a basic aspect of who occupational therapy practitioners are, and student demographics are one reflection of the diversity of future occupational therapy practitioners. Limiting diversity in the profession was initially intentional as a way to supposedly promote the professionalization of occupational therapy; however, such practices set up a potentially exclusionary dynamic that current occupational therapy educators continue to struggle against.

Occupational therapy was originally created as a profession for women, and recruitment for occupational therapy students has a history of being strongly gendered. The U.S. government set qualifications for women to become reconstruction aides during World War I, and occupational therapy educators recruited upper-class, well-educated, White women to the profession (Quiroga, 1995). In the 1920s, occupational therapy educators emphasized the importance of an individual's character and personality because they sought students who matched their ideas of professional women (Quiroga, 1995). By the 1930s, there was a more concerted effort to recruit men into the profession, although the St. Louis School of Occupational Therapy (now Washington University) was the only program that accepted men until the 1940s (Black, 2002; Klinefelter, 1938, 1939). Tracking the number of men in educational programs was one way that AOTA monitored the diversity of the profession, and in the 1950s and 1960s, AOTA encouraged the recruitment of men to stabilize the workforce because many women left the field when they married (Black, 2002). This resulted in what Clare Spackman reported as occupational therapy's "matrimonial death rate" (Foley, 1962). These early patterns of recruitment and dominance of women in the field have persisted, and men continue to be a significant minority among occupational therapy practitioners to this day (Maxim & Rice, 2018).

Although lesbian women have likely not been underrepresented in occupational therapy, their presence has been hidden. Students and practitioners who challenged heterosexual and gender norms have not been consistently welcomed into the field. There is evidence that some lesbian occupational therapists created life partnerships in the 1950s through 1970s and even earlier; however, lesbian or gay identity was not openly discussed or accepted in the professional realm during this time (Peters, 2013). Although societal acceptance of the range of sexual orientations and gender identities is improving, many current occupational therapy practitioners continue to express caution about being open about their personal life while in professional settings, and the educational setting can reinforce these dynamics for students (Falzarano & Pizzi, 2015; Jackson, 2000; Murphy, 2014).

Racial diversity has been limited in occupational therapy, and occupational therapy recruitment often reflected structural discrimination present in the larger society. The first African American occupational therapists graduated in 1946, and they were expected to fit in with the dominant White, middle-class culture of occupational therapy (Black, 2002). Lela Llorens, an African American occupational therapist who graduated in 1953, reported that she felt that occupational therapy education programs may have been hesitant to recruit African American students because "they won't get jobs … [or they will] be rejected by patients who wouldn't want an African American working with them" (Peters, 2013, p. 124). This protectionist view may have perpetuated racial discrimination in occupational therapy. The founding of the Black Caucus group in the mid-1970s, 20 years before other diversity-based occupational therapy groups, was a concerted effort to counter this discrimination and support African American occupational therapy students and practitioners (Black, 2002; Peters, 2013). At the same time that the Black Caucus formed, Naomi Wright, one of the first African American occupational therapists, became the founding director at Howard University, the first historically black college or university with an occupational therapy program, another mechanism to support professional diversity (AOTA, 1976; Black, 2002).

Including individuals with disabilities in occupational therapy education programs has been a source of long-running debate in the profession. Although there was not universal agreement, in the 1940s, AOTA's education subcommittee took a protectionist stance toward individuals with disabilities that was similar to practices for racial minorities. Bea Wade, chairman of AOTA's education subcommittee, wrote that the committee considered it "advisable that applicants with marked handicaps should be excluded" (AOTA, 1948). Such blatant discrimination ended by the 1970s with federal legislation (Section 504, Rehabilitation Act of 1973) that prohibited higher education institutions from discriminating against people with disabilities. However, occupational therapy students and practitioners with disabilities continue to experience attitudinal barriers and issues with reasonable accommodations (Gitlow, 2001; Velde, Chapin, & Wittman, 2005).

The only diversity information AOTA requested from occupational therapy education programs in the 1940s and 1950s was sex and African American race (Black, 2002). In 1955, they stopped collecting race information and began asking about foreign students, likely prompted by the international expansion of occupational therapy and the formation of the World Federation of Occupational Therapists. In the 1940s through 1960s, occupational therapy education in the United States was a source of international growth and development of the profession as individuals attended school in the United States and returned to start occupational therapy educational programs in other countries such as India, Israel, the Philippines, and Japan (Bondoc, 2005; Nimbkar, 1980; Sachs & Sussman, 1995; Suzuki, 1982).

Sex, sexual orientation, race, and country of origin do not sufficiently reflect the diversity of occupational therapy even in these earlier time periods, but it was not until the 1980s that there was an effort at the national level to begin to challenge the structures that encouraged limited diversity among occupational therapists (Black, 2002). This struggle continues to the present, and the effects on diversity with the emphasis on entry-level doctoral education is unknown (Brown et al., 2015).

Shared Vision

Although debate within the broader profession is healthy for development, at the level of the individual educational programs, there needs to be sufficient agreement among the educators to develop a shared vision of how the program hopes to see the field evolve and who the program wants occupational therapy practitioners to become. This challenge to create a common vision for the occupational therapy education program involves negotiating the beliefs, values, and priorities of individual faculty, educational institutions, and environments where graduates will work.

Educational Systems

Education is the means of creating the occupational therapy practitioner of the future, and educational systems are the primary mediator between the profession's internal view of itself and the health care and community environments where occupational therapy practitioners provide services.

Educational Philosophy

Occupational therapy formed at a time of educational reform that influenced the development of the emerging profession and occupational therapy education (Schwartz, 1992; Townsend & Friedland, 2016). In addition to structuralism and pragmatism discussed earlier that inform how occupational therapists teach and practice, occupational therapy has been strongly influenced by the educational philosophy of learning by doing (Schwartz, 1992; Townsend & Friedland, 2016).

Although this philosophy was adopted at the profession's inception, the clearest example of the implementation of learning through doing in occupational therapy education is the inclusion of fieldwork as an essential aspect of entry-level preparation. In addition to modeling nursing and medicine to include clinical education, fieldwork education provided a mechanism to implement the educational philosophy of learning through doing. While embracing this educational philosophy, it also set up a potential conflict for occupational therapy's goal to become a profession because technical, skill-based training or apprenticeship are hallmarks of trades more so than professions (Grant, 1986).

Educational Institutions

Once housed in a college or university, each occupational therapy program had to negotiate another layer of influence to consider its contributions to the educational institution and how to advance the mission of the institution. Recognizing the potential for competing interests, the 1973 standards provided latitude to defer aspects of program requirements to the institution while ensuring protections for sufficient university resources for the program, such as space, equipment, and direct involvement with program budgeting (AOTA, 1975). Occupational therapy programs found their institutional home in a wide array of settings, including medical schools, liberal arts colleges, schools of education, and new allied health schools (Yerxa, 1994).

PSOT provides a key historical example of a cautionary tale of a program that did not sufficiently anticipate changes in its educational institution or ensure that the program goals were consistent with the goals of the university (Peters et al., 2017). PSOT began in 1918 in response to the World

War I emergency and was one of the original occupational therapy programs to meet the first educational standards. The program affiliated with the University of Pennsylvania School of Education in the 1940s as a way for students to earn a bachelor's degree in education and a certificate in occupational therapy, but PSOT remained an independent institution. PSOT became part of the University of Pennsylvania in 1950 as part of the newly formed School of Auxiliary Medical Services. As early as 1953, the dean explained to university administration that allowances needed to be made for faculty credentials and scholarship because occupational therapy and other programs in the school were relatively new fields with few scholars (Hutchinson, 1953; Peters et al., 2017). This early indication of a conflict between the program and the institution did not prompt changes in the program, although the protection of an understanding dean and powerful physicians on the program advisory board safeguarded the school for many years. When the university experienced financial constraints in the 1970s and reconsidered its strategic plan in light of national issues in higher education, the rift between the purpose of the occupational therapy program to produce strong occupational therapists and the purpose of the university to foster scholarship consistent with an Ivy League research university became insurmountable (Peters et al., 2017). Despite an outcry from many stakeholder groups, the Board of Trustees voted in 1977 to close the School of Allied Medical Professions, as it had been renamed, and one of the original occupational therapy programs that had produced many leaders in the field closed in 1981 (Peters et al., 2017).

Different types of universities prioritize external funding, research production, teaching, and service to varying degrees. Occupational therapy programs need to monitor and respond to the explicit and implicit expectations of their institutional home to proactively anticipate changes that may be required. Furthermore, occupational therapy programs must clearly align the program goals with the educational institution's goals and mission. The responsibility for the closure of PSOT does not solely lie with the occupational therapy program, but the lesson for current educators is to work to ensure philosophical and strategic consistency between their own programs and their institutional home.

Health Care and Societal Systems

The health care and community systems where occupational therapists provide services expect education programs to produce good occupational therapists who can meet clients' needs and fit into their organizations. Occupational therapy educators and programs have to negotiate the external demands from the health care system, legal requirements, and societal expectations and opportunities with the internal demands of who the profession is and wants to become. As the profession of occupational therapy moved beyond medical settings, community agencies and society at large have become important stakeholders that influence occupational therapy education. This phenomenon that began in the 1970s with the passage of special education legislation and increased interest in community practice has not yet been the subject of historical analysis in occupational therapy. However, occupational therapy's relationship in the health care system and with medicine, in particular, has been a factor in occupational therapy education since the beginning of the field.

Occupational therapy founders disagreed about the relationship occupational therapy should have with medicine. Susan Tracy insisted that occupational therapy should be a nursing specialty, and her primary professional identity as a nurse led her to disengage from occupational therapy in the early 1920s (Quiroga, 1995). The early departure from the fields of education and vocational rehabilitation were attempts to legitimize occupational therapy as a medical profession (Quiroga, 1995). The decision to continue independent schools of occupational therapy meant that occupational therapists could not claim the same emerging professional status as teachers who were educated in colleges, but this early push for autonomy set the stage for the tension in occupational therapy's relationship with medicine.

Occupational therapy's relationship with medicine has existed as a range between autonomy and protection. The independent schools of occupational therapy and AOTA's national registry were attempts to ensure the autonomy of the burgeoning profession from medicine. However, to legitimize occupational therapy as a medical field with the goal of developing into a health care profession, occupational therapy sought protection through physicians and an alliance with the AMA.

Occupational therapy initially promoted itself as a medical field by insisting that occupational therapy services be provided only under a physician's orders, a practice that continued for many years (Quiroga, 1995; Spackman, 1971). The official 1972 definition of occupational therapy no longer included this protection from a physician and specified that occupational therapists "both receive from and make referrals to [a wide range of] health, education, or medical specialists" (AOTA, 1972, p. 205). However, as states enacted licensure laws, some included requirements for physician referrals despite occupational therapy's stance that this protection was no longer necessary (Davy & Peters, 1982).

A historical example of the impact of the health care system on occupational therapy education is illustrated by physical medicine's attempt to take over occupational therapy in the 1940s (Colman, 1992b; West, 1992; Yerxa, 1994). The relationship between medicine and occupational therapy up to that point was amicable, and occupational therapy generally deferred to medicine (West, 1992). As physical medicine developed as a new medical specialty, it sought to define a scope of influence that included physical therapy and occupational therapy (Colman, 1992b). The first indication that this was a threat came from Bea Wade, an occupational therapy educator at the University of Illinois, who experienced issues with physical medicine at her university (Colman, 1992b; West, 1992). Some occupational therapy leaders felt that closely aligning with physical medicine would protect the field from competition from physical therapy as well as increase recognition for occupational therapy's still developing role in physical rehabilitation. However, others feared this would negatively impact occupational therapy's role in psychiatric practice and decrease the field's autonomy. When AOTA representatives met with the Baruch Commission on Physical Medicine in the late 1940s, it became clear the physicians planned to control occupational therapy education and the national registry (Colman, 1992b; West, 1992). Because of the early warnings from Bea Wade, who recognized the national implications of an issue at her university, and the work of other occupational therapy leaders, occupational therapy predicted that the potential protections offered by an alliance with physical medicine would result in too much loss of autonomy of the profession. The potential loss included limiting occupational therapy clients to those with physical disabilities and restricting occupational therapy's knowledge development (Yerxa, 1994). In addition to demonstrating the potential impact of medicine on occupational therapy education, this example demonstrates how educators may recognize threats within their own institutions that have national implications for the profession and occupational therapy education.

CONCLUSION

The overarching tension prompting changes in occupational therapy education over time has been the aim to professionalize occupational therapy. This goal to become a profession has led to debates between the primacy of art or science, competing educational philosophies, and changes in student recruitment and acceptance of diversity. Occupational therapy education programs have to manage distinct expectations from the profession, educational institutions, and health care and societal systems. Debate can be healthy for professional growth and development, and it can be helpful to explore underlying assumptions that likely connect to views about what occupational therapy is and should become. Determining if different positions are based on divergent visions for the profession or separate ways to reach a shared vision can make debate more productive. In addition to negotiating internal factors within the profession, occupational therapy educators and practitioners need to monitor external expectations from educational and practice settings as well as sociopolitical and policy changes to anticipate and address potential challenges to occupational therapy practice and education. The examples from occupational therapy history presented in this chapter can help educators recognize the ongoing impact of these competing forces and navigate a path through them that continues to foster growth of occupational therapy as an autonomous profession building knowledge about and addressing society's occupational needs.

Implications for Occupational Therapy Education

- Occupational therapy educators need to consider their own professional identity as occupational therapy practitioners, how their views influence what they want occupational therapy to become, and how their teaching practices implicitly and explicitly encourage or restrict this vision.
- Occupational therapy educational programs may inadvertently perpetuate undesirable patterns with strong historical roots, such as limited diversity of occupational therapy students, unless they challenge the structures and assumptions underlying their practices.
- Educators can watch for and address challenges and opportunities from occupational therapy education's external forces including educational, societal, and health care systems.

Key Reflection Questions

1. How do your teaching practices promote the type of occupational therapy practitioner you want to see your students become in the future? How do you analyze your own assumptions about knowledge, and how do you help students to do this?
2. What do you see occupational therapy as now, and what would you like to see it become? How do your views influence how you foster occupational therapy students' professional identity?
3. What changes have you seen in the educational system that have influenced occupational therapy education? How did you anticipate and/or respond to these changes?
4. How have you seen changes in the occupational therapy role within the health care system and society at large influence occupational therapy education?

What led you to become an occupational therapy educator?

I knew that I wanted to become an occupational therapy educator from the time that I was a student in an entry-level master's degree program in the late 1990s. I have always been interested in teaching, research, and community-based practice, and becoming an educator was a way to do all of these. While pursuing my doctoral degree, I received the helpful advice to wait until I finished my degree to transition from full-time clinical practice to become a faculty member. I love fostering learning and excitement for our profession, and working with students first as a fieldwork educator and later as a faculty member has allowed me to become a better occupational therapist and teacher. I am passionate about promoting theory-based, occupation-centered practice and influencing the profession through interactions with future occupational therapists. My role as an educator supports my work to enhance the occupational lives of children and adults with developmental disabilities through practice and research, and I appreciate how studying history has strengthened my own professional identity and provided examples to encourage my students as they develop their professional identities. Being an occupational therapy educator is challenging in the way that all worthwhile things are, and my initial goal to combine teaching, research, and community-based practice in a career I love has certainly been met.

Wanda J. Mahoney, PhD, OTR/L

ACKNOWLEDGMENTS

The author thanks Teague Murphy, Laura Dunne, and Sara Kopera, Midwestern University occupational therapy students, for research assistance to prepare this chapter.

REFERENCES

Accreditation Council of Occupational Therapy Education. (2012). 2011 Accreditation Council of Occupational Therapy Education (ACOTE) standards and interpretive guide. *American Journal of Occupational Therapy, 66*, S6-S74. doi:10.5014/ajot.2012.66S6

American Medical Association. (1935). Essentials of an acceptable school of occupational therapy. *JAMA: The Journal of the American Medical Association, 104*, 1632-1633.

American Occupational Therapy Association. (1924). Minimum standards for courses of training in occupational therapy. *Archives of Occupational Therapy, 3*(4), 295-298.

American Occupational Therapy Association. (1930). *Minimum standards for courses of training in occupational therapy.* New York, NY: Author.

American Occupational Therapy Association. (1948). Meeting of the sub-committee on schools and curriculum, March 1948. American Occupational Therapy Association Archives (Box 42, Folder 283). Wilma West Library, Bethesda, MD.

American Occupational Therapy Association. (1950). Schools offering courses in occupational therapy. *American Journal of Occupational Therapy, 4*(3), 142.

American Occupational Therapy Association. (1960). Colleges and universities offering courses in occupational therapy. *American Journal of Occupational Therapy, 14*(6), back cover.

American Occupational Therapy Association. (1963). *Occupational therapy curriculum study.* New York, NY: Author.

American Occupational Therapy Association. (1967). *Guidelines for the utilization of the essentials of an accredited curriculum in occupational therapy.* New York, NY: Author.

American Occupational Therapy Association. (1970). Occupational therapy curricula. *American Journal of Occupational Therapy, 24*(2), 144-145.

American Occupational Therapy Association. (1972). Occupational therapy: Its definition and functions. *American Journal of Occupational Therapy, 26*(4), 204-205.

American Occupational Therapy Association. (1975). Essentials of an accredited educational program for occupational therapists. *American Journal of Occupational Therapy, 24*, 485-496.

American Occupational Therapy Association. (1976). Occupational therapy educational programs. *American Journal of Occupational Therapy, 30*(10), 650-654.

American Occupational Therapy Association. (1983a). Essentials of an accredited educational program for the occupational therapist. *American Journal of Occupational Therapy, 37*(12), 817-823. doi:10.5014/ajot.37.12.817

American Occupational Therapy Association. (1983b). Listing of educational programs in occupational therapy. *American Journal of Occupational Therapy, 37*(11), 773-780. doi:10.5014/ajot.37.11.773

American Occupational Therapy Association. (1990). Listing of educational programs in occupational therapy. *American Journal of Occupational Therapy, 44*(12), 1104-1112. doi:10.5014/ajot.44.12.1104

American Occupational Therapy Association. (1991). Essentials and guidelines for an accredited educational program for the occupational therapist. *American Journal of Occupational Therapy, 45*(12), 1077-1084. doi:10.5014/ajot.45.12.1077

American Occupational Therapy Association. (1998). Listing of educational programs in occupational therapy. *American Journal of Occupational Therapy, 52*(10), 885-903. doi:10.5014/ajot.52.10.885

American Occupational Therapy Association. (1999). Standards for an accredited educational program for the occupational therapist. *American Journal of Occupational Therapy, 53*(6), 575-582. doi:10.5014/ajot.53.6.575

American Occupational Therapy Association. (2000). Listing of educational programs in occupational therapy. *American Journal of Occupational Therapy, 54*(6), 649-660. doi:10.5014/ajot.54.6.649

American Occupational Therapy Association. (2010). List of educational programs in occupational therapy. *American Journal of Occupational Therapy, 64*(Suppl. 2), S146-S158. doi:10.5014/ajot2010.64S146

American Occupational Therapy Association. (2016). History of AOTA accreditation. Retrieved from http://www.aota.org/education-careers/accreditation/overview/history.aspx

American Occupational Therapy Association. (2017). ACOTE mandate 2027 background materials. Retrieved from https://www.aota.org/~/media/Corporate/Files/EducationCareers/Accredit/ACOTE-2027-Mandate-Background-Materials.pdf

American Occupational Therapy Association. (2018). List of educational programs in occupational therapy. *American Journal of Occupational Therapy*, 72(S2), 7212420025p1-7212420025p18. doi:10.5014/ajot.2018.72S214

American Occupational Therapy Association [AOTA], & Accreditation Council of Occupational Therapy Education [ACOTE]. (2019). Joint AOTA-ACOTE statement on entry-level education. OT Practice, 24(5), 4.

American Occupational Therapy Association State Affairs Group. (2017). Occupational therapists–Licensure requirements. Retrieved from https://www.aota.org/~/media/corporate/files/secure/advocacy/licensure/stateregs/qualifications/ot-qualifications-licensure-requirements-by-state.pdf

Black, R. M. (2002). Occupational therapy's dance with diversity. *American Journal of Occupational Therapy*, 56(2), 140-148. doi:10.5014/ajot.56.2.140

Bondoc, S. (2005). Occupational therapy in the Philippines: From founding years to the present. *Philippine Journal of Occupational Therapy*, 1(1), 9-22.

Brandt, H. (1956). The AOTA registration examination. *American Journal of Occupational Therapy*, 10(6), 281-287, 309.

Brown, T., Crabtree, J. L., Mu, K., & Wells, J. (2015). The next paradigm shift in occupational therapy education: The move to the entry-level clinical doctorate. *American Journal of Occupational Therapy*, 69, 1-6. doi:10.5014/ajot.2015.016527

Colman, W. (1986). History of the formation of educational values in occupational therapy. In *Occupational therapy education: Target 2000 proceedings* (pp. 12-18). Rockville, MD: American Occupational Therapy Association.

Colman, W. (1990). Evolving educational practices in occupational therapy: The war emergency courses, 1936-1954. *American Journal of Occupational Therapy*, 44(11), 1028-1036. doi:10.5014/ajot.44.11.1028

Colman, W. (1992a). Exploring educational boundaries: Occupational therapy and the multiple-entry-route system, 1970-1982. *American Journal of Occupational Therapy*, 46(3), 260-266. doi:10.5014/ajot.46.3.260

Colman, W. (1992b). Maintaining autonomy: The struggle between occupational therapy and physical medicine. *American Journal of Occupational Therapy*, 46(1), 63-70. doi:10.5014/ajot.46.1.63

Cottrell, R. P. F. (2000). COTA education and professional development: A historical review. *American Journal of Occupational Therapy*, 54(4), 407-412. doi:10.5014/ajot.54.4.407

Council on Medical Education and Hospitals. (1943). Essentials of an acceptable school of occupational therapy. *JAMA: The Journal of the American Medical Association*, 122(8), 541-543. doi:10.1001/jama.1943.02840250041017

Council on Medical Education and Hospitals. (1950). Essentials of an acceptable school of occupational therapy. *American Journal of Occupational Therapy*, 4(3), 125-128.

Craddock, L. (2008). Good moral character as a licensing standard. *Journal of the National Association of Adminstrative Law Judiciary*, 28(2), 449-469.

Davy, J. D., & Peters, M. (1982). Nationally speaking: State licensure for occupational therapists. *American Journal of Occupational Therapy*, 36(7), 429-432. doi:10.5014/ajot.36.7.429

Dunton, W. R. (1947). History and development of occupational therapy. In H. S. Willard & C. S. Spackman (Eds.), *Principles of occupational therapy* (1st ed., pp. 1-9). Philadelphia, PA: J. B. Lippincott Company.

Falzarano, M., & Pizzi, M. (2015). Experiences of lesbian and gay occupational therapists in the healthcare system. *Journal of Allied Health*, 44(2), 65-72.

Fisher, G. S. (2000). The status of occupational therapy education in the 90's. *Occupational Therapy in Health Care*, 12(1), 1-15. doi:10.1080/J003v12n01_01

Foley, E. (1962). Occupational therapists hold global meeting here, Philadelphia Bulletin newspaper article, October 21, 1962. University Archives and Records Center, University of Pennsylvania (UPC 6.11, Box 2, Folder 112), Philadelphia, PA.

Gitlow, L. (2001). Occupational therapy faculty attitudes toward the inclusion of students with disabilities in their educational programs. *Occupational Therapy Journal of Research*, 21(2), 115-131.

Grant, H. K. (1986). The role of education in the development of a profession. In *Occupational therapy education: Target 2000 proceedings* (pp. 6-11). Rockville, MD: American Occupational Therapy Association.

Grant, H. K. (1991). Education then and now: 1949 and 1989. *American Journal of Occupational Therapy*, 45(4), 295-299. doi:10.5014/ajot.45.4.295

Hooper, B. (2006). Epistemological transformation in occupational therapy: Educational implications and challenges. *OTJR: Occupation, Participation & Health*, 26(1), 15-24. doi:10.1177/153944920602600103

Hooper, B., & Wood, W. (2002). Pragmatism and structuralism in occupational therapy: The long conversation. *American Journal of Occupational Therapy*, 56(1), 40-50. doi:10.5014/ajot.56.1.40

Hutchinson, W. G. (1953). Letter to Dr. Paul W Bruton, October 28, 1953. University Archives and Records Center, University of Pennsylvania (UPC 7.4, Box 2, Folder 37), Philadelphia, PA.

Jackson, J. (2000). Understanding the experience of noninclusive occupational therapy clinics: Lesbians' perspectives. *American Journal of Occupational Therapy*, 54(1), 26-35. doi:10.5014/ajot.54.1.26

Klinefelter, L. M. (1938). *Medical occupations available to boys when they grow up*. New York, NY: E. P. Dutton & Co., Inc.

Klinefelter, L. M. (1939). *Medical occupations for girls: Women in white*. New York, NY: E. P. Dutton & Co., Inc.

Linker, B. (2005). Strength and science: Gender, physiotherapy, and medicine in the United States, 1918-35. *Journal of Women's History, 17*(3), 106-132. doi:10.1353/jowh.2005.0034

Low, J. F. (1992). Another look at licensure: Consumer protection or professional protectionism? *American Journal of Occupational Therapy, 46*(4), 373-376. doi:10.5014/ajot.46.4.373

Lucci, J. A. (1974). Basic master program. *American Journal of Occupational Therapy, 28*(5), 292-295.

MacDonald, K. M. (1995). *The sociology of the professions*. London, England: Sage.

Maxim, A. J. M., & Rice, M. S. (2018). Men in occupational therapy: Issues, factors, and perceptions. *American Journal of Occupational Therapy, 72*(1), 7201205050p1-7201205050p7. doi:10.5014/ajot.2018.025593

Murphy, M. (2014). Hiding in plain sight: The production of heteronormativity in medical education. *Journal of Contemporary Ethnography, 45*(3), 1-34. doi:10.1177/0891241614556345

Nimbkar, K. V. (1980). *A new life for the handicapped: A history of rehabilitation and occupational therapy in India*. Bombay, India: Nimbkar Rehabilitation Trust.

Peters, C. O. (2013). *Powerful occupational therapists: A community of professionals, 1950-1980*. New York, NY: Routledge.

Peters, C. O., Martin, P. M., & Mahoney, W. J. (2017). The Philadelphia School of Occupational Therapy: A centennial lesson. *Journal of Occupational Therapy Education, 1*(1), 1-18. doi:10.26681/jote.2017.010108

Philadelphia School of Occupational Therapy. (1941). *Healing by work: Philadelphia School of Occupational Therapy brochure*. Philadelphia, PA: PSOT.

Quiroga, V. A. M. (1995). *Occupational Therapy: The first 30 years, 1900 to 1930*. Bethesda, MD: American Occupational Therapy Association.

Sachs, D., & Sussman, N. (1995). Historical research: The first decade of occupational therapy in Israel: 1946-1956. *Occupational Therapy International, 2*(4), 241-256.

Schwartz, K. B. (1992). Occupational therapy and education: A shared vision. *American Journal of Occupational Therapy, 46*(1), 12-18. doi:10.5014/ajot.46.1.12

Spackman, C. S. (1971). Coordination of occupational therapy with other allied medical and related services. In H. S. Willard & C. S. Spackman (Eds.), *Occupational therapy* (4th ed., pp. 1-12). Philadelphia, PA: J. B. Lippincott Company.

Suzuki, A. K. (1982). *History of Japanese occupational therapy education, 1963-1981*. Wayne State University, Detroit, MI.

Townsend, E., & Friedland, J. (2016). 19th & 20th century educational reforms arising in Europe, the United Kingdom, and the Americas: Inspiration for occupational science? *Journal of Occupational Science, 23*(4), 488-495. doi:10.1080/14427591.2016.1232184

Velde, B. P., Chapin, M. H., & Wittman, P. P. (2005). Working around "it": The experience of occupational therapy students with a disability. *Journal of Allied Health, 34*(2), 83-89.

West, W. L. (1992). Ten milestone issues in AOTA history. *American Journal of Occupational Therapy, 46*(12), 1066-1074. doi:10.5014/ajot.46.12.1066

Yerxa, E. J. (1994). Who is the keeper of occupational therapy's practice and knowledge? *American Journal of Occupational Therapy, 49*(4), 295-299. doi:10.5014/ajot.49.4.295

Section II

Present

3

Occupational Therapy Education in a Changing Health Care System
Current Issues and Trends

Tina DeAngelis, EdD, OTR/L; Giulianne Krug, PhD, OTR, CLA;
and Bridgett Piernik-Yoder, PhD, OTR

Chapter Objectives

By the end of this chapter, the reader will be able to:

1. Understand the trajectory of the occupational therapy accreditation process for the occupational therapy degree.
2. Develop knowledge regarding the occupational therapy profession's move to the entry-level master's and entry-level doctorate degrees.
3. Identify the ongoing impact of social, political, and economic factors influencing occupational therapy educational requirements.

EDUCATIONAL REQUIREMENTS FOR OCCUPATIONAL THERAPY PRACTICE

The evolution of educational standards used to inform occupational therapy curricula in the United States has progressed significantly over the past 100 years (Table 3-1). In 1917, when the National Society for the Promotion of Occupational Therapy was established, no formal educational standards were in existence. At this time, there were five institutions teaching short but intensive courses in the use of occupation (Kearney, 2004). These previously termed *reconstruction programs* became occupational therapy programs in 1918 and evolved to include mandatory training in crafts, lectures in topics related to psychology, kinesiology, working with "invalids," and hospital-based practice. These early programs were not degree programs but were training programs to meet a specific need (McDaniel, 1968).

In 1923, the National Society for the Promotion of Occupational Therapy became the American Occupational Therapy Association (AOTA). That same year, in response to the advice of well-respected

Taff, S. D., Grajo, L. C., & Hooper, B. R. (Eds.). *Perspectives on*
Occupational Therapy Education: Past, Present, and Future (pp. 31-44).
© 2020 Taylor & Francis Group.

Table 3-1

TRAJECTORY OF AMERICAN OCCUPATIONAL THERAPY ASSOCIATION ACCREDITATION: 1923 TO 2018

1917	National Society for the Promotion of Occupational Therapy established in District of Columbia (no standards established for the profession).
1923	The now-termed AOTA (1921) develops minimum occupational therapy training program standards.
1935	The AOTA and the Council on Medical Education of the American Medical Association (AMA) collaborate to further refine educational standards for entry-level occupational therapy practice termed "Essentials of an acceptable school of occupational therapy."
1964	AOTA/AMA relationship is acknowledged by the National Commission on Accreditation.
1994	AOTA Accreditation Committee name is changed to the AOTA Accreditation Council for Occupational Therapy Education (ACOTE) and becomes independent of the AMA.
1998	ACOTE develops a position statement regarding draft accreditation standards, "given the demands, complexity and diversity of contemporary occupational therapy practice ... standards are most likely to be achieved in post-baccalaureate degree programs" (AOTA, n.d.).
1999	"Resolution J" passed by Representative Assembly of the AOTA, moving to approve postbaccalaureate as a requirement for entry-level occupational therapy practice by 2007. Creighton University establishes the nation's first entry-level doctor of occupational therapy program (https://spahp.creighton.edu/future-students/doctor-occupational-therapy).
2006	ACOTE "formally adopted Accreditation Standards for a Doctoral-Degree-Level Educational Program for the Occupational Therapist" with an effective date of January 1, 2008" (AOTA, n.d.).
2007	ACOTE mandate that all entry-level occupational therapy programs be offered at the postbaccalaureate level only.
2015	ACOTE "determined that the entry-level-degree requirement for the occupational therapist will remain at both the master's and the doctoral degree" (AOTA, n.d.).
2017	ACOTE revealed that "the entry-level degree requirement for the occupational therapist will move to the doctoral level by July 1, 2027" (https://www.aota.org/Education-Careers/Accreditation/acote-doctoral-mandate-2027.aspx).

physicians and hospital administrators alike, standards for occupational therapy education were approved that reflected the postwar movement toward increased education, inclusive of not only concepts of moral treatment but also the biomedical perspective (Kearney, 2004). These "basic educational standards" in occupational therapy programming across the country served to protect the consumer from incompetent or ill-prepared practitioners (Gordon, 2009; AOTA, 2017a).

The transition of some of occupational therapy's primary areas of employment from psychiatric facilities to acute care/hospital-based and rehabilitation settings brought about change to a medical model approach in the profession. This shift was primarily due to the result of injured soldiers returning to the United States in need of orthopedic care. This change in need resulted in an official affiliation between the AOTA and the American Medical Association (Kearney, 2004). Programs were significantly expanded both in terms of breadth and depth (Table 3-2).

The next major contributor to changes in occupation therapy education standards was World War II. Although the restoration aides and early occupational therapists (and hence occupational therapy education) focused primarily on mental health, World War II brought about increased attention to the physical sequelae of battle. Consequently, the 1940s and 1950s were a time of proliferation for occupational therapists specializing in physical rehabilitation. Reductionist scientific principles filled the occupational therapy literature, and the medical model became the archetype for the direction of occupational therapy theory and practice models (Gillette & Kielhofner, 1979).

The time between 1949 and 1965 was one of continued increase in the specialization of occupational therapy practice. The occupational therapy profession entered a period in which emerging practice areas included prosthetics, pediatrics, and neurology (that extended beyond the traditional physical disability and mental health settings) (Crepeau, Cohn, & Boyt Schell, 2003). The reductionist paradigm became an accepted treatment; hence, education focus shifted to diagnosis and age. The AOTA/American Medical Association collaborative was eventually recognized in the 1960s by the esteemed National Commission on Accreditation, further strengthening the profession's value to its constituents and society. During this time, accreditation standards were also developed for the occupational therapy assistant (see Table 3-2).

The 1965 revision of the Essentials for occupational therapist education mandated the following new components: the inclusion of both psychosocial and physical rehabilitation clinical experiences, specific minimum credit requirements in occupational therapy evaluation and treatment in psychosocial and physical rehabilitation, and the inclusion of administrative content and scientific methodology (Gillette & Kielhofner, 1979).

In 1973, the Essentials were changed to no longer include mandated semester hours for any content area. This allowed individual programs to establish their own curriculum design inclusive of the basic sciences, human development, specific occupations, the health continuum, and occupational therapy theory and practice. Ten years later, the Essentials were again revised to include standards in research and professional development as well as to add Level I fieldwork requirements during coursework to enhance student learning. Interestingly, this iteration also included removal of the requirement that the program director be an occupational therapist, a decision that was reversed again in 1991 (the primary change evident in the 1991 Essentials).

The arrival of managed care in the 1980s prompted a decrease in hospital-based programming, facilitating the movement of practitioners working in traditional settings to more community-based programs. As the profession continued to grow and reach new areas of practice such as school-based practice, skilled nursing facilities, and community mental health settings, the Accreditation Council for Occupational Therapy Education (ACOTE) was formally recognized by the U.S. Department of Education, a national agency that acknowledges professional programs.

The 1990s brought about changes to occupational therapy education reflective of a shift in epistemology away from the reductionism of the medical model and toward higher-level thought, knowledge, and application (Hooper, 2006). This shift was dramatic and resulted in the separation from oversight of education standards by the American Medical Association and the development of ACOTE in 1999. In 1997, in light of ongoing demands placed on occupational therapy practitioners, the Commission on Education Entry-Level Education Task Force concluded that the occupational therapy profession would better serve the public if future occupational therapists were educated at the postbaccalaureate level (Hughes Harris, Brayman, Clark, Delaney, & Miller, 1998). One of the many factors that prompted this decision was the reality that clinicians were being tasked with the responsibility of making critical decisions (consultation needs/early discharge plans for clients)

Table 3-2

Timeline of the Development of Curriculum and Accreditation Standards for Occupational Therapy Entry-Level Education

YEAR	ACCREDITATION ACTION/ STANDARDS	DEGREE LEVEL(S) ACCREDITED	FACULTY EDUCATION REQUIREMENTS
1918	The Surgeon General's office proposed standards to separate training in occupation from nursing were initiated and revised in 1918.	Final 1918 version was a 12- to 16-week course including 264 hours training in crafts; 64 hours of lecture in topics such as psychology, kinesiology, and working with the "invalid"; and 24 hours of hospital practice (McDaniel, 1968).	
1923	The AOTA develops minimum occupational therapy training program standards.	12-month course of training expanded to 18 months in 1930 (no documented change in standards) (Gordon, 2009), including at least 3 months of hospital training.	
1935	The AOTA and the Council on Medical Education of the AMA collaborates to further refine educational standards for entry-level occupational therapy practice, termed "Essentials of an Acceptable School of Occupational Therapy."	A minimum of 100 weeks of full-time training, including 30 semester hours of didactic training in the biological sciences, social sciences, occupational therapy theory, clinical conditions, activity training, and electives and a minimum of 36 weeks of hospital-based training.	
1943 and 1949	Revisions of "Essentials of an Acceptable School of Occupational Therapy."	Revisions increased semester hours for specific coursework and change in clinical training requirements.	

continued

Table 3-2 (continued)

TIMELINE OF THE DEVELOPMENT OF CURRICULUM AND ACCREDITATION STANDARDS FOR OCCUPATIONAL THERAPY ENTRY-LEVEL EDUCATION

YEAR	ACCREDITATION ACTION/ STANDARDS	DEGREE LEVEL(S) ACCREDITED	FACULTY EDUCATION REQUIREMENTS
1965	Revisions of "Essentials of an Acceptable School of Occupational Therapy."	Revisions included mandatory psychosocial and physical rehabilitation clinical training and a reduction to 24 weeks (from 36) of clinical training.	
1973	Revisions of "Essentials of an Acceptable School of Occupational Therapy."	Revisions included the elimination of required semester hours for specific content; no change in clinical training requirement.	
1983	AOTA in collaboration with AMA: Revised "Essentials of an Accredited Educational Program for the Occupational Therapist" published (AOTA, 1983).	Baccalaureate or postbaccalaureate entry-level acknowledged. Research and professional development standards added. Level I fieldwork was added to be concurrent with coursework.	Director should hold a master's or doctoral degree (or equivalent qualifications). Does NOT need to be an occupational therapist. Faculty should meet the standards of the sponsoring institution for their academic preparation (no minimum standard imposed by AOTA).
1991	Accreditation Committee of the AOTA: Revised "Essentials and Guidelines for an Accredited Educational Program for the Occupational Therapist" published (AOTA, 1991).	Baccalaureate or postbaccalaureate entry-level (same standards apply); little change from 1983.	Director should be an initially licensed occupational therapist, hold a minimum of a master's degree, or have equivalent educational qualifications. Faculty must collectively have academic and experiential qualifications and background appropriate to meet program objectives.

continued

Table 3-2 (continued)

TIMELINE OF THE DEVELOPMENT OF CURRICULUM AND ACCREDITATION STANDARDS FOR OCCUPATIONAL THERAPY ENTRY-LEVEL EDUCATION

YEAR	ACCREDITATION ACTION/ STANDARDS	DEGREE LEVEL(S) ACCREDITED	FACULTY EDUCATION REQUIREMENTS
1999	Independent of the AMA, established by ACOTE: Revised "Standards for an Accredited Educational Program for the Occupational Therapist" published (AOTA, 1999). Effective July 1, 2000.	Baccalaureate or postbaccalaureate entry-level (same standards apply). Director shall be an initially licensed occupational therapist with academic qualifications comparable with other administrators who manage similar programs within institutions. Director and faculty must possess the necessary academic and experiential qualifications and backgrounds to meet program objectives.	
2006	ACOTE formally adopted "Accreditation Standards for a Doctoral-Degree-Level Educational Program for the Occupational Therapist" (AOTA, n.d.). Effective January 1, 2008.	Entry-level doctoral degree (optional entry-level degree).	Director must be an initially licensed occupational therapist with a doctoral degree. All full-time faculty must hold a doctoral degree.

continued

Table 3-2 (continued)

TIMELINE OF THE DEVELOPMENT OF CURRICULUM AND ACCREDITATION STANDARDS FOR OCCUPATIONAL THERAPY ENTRY-LEVEL EDUCATION

YEAR	ACCREDITATION ACTION/ STANDARDS	DEGREE LEVEL(S) ACCREDITED	FACULTY EDUCATION REQUIREMENTS
2006	"Accreditation Standards for a Master's-Degree-Level Educational Program for the Occupational Therapist" published (AOTA, 2007). Effective January 1, 2008.	Entry-level master's degree (mandatory entry-level degree).	Director must be an initially licensed occupational therapist with academic qualifications comparable with the majority of other program directors within the institutional unit. By July 1, 2012, the program director must hold a doctoral degree. All full-time faculty must hold a minimum of a master's degree. By July 1, 2012, the majority of all full-time faculty who are occupational therapists must hold a doctoral degree.
2011	"2011 ACOTE Standards" including master's and doctoral degree level standards published. Effective July 31, 2013.	Entry-level master's (mandatory) and doctoral degree (optional).	Master's: Director must be an initially licensed occupational therapist with a doctoral degree. The majority of full-time faculty must hold a doctoral degree, minimum of master's degree. Doctoral: Director must be an initially licensed occupational therapist with a doctoral degree. All full-time faculty must hold a doctoral degree.

continued

Table 3-2 (continued)

TIMELINE OF THE DEVELOPMENT OF CURRICULUM AND ACCREDITATION STANDARDS FOR OCCUPATIONAL THERAPY ENTRY-LEVEL EDUCATION

YEAR	ACCREDITATION ACTION/ STANDARDS	DEGREE LEVEL(S) ACCREDITED	FACULTY EDUCATION REQUIREMENTS
2017	Third draft of the proposed 2018 ACOTE standards is in process.		Degree requirements for full-time faculty are highly debated.
2018	2018 ACOTE standards are approved. Effective July 31, 2020.	Entry-level master's (mandatory) and doctoral degree (optional).	Master's: At least 50% of full-time core faculty must hold a doctoral degree. The program director is counted as a faculty member. At least 25% of full-time core faculty must have a postprofessional doctorate. Doctoral: All full-time core faculty who are occupational therapy practitioners teaching in the program must hold a doctoral degree. At least 50% of full-time core faculty must have a postprofessional doctorate.

that were formally made by seasoned professionals. These factors and more led to the development and eventual approval of Resolution J, requiring the transition of occupational therapy education move from the baccalaureate to the postbaccalaureate for entry-level occupational therapy practice by 2007 (DeAngelis, 2006). During this time, Runyon, Aitken, and Stohs (1994) also suggested that the profession of occupational therapy had evolved so greatly in its depth and breadth of required knowledge that it had practically grown out of its traditional master's degree. While these discussions were occurring in the profession, in 1999, Creighton University launched the nation's first entry-level doctor of occupational therapy program.

EDUCATIONAL ADVANCEMENT IN THE MILLENNIUM

The decade from 2000 to 2010 was quite prolific in terms of the advancement of occupational therapy education and the development of new entry-level standards for both the entry-level master's degree as the minimum degree required and the entry-level doctoral degree (occupational therapy doctorate) as a postbaccalaureate option. As of 2006, there were five accredited entry-level occupational therapy doctorate programs in the United States. However, the amount of accredited occupational therapy entry-level programs would remain at this number because of the AOTA Accreditation Group's "press report" of 2004 announcing that a vote had been passed to defer accreditation to any newly developing entry-level occupational therapy programs (DeAngelis, 2006). The AOTA accreditation moratorium was eventually lifted, and in 2006 "ACOTE formally adopted Accreditation Standards for a Doctoral-Degree-Level Educational Program for the Occupational Therapist" with an effective date of January 2008 (AOTA, n.d.). Since this time, both the master's and doctoral degrees have continued to be considered acceptable for entry-level occupational therapy practice.

A challenge to degree advancement in occupational therapy education was, and remains, the paucity of occupational therapists who have adequate educational qualifications for the academic environment. The initial ACOTE standards for the occupational therapy master's degree required the program director academic qualification be defined by those in comparable positions in the institution; it was mandated that "[by] July 1, 2012, the program director must hold a doctoral degree" (AOTA, 2007). Similarly, although initially all full-time faculty of master's-level occupational therapy programs were required to hold a minimum of a master's degree, at least half of the full-time faculty were required to hold a doctoral degree as of July 1, 2012. The program director and all full-time faculty in entry-level doctoral programs were required to hold doctoral degrees by ACOTE at the time of the initial standards; the type of doctoral degree (research vs clinical) was not designated. At the time of the writing of this chapter, there are considerably more unfilled occupational therapy faculty positions than qualified faculty available to fill them.

The AOTA Board of Directors position statement on entry-level degrees for the occupational therapist (AOTA, 2013) expressed that "a single point of entry-level degree clearly articulates the entry-level competencies and educational requirements to all stakeholders." The position statement also spoke to the need for increased practice-based research and scholarship while increasing opportunities for specialization, primary care, and interprofessional education.

In August 2017, ACOTE announced the entry-level degree requirement would be a doctor of occupational therapy after 2027. In December 2017, ACOTE released an announcement reaffirming this position, stating that after much deliberation it was determined that the entry to practice for the occupational therapist will be at the doctorate level as of 2027. ACOTE stated, "given the deliberate process undertaken to ensure input from stakeholder groups in determining the mandate that the entry-level degree requirement for the occupational therapist will move to the doctoral level by July 1, 2027" (AOTA, 2017b). The ACOTE 2011 and 2018 doctoral-level accreditation standards include requirements for the development of advanced skills beyond the generalist level in one or more of the following areas: clinical practice, research, administration, leadership, program and policy development, advocacy, education, or theory development. As mentioned in this chapter, these recommendations were developed in response to a call from key stakeholders. However, in August 2018, AOTA placed this mandate in abeyance, and further deliberation continues on this issue. Only time will reveal the impact of the final position with regard to entry-level education requirements, but until then the profession continues to aspire to the pillars set forth in the AOTA's Vision 2025 (AOTA, 2017b) for occupational therapists to be evidence and outcomes based, client centered, cost-effective, influential, and culturally responsive to the needs of individuals, populations, and communities.

PREPARING FUTURE PRACTITIONERS FOR EMERGING TRENDS IN HEALTH CARE

It is essential that occupational therapy curricula respond to the ever-changing health care needs and trends throughout the country to prepare entry-level practitioners for current practice. At the time of the writing of this chapter, one of the most prominent examples of such a growing area of health care is primary care. According to the AOTA, "the concept of primary health care includes interprofessional collaboration and practice to more efficiently improve health and access to services while reducing costs and improving general satisfaction for clients and health care providers" (AOTA, 2018a, p. 1). Occupational therapists are key players for health promotion and prevention, particularly in regard to safe and satisfactory engagement in valued occupations. In the primary care setting, occupational therapists are in a position to screen all primary health patients for impairments or risk thereof in regard to "daily activities (roles), age-level development, exploration of social networks, evaluation of environmental hazards, and the combined performance skills that might affect safety at work and home" (AOTA, 2018a, p. 2). Curricular standards in occupational therapy education fully support the role of occupational therapy in primary care. Relevant themes throughout the ACOTE standards for master's and doctoral programs include occupational performance, health and well-being, self-care and self-management training, functional and community mobility, home and community programming, and interprofessional practice, among others.

Interprofessional practice is essential to positive patient outcomes not only in primary care but also throughout the health care continuum and in most nonmedical occupational therapy practice settings (AOTA, 2015). Accordingly, an education standard specific to interprofessional education (IPE) was added in the 2011 ACOTE educational standards (B.5.21) that requires that students will be able to "effectively communicate, coordinate, and work interprofessionally with those who provide services to individuals, organizations, and/or populations in order to clarify each member's responsibility in executing components of an intervention plan" (ACOTE, 2012, p. S48). IPE is essential for occupational therapy students to learn to communicate about occupational therapy and learn disciplinary similarities, differences, and collaborative strategies. Through IPE activities such as simulations, service learning, and student-run clinics, students learn about their own professional roles, valuable communication skills, and how the various professionals on the team work together for the common good of the client.

THE CALL TO ACTION FOR CHANGES IN ENTRY-LEVEL DEGREE REQUIREMENTS

Many factors in the practice settings have resulted in professional programs increasing entry-level requirements, including clinical doctorates due to an increased knowledge base in most professions; technological advances; the need to prepare graduates to enter the complex, dynamic, and interprofessional practice settings; and increasing accreditation standards across professions (Royeen & Lavin, 2007). Therefore, because some professions such as pharmacy, audiology, and physical therapy have moved to clinical doctorates as the entry-level degree for the profession, occupational therapy has evaluated a similar progression (Wells & Crabtree, 2012). The December 2017 announcement that the occupational therapy doctorate will be the required entry-level degree as of 2027 was a defining statement after more than 10 years of consideration of the anticipated benefits and challenges of moving to this single point of entry-level degree for the profession (AOTA, 2017a). Factors that support the rationale to move to a single point of entry of the occupational therapy doctorate include the need to enhance areas in curricula to prepare graduates for advanced practice, such as primary care, and professional roles, such as consultation and advocacy.

In order to fully explore the call to action for changes in the entry-level degree requirements, it is important to consider the trajectory of events that transpired to conclude with the mandate, the rationale for the move to the occupational therapy doctorate as the single point of entry to the profession, and the remaining concerns with the requirement to move to an entry-level doctoral degree requirement.

In response to a request for the information regarding the decision, ACOTE in November 2017 released an 897-page compiled document that consisted of various reports, meeting notes, committee activities, surveys, and other publications (AOTA, 2017a) related to the proposed change in required entry-level education. It is important to note that this document is a compendium of a multitude of AOTA documents and was not presented with any interpretation, index, or consistent chronological order. In order to fully appreciate the circuitous route to the final mandate, it is useful to consider key points of the process en route to the final decision being issued.

As indicated in the ACOTE entry-level degree mandate timeline, an ad hoc committee was established in February 2011 to examine the future of occupational therapy education (AOTA, 2017b, p. 3). In February 2013, this committee presented a list of 19 recommendations based on their findings. These recommendations included establishing a research agenda for occupational therapy education, identifying signature pedagogies in occupational therapy education, strengthening opportunities to disseminate research and scholarship on occupational therapy education, supporting pathways to the professoriate in occupational therapy education including doctoral fellowships, and supporting an interprofessional coalition to address factors impacting clinical education. Specifically, the 16th recommendation in the committee's final report calls on AOTA to "adopt a mandate that entry-level degree for practice as an occupational therapist to be a doctorate in 2017 with a requirement for all academic programs to transition to the doctorate by 2020" (AOTA, 2017b, p. 8).

It is interesting to note the move to doctoral entry level is referred to in other committee reports as well. For example, in an undated report from the Maturing of the Profession Task Group (AOTA, 2017b, pp. 155-263), it appears the eventual move to doctoral entry level is accepted, but the lingering question was when the move would occur. This committee report posits that "pragmatic concerns and occupational therapy's tendency to cling to the status quo" had kept the move in limbo (AOTA, 2017a, p. 160). Citing that the profession's slow move to the master's degree resulted in decreased competitiveness in some practice settings such as mental health, the authors seem to suggest the opportunity cost of not moving to doctoral entry level is perhaps more detrimental to the professional than any negative consequences of doing so.

In February 2013, the AOTA Board of Directors voted in favor of a motion to support the Future of Occupational Therapy Education Ad Hoc Committee's recommendation to move to doctoral entry level but with a proposed target start date of 2025 (AOTA, 2017b). In April 2014, the AOTA Board of Directors released several documents that outlined the rationale for this decision, as well as the pros and cons of the move to doctoral entry level. The rationale included a multitude of factors, including that a doctoral level of preparation is what will be needed in the future to support graduates' evidence-based practice skills to meet the occupational needs of society in increasingly complex care delivery models and demonstrate professional autonomy and leadership roles in the health care delivery system, interprofessional teams, and specialized practice settings. Other factors cited include the move to doctoral entry level by many other health-related professions and this potential to impact hiring practices and leadership opportunities, as well as the potential confusion for all stakeholders to maintain two entry-level degrees (AOTA, 2017b, p. 209).

It was recognized by the AOTA Board of Directors that the move to doctoral entry level entails several hypothesized areas of concern with the potential for negative impact in the profession. These include the additional cost to students and the amount of student debt, a potentially negative impact on diversity in the field, and many unknowns such as the impact on quality of practice, reimbursement, and the impact on the faculty workforce. However, it was also noted that it is important to consider the additional tuition cost to students relative to the credit-intensive master's degrees offered at most occupational therapy education programs, and the move to the entry-level master's degree did not reduce the diversity of those entering the profession.

Following the AOTA Board of Directors' position statement supporting the move to doctoral entry level, ACOTE appointed a task group in April 2014 to consider the entry-level degree requirement. The move to a baccalaureate entry level for occupational therapist assistants was also being deliberated during this process. The task force conducted numerous meetings and work activities, including a survey of the professions in which there were approximately 2,800 respondents. Although 70% of respondents indicated they favored a single point of entry for occupational therapy, the survey did not include a specific question about the support for the move to doctoral entry level (AOTA, 2017b, pp. 415-420). Results of a survey of program directors conducted in May 2015 with 86% of program directors responding revealed 61% of programs were planning to transition to the entry-level doctorate within 5 years. The committee presented the findings at the August 2015 ACOTE meeting, which consisted of numerous other reports and roundtable discussions regarding the benefits and concerns of requiring doctoral entry level. However, at the end of the meeting, the motion that ACOTE mandate a single point of entry at the doctoral level was defeated. Although a comparable motion that the baccalaureate degree becomes the entry-level degree for occupational therapist assistants was also defeated, a motion to allow two points of entry for occupational therapy assistants was adopted (AOTA, 2017b, p. 407).

ACOTE continued reviewing feedback received from stakeholders at their next meeting held in December 2015. It was noted that the majority of the feedback received addressed the potential impact on academic programs, diversity, and cost (AOTA, 2017b, p. 3). At this meeting, ACOTE appointed a task group to review the potential impact of the move to doctoral entry level to prepare graduates to meet the changing demands of the health care system. Multiple forums were held at the 2016 AOTA Annual Conference and the Academic Leadership Council meetings to continue the discussions and garner feedback. However, a motion for a single point of entry was once again defeated.

Interestingly, this was not the first time the occupational therapy profession had engaged in a protracted internal debate regarding entry-level standards for education. ACOTE documents reveal the initial call to move from a bachelor's degree to a master's degree as entry level began nearly 40 years before the decision was made to do so. In the years preceding the move, supporters cited changes in the health care environment, the evolving nature of the profession and length of time required to meet curriculum requirements, and the need to achieve equal educational status with other professions on our same arenas to support pay equity and leadership opportunities as being key issues to warrant the move. However, reasons against the move included the possibility that there would be no difference in practice outcomes and that the focus of the curriculum would shift too far from practice skills. Such a move was only being proposed to keep up with other professions, and the increased educational requirements would make it even more difficult to attract diverse representation into the profession (AOTA, 2017b, pp. 297-302).

The fall 2016 and spring 2017 ACOTE meetings provided forums for receipt and review of additional reports and updates regarding the mandate from the various task groups and ad hoc committees. ACOTE reviewed reports, data, and other information during the August 2017 meeting and reviewed the information collected since 2013. A motion to mandate the doctoral entry-level degree was adopted at this meeting. Additionally, a motion to mandate a bachelor's entry-level degree for occupational therapy assistants was also adopted at this meeting. However, ACOTE voted to hold the bachelor's entry-level degree for occupational therapy assistants in abeyance because of the substantial amount of feedback they received expressing concerns about this mandate. As previously stated, in August 2018, AOTA issued a statement to place the decision to move to the occupational therapy doctorate in abeyance, and ACOTE issued its own statement to the same effect in October 2018, indicating a task force will examine the issues affecting entry-level education in the profession (AOTA, 2018b).

CONCLUSION

The issues and trends that impact occupational therapy education remain varied and complex. Changes in the health care environment and reimbursement systems, evolving accreditation standards, and increasing curriculum requirements all indicate the need for educators to be well informed in order to shape and adapt the delivery of occupational therapy education. However, the current abeyance to hold on the mandate move to doctoral entry-level education after 2027 will undoubtedly set the trajectory for occupational therapy education and practice for years to come as education programs work to meet the changes in requirements and accreditation. Supporters and critics of the mandate will undoubtedly closely monitor the outcomes of the eventual decision on the mandate's abeyance and its impact on education and the profession.

Implications for Occupational Therapy Education

- Only time will reveal the impact of the final position with regard to entry-level education requirements, but until then, the profession continues to aspire to the pillars set forth in the AOTA Vision 2025 (AOTA, 2017a) for occupational therapists to be evidence and outcomes based, client-centered, cost effective, influential, and culturally responsive to the needs of individuals, populations and communities.

Key Reflection Questions

1. How have historical events influenced changes in accreditation over the past 100 years?
2. What are potential opportunities and barriers associated with the ACOTE abeyance regarding the entry-level doctorate?
3. Why are many of the strengths and challenges associated with the doctoral entry level similar to those raised at the time of the move to the master's entry level?

What led you to become an occupational therapy educator?

I entered my career as an occupational therapy assistant; desiring to acquire more knowledge, I continued to pursue my bachelor's and master's in occupational therapy. I later pursued a doctorate degree in higher education leadership in order to share my passion for occupational therapy with future practitioners.

Tina DeAngelis, EdD, OTR/L

As an occupational therapy student, my professors were excellent role models. I was inspired by their passion not only for occupational therapy but also for advancing their own knowledge through research and education. I knew when I completed my bachelor of science in occupational therapy that I wanted to teach one day, so I began guest lecturing as soon as I felt adequately competent. I knew immediately it was my calling to teach occupational therapy and have been very blessed by the opportunities I have been given to learn with those I teach every day.

Giulianne Krug, PhD, OTR, CLA

I became interested in a career as an occupational therapy educator while I was completing my occupational therapy degree. The thought of teaching in the profession that I was very passionate about intrigued me. I began volunteering to provide guest lectures within a few years of graduating and then became adjunct faculty. These experiences only reinforced my interest to pursue a path to become a full-time educator. Being an occupational therapy educator is rewarding, demanding, and exhilarating, and it is with an extraordinary sense of gratitude that I have been able to make my life's work that of an educator of future occupational therapists.

Bridgett Piernik-Yoder, PhD, OTR

REFERENCES

Accreditation Council for Occupational Therapy Education. (2012). 2011 Accreditation Council for Occupational Therapy Education (ACOTE) standards. *American Journal of Occupational Therapy, 66*, S6-S74. doi:10.5014/ajot.2012.66S6

American Occupational Therapy Association. (n.d.) History of OT education. Retrieved from https://www.aota.org/Education-Careers/Accreditation/Overview/History.aspx

American Occupational Therapy Association (1983). Essentials of an accredited educational program for the occupational therapist. *American Journal of Occupational Therapy, 37*(12), 817-823. doi: 10.5014/ajot.37.12.817

American Occupational Therapy Association (1991). Essentials and guidelines for an accredited program for the occupational therapist. *American Journal of Occupational Therapy, 45*, 1077-1084. doi: 10.5014/ajot.45.12.1077

American Occupational Therapy Association (1999). Standards for an accredited educational program for the occupational therapist. *American Journal of Occupational Therapy, 53*, 575-582. doi:10.5014/ajot.53.6.575

American Occupational Therapy Association (2007). Accreditation standards for a master's-degree-level educational program for the occupational therapist. *American Journal of Occupational Therapy, 61*, 652-661. doi: 10.5014/ajot.61.6.652

American Occupational Therapy Association. (2013). Future of education ad hoc report. Bethesda, MD: Retrieved from https://www.aota.org/AboutAOTA/Get-Involved/BOD/OTD-Statement.aspx

American Occupational Therapy Association. (2015). Importance of interprofessional education in occupational therapy curricula. *American Journal of Occupational Therapy, 69*(Suppl. 3), 691341020. doi:10.5014/ ajot.2015.696S02

American Occupational Therapy Association. (2017a). ACOTE 2027 mandate and FAQs. Retrieved from https://www.aota.org/Education-Careers/Accreditation/acote-doctoral-mandate-2027/ACOTE-responds-to-requests-for-an-abeyance-of-the-OTD-mandate.aspx

American Occupational Therapy Association. (2017b). Vision 2025. *American Journal of Occupational Therapy, 71*, 7103420010. Retrieved from https://doi.org/10.5014/ajot.2017.713002

American Occupational Therapy Association. (2018a). Importance of primary care education in occupational therapy curricula. *American Journal of Occupational Therapy, 72*(Suppl. 2), 7212410040. Retrieved from https://doi.org/10.5014/ajot.2018.72S202

American Occupational Therapy Association. (2018b). Task force to determine external issues affecting entry-level education. Retrieved from https://www.aota.org/AboutAOTA/Get-Involved/BOD/News/2018/Task-Force-to-Determine-External-Issues-Affecting-Entry-Level-Education.aspx

Crepeau, E., Cohn, E., & Boyt Schell, B. (2003). *Willard & Spackman's occupational therapy* (10th ed). Philadelphia, PA: Lippincott Williams & Wilkins.

DeAngelis, T. M. (2006). Elite occupational therapists attitudes regarding the entry level clinical occupational therapy doctorate degree (Doctoral dissertation, Widener University). Retrieved from http://www.worldcat.org/title/elite-occupational-therapists-attitudes-regarding-the-entry-level-clinical-occupational-therapy-doctorate-degree/oclc/68039075

Gordon, D. (2009). The history of occupational therapy. In Crepeau, E.B., Cohn, E.S. and Boyt Schell, B.A. (Eds), *Willard & Spackman's Occupational Therapy* (11th ed.), pp. 202-215. Philadelphia: Lippincott, Williams & Wilkins.

Gillette, N., & Kielhofner, G. (1979). The impact of specialization on the professionalization and survival of occupational therapy. *American Journal of Occupational Therapy, 33*(1), 20-28.

Hooper, B. (2006). Epistemological transformation in occupational therapy: Educational implications and challenges. *Occupational Therapy Journal of Research: Occupation, Participation and Health, 26*(1), 15-24.

Hughes Harris, C., Brayman, S., Clark, F., Delaney, J., & Miller, R. (1998, March 12). COE recommends postbaccalaureate OT education. *OT Week, 12*(11), 18.

Kearney, P. (2004). The influence of competing paradigms on occupational therapy education: A brief history. Retrieved from https://www.newfoundations.com/History/OccTher.html

McDaniel, M. (1968). Occupational therapists before World War II (1917-1940). In H. S. Lee & M. L. McDaniel (Eds.), *Army Medical Specialist Corps* (p. 69). Washington, DC: U.S. Government Printing Office.

Royeen, C., & Lavin, M. (2007). A contextual and logical analysis of the clinical doctorate for health practitioners: dilemma, delusion, or de facto? *Journal of Allied Health, 36*, 101-106.

Runyon, C. P., Aitken, M. J., & Stohs, S. (1994). The need for a clinical doctorate in occupational therapy. *Journal of Allied Health, 23*(2), 57-63.

Wells, J., & Crabtree, J. (2012). Trends affecting entry level occupational therapy education in the United States of American and their probable global impact. *Indian Journal of Occupational Therapy, 44*(3), 17-22.

4

Signature Pedagogies and Learning Designs in Occupational Therapy Education

Patricia Schaber, PhD, OTR/L, FAOTA
and Catherine Candler, PhD, OTR, BCP

Chapter Objectives

By the end of this chapter, the reader will be able to:

1. Explore the origins of signature pedagogies in the scholarship of teaching and learning.
2. Connect learning designs from other fields, including educational psychology, that support signature pedagogies in occupational therapy education.
3. Examine proposed signature pedagogies in occupational therapy education and connect to antecedent learning designs.
4. Summarize challenges and opportunities in designing learning models for the future of occupational therapy education.

INTRODUCTION TO SIGNATURE PEDAGOGIES

What is good teaching in occupational therapy education? This is a question that resonates with academic instructors hired to provide education to occupational therapy students. The debate between content experts vs. course design experts extends through every discipline; should good teaching focus on quantities of knowledge or methods of teaching targeting student learning? For most professors, the tendency is to believe the best way to teach is the way one has been taught, using the default pedagogies found in the classroom. The humbling part of this assumption is that learning is impacted by an evolving generational consciousness. Each generation of students brings a vastly different student experience into the classroom. Teaching the same way one has been taught does not move the practice forward into the context of today.

As disciplines wrestle with this challenge, there has been an increased focus on the scholarship of teaching and learning (SoTL) in an attempt to study pedagogical principles and approaches that provide evidence of teaching effectiveness. Out of this new field of scholarship, a realization has emerged

Taff, S. D., Grajo, L. C., & Hooper, B. R. (Eds.). *Perspectives on Occupational Therapy Education: Past, Present, and Future* (pp. 45-53).

that good teaching and learning designs are not universal. Disciplinary educational practices can be distinguished by their ability to teach and train students for a particular career pathway, and not all educational approaches yield the same outcomes. Thus, each discipline tends to teach in its own way.

The term *signature pedagogy* was introduced by Shulman (2005) in response to a wave of experts who applied disciplinary practices that were actualized in the classroom, had historic value in preparation of students, and were part of shared values and beliefs uniquely emphasized in the discipline. According to Shulman, identifying signature pedagogies is a metacognitive exercise in which a discipline examines itself, reflecting on its own teaching and learning practices to find those that uniquely distinguish its field of study from another. These distinguishing characteristics have been termed *signature pedagogies.*

Shulman (2005) defines signature pedagogies as "the types of teaching that organize the fundamental ways in which future practitioners are educated for their new professions" (p. 52). Signature pedagogies consist of three structures: surface, deep, and implicit. *Surface structures* are those that can be seen. For example, a visitor walking into an occupational therapy classroom may find the students gathered around a learning object, exploring and questioning. The instructor has likely given an explanatory introduction to the meaning and function of the object and has now taken a guiding role, facilitating the students' exploration and understanding. *Deep structures* consist of the assumptions adopted by the discipline on how "what needs to be known" can best be taught. In our example, this is reflected in the rationale that underlies the instructor's actions. The instructor has explained the object. This indicates his or her assumption that the students need to be provided some basic information for their understanding of its relevance, purpose, and use. Given that understanding, the instructor has now assumed that deeper learning must come from the students' own explorations; thus, he or she has stepped back and, rather than direct, now guides their discovery. Surface and deep structure pedagogies are methods to teach content and develop skills. *Implicit structures* go beyond this and encompass professional identity (i.e., the attitudes, values, and beliefs of the profession). Often, in addition to direct teaching of the profession's mission, ethics, and philosophy, this is modeled by an instructor's personal conduct when teaching and designing self-reflective experiences that transmit values and beliefs. For example, the instructor models respect for students in the same way respect should be afforded to clients. This action demonstrates professional collegiality in the face of conflict or models assertiveness when encountering injustice.

Signature pedagogies have been explored by many professions. Emerging from an initiative by the Carnegie Foundation, disparate pedagogies have been identified for clergy (Foster, Dahill, Golemon, & Wang Tolentino, 2005), lawyers (Sullivan, Colby, Welch Wegner, Bond, & Shulman, 2007), engineers (Sheppard, Macatangay, Colby, & Sullivan, 2008), nurses (Benner, Sutphen, Leonard, & Day, 2009), and physicians (Cooke, Irby, & O'Brien, 2010). Occupational therapy is initiating the exploration of its own signature pedagogies.

TEACHING-LEARNING DESIGNS FROM EDUCATIONAL PSYCHOLOGY

Early and Midcentury Learning Designs

Occupational therapy educators' methods of teaching and learning have not developed in isolation. Occupational therapy teaching practices have parallel trends with other health care disciplines in higher education. Historically, in its inception, occupational therapy education occurred in authentic settings, such as psychiatric institutions or hospitals (Meyer & Haworth Continuing Features Submission, 1983). Education was moved to university settings following the demand for rehabilitation services after World War II. The trend was tabula rasa, an approach in which the learner assumes a passive role. This was actualized as lecture combined with clinical apprenticeship and was standard practice with many health care professional programs.

In the latter part of the 19th century, the field of educational psychology influenced and informed teaching practices in higher education. In 1956, Benjamin Bloom, an educational psychologist, proposed a taxonomy that presented learning as hierarchical and progressive in three domains: cognitive, affective, and psychomotor. Rather than mere knowledge transfer, higher-level learning in the cognitive domain required analysis, synthesis, and, ultimately, evaluation of information (Bloom, 1956). This shift of emphasis to the student learning experience paved the way for adult learning models, emphasizing the role of the learner taking responsibility for the experience. In the late 1960s, educator Malcolm Knowles (1968, 1970) presented the notion of classic *andragogy*, which draws from the natural curiosity of the adult learner to explore phenomena of interest. This learning approach uses experiences in and out of the classroom in which the learner is stimulated and challenged with real-world problems that can be solved. Often referred to as an extension of andragogy, *heutagogy*, or self-determined learning, focuses on building flexibility in learning. When successful, learners increase their adaptability to environmental changes, molding responses through practicing those responses along with variations to those responses. They develop new ways to process content, enabling learners to make sense of their worlds by focusing on learning "how to learn" rather than teaching content (Hase & Kenyon, 2007).

The redirected focus on student learning capacity led to the development of metacognitive learning strategies (Mezirow, 1997) or, simply, "thinking about thinking." The main concepts of metacognition that are emphasized are metamemory (the intuitive knowledge of one's memory capabilities and strategies to improve it), metacomprehension (our ability to assess our own skills, knowledge, learning, or depth of understanding), problem solving, and critical thinking. These concepts foster critical thinking through a range of learning activities, including role-playing, simulations, problem-based learning, use of patient cases/scenarios, and Socratic methods of probing and questioning.

Along with learning capacity, attention was directed to student learning characteristics or personal attributes in taking in and processing information. During this era, sociologist Jack Mezirow (2000) focused his work on student values and beliefs. He perceived the educational experience as one that transformed the learner by internally changing his or her ways of thinking, feeling, believing, and doing. By experiencing a critical reflection on self, students build the skills to guide others in this transformative process. Learning is through "meaning making" activities in which personal beliefs, schemes, perspectives, and values are recreated. Students critically reflect on their assumptions and beliefs about the world around them and create new ways of being. The intent was to elevate the student's higher-order thinking processes by bringing into awareness the students learning style, guiding reflection on personal performance, and provoking new ways of thinking. Mezirow incorporated these learning strategies into a theory of transformation in which the learner strives to understand experiences that shape perceptions and define the world around him or her. It propels the student toward an autonomous thinker who self-reflects and critiques "habits of mind" that influence assumptions.

A pivotal text that stimulated the conversation around teaching methodologies and influenced occupational therapy education was philosopher Donald Schön's (1987) book titled *Educating the Reflective Practitioner: Toward a New Design for Teaching and Learning in the Professions*. This challenged academics to incorporate the reflection-in-action approach and challenged students to apply theory and technique to solve concrete problems. Schön's was one of the first learning theories to guide health care education specifically; it challenged acquisition of knowledge to application of knowledge in grooming professionals for practice. Teaching occurred through guided reflection after active engagement with the patient. Learning through guided reflection stems from a trusting relationship between the teacher and student, nurtured through a connected learning community. With an emphasis on grooming the student into the consummate professional, therapy professionals were role models to students, offering guided reflection, insight, and questioning.

During the same midcentury era, psychologist Albert Bandura (1971) promoted ideas around social learning. Education was social in nature, and job skills were gained through attention or exposure to behaviors, retention or remembering behaviors, reproduction or reproducing behaviors, and motivation to perform the behavior well. The teacher provided a model of behavior and verbal feedback about behavior, and students practiced those behaviors in a safe environment. Learning was most effective in the presence of disciplinary experts who provided corrective feedback in real time and discussed how to change, grow, and master professionalism. With emphasis on the social context, learning is designed in a social milieu with methodologies tested across time involving small group problem-solving or adviser-guided investigations.

Contemporary and Emerging Learning Designs

At the turn of the century and as teaching technologies expanded, academics coined new strategies in teaching and learning that built on learning methods of the latter 1900s. Contemporary learning designs depend on the adult learner to take responsibility and organize the learning experience independent of external environments. Defined borders that delineate learning from nonlearning experiences disappear; social learning can be distant via virtual connections. The student-centered approaches presaged in the prior century have come to fruition today but in a way not forewarned.

Professional programs have been contained with increasingly rigorous accreditation standards with expectations of measuring competency in shorter time periods. With the emphasis on outcomes, educators incorporated competency-based learning where students must master each competency to move forward in the learning process. Learning is self-paced with individualized timing so each student can focus on learning the competency with repetition or acceleration. This opened the opportunity for technology-enhanced learning, online learning, and hybrid learning formats. Blended or hybrid learning uses Web-based technology to guide the learners through their learning experience balanced with face-to-face experiential learning (Allen & Seaman, 2013). This approach reduces the amount of face-to-face time and effort for which the student is responsible and increases the preparation time. Although there are many models for hybrid teaching and learning, the flipped learning model is used in class sessions for direct student engagement by incorporating flexible timelines and spaces that enable students to reflect, synthesize, and learn in their own style and pace; active learning in which students learn by doing and skills learning is immersive and hands-on in the classroom (example, simulations, role playing, demonstrations, and labs); and instructional content to maximize student-centered learning.

In addition, metacognitive learning strategies provided a foundation for academic controversy that increased intellectual conflict and challenged students with solving actual problems; these strategies set the stage for problem-based learning and authentic learning, which connected students with community leaders to bridge disciplinary content with real-world application. The reflective practitioner and social learning theories foretasted learning communities, aligning expert with student and student to student in small group experiences. These enhanced teaching and learning strategies revealed the dynamic evolutionary nature of higher education and the importance of adaptation and change.

Effect on Occupational Therapy Education

Occupational therapy education continues to build on learning designs from higher education. Classroom lectures continue to be a standard methodology despite the limitations of going beyond knowledge dissemination. Bloom's taxonomy (Bloom, 1956) and iterations of the taxonomy are still widely used in scaffold learning (Krathwohl, 2002). The commitment to lifelong learning is built into the certification and licensure requirements, and it is widely recognized that learners must be groomed to be highly autonomous and self-determined to meet the complexities of today's workplace (Blaschke, 2012). Throughout decades, occupational therapy educators have innovatively designed active learning experiences and expanded authentic learning to diverse settings such as prisons, crisis centers, shelters, and free clinics. This potpourri of instructional methodologies offers a rich arena from which to develop curricula and test effective teaching and learning practices. Yet, which of these multiple approaches are central to occupational therapy education? The national Accreditation Council for Occupational Therapy Education's outlined blueprint for occupational therapy education requires a design of a creative and cohesive educational experience for student learning. There appears to be a need to identify a common center, a cluster of methods that portray an identity unique to occupational therapy education, what we may refer to as signature pedagogies that guide and protect vital disciplinary teaching and learning practices.

SEARCHING FOR SIGNATURE PEDAGOGIES IN OCCUPATIONAL THERAPY EDUCATION

At present, the search for the signature pedagogies in occupational therapy is in its infancy. Regina Doherty, an occupational therapist educator, made the case for clinical reasoning as signature pedagogy at the 2015 AOTA Education Summit (Doherty, 2015). Hooper, King, Wood, Bilics, and Gupta (2013) have suggested that integrative learning, learning paradigms, complexities of practice, and student reasoning could serve as a starting point for reforming occupational therapy education based on educational research, with integrative learning as a signature pedagogy. These epitomes of learning, clinical reasoning and integrative learning, are not unique to occupational therapy. Approaching the search for signature pedagogies using a qualitative method, Schaber, Marsh, and Wilcox (2012) conducted an observational analysis and investigative review of academic teaching articles in *The American Journal of Occupational Therapy*. Guided by Shulman's (2005) blueprint to explore signature pedagogies, finding the surface structure or observed acts of how the discipline teaches and learns began with classroom observations by experts from the Center for Educational Innovation at the University of Minnesota. The deep structure, or how the underlying knowledge is imbued, was uncovered by delving into the literature for the published lessons learned through instructional methods used to stimulate deeper thought and reflection. The implicit structure was detected in articles on ethical standards, core values, and beliefs that drew the moral plumb line and were found in honored lectures and professional white papers. Among these sources emerged three consistent pedagogies: *relational learning* or learning that occurs through human connection; *affective learning* or learning that transforms personal identity exemplified by a change in attitudes, beliefs, and values; and *highly contextualized, active engagement* referring to learning that occurs through doing. Looking broadly at this tripartite schema, remnants of learning designs from the field of educational psychology are active and flourishing. In combination, at the crux, they seem to embody occupational therapy education's unique aspiration for training future professionals.

Relational Learning

Occupational therapy education has, up until the past decade, emphasized the human connections in teaching and learning. The profession embraced an "it takes a village" approach, and academic instructors, practitioners, clinicians, client instructors, fieldwork supervisors, and others all strongly contributed to the student learning experience. Gail Fidler (1966), in her Eleanor Clark Slagle lecture, promoted the idea that supervising occupational therapy students was at its core building a relationship as a "dynamic, interactional growth process" (pp. 5-8). The teacher-to-student connection was a model for the therapist to client connection in the student transformational process. There is emphasis in teaching on sharing stories, either clinical cases or reasoning processes. Educators personify the attitudes, values, and behaviors of a therapy practitioner and design opportunities for students to try on these new roles. Modeling therapeutic relationships and reasoning processes, students acquire the skills to act in a similar fashion. Teaching through relationship building echoes the premises of social learning theories, with the expert as the gold standard. More importantly, the expert guides the student experience by reflection in action, stimulating reflection, and providing feedback on student responses and behaviors. The relationship serves a prime motivator for student learning. Beyond the relationships between instructor and student, the learning community approach draws from the power of student relationships in small group work.

Affective Learning

The goal of the professional program is to transform the occupational therapy student emotionally to fit into a cultural ethos embraced by the profession (Peloquin, 2005). This affective learning involves becoming vulnerable in the student community in examining and altering attitudes, values, and beliefs to conform to the large occupational therapy community. These beliefs include supporting the rights of each person to determine his or her occupational choices, acknowledging the dignity of every person at every stage of life, and the belief in the power of "doing" to facilitate change. Hooper (2006) called this identity formation impacting the students "ways of knowing and ways of seeing" (p. 228). Targeting core values, affective learning resonates with transformational learning theories in which the student emerges from the learning experience transformed into a person exemplifying professional ethics and core values. This gradual conversion impacts the student ways of being in the workplace and beyond. Krathwohl, Bloom, and Masia (1956) identified that learning encompassed an affective domain, which must have a "systematic method for appraising the extent to which students grow in the desired ways" or affective objectives "are meaningless" (p. 23). Occupational therapy education formatively evaluates student's affective growth toward the standards of an entry-level practitioner throughout the didactic and experiential program.

Highly Contextualized, Active Learning

The fieldwork experience is a highly contextualized, actively engaged "learning through doing" pedagogy. Throughout the past century, occupational therapy practitioners have been trained in authentic contexts to learn the skills. Case in point, the profession began in a mental health unit with students learning the discipline on-site before moving into academic institutions. Many of the academic studies examined the impact of a variety of practice settings on the learning experience of the student including prisons, schools, community centers, and medical clinics. Adult learning theories set the stage for the learner to take on responsibility for learning experience and paved the way for authentic learning through public and professional engagement opportunities. New formats, such as hybrid learning designs, incorporate mastery of online content that prepare the student for active learning in classroom laboratories and clinical and community spaces. The apprenticeship or internship model has pervaded higher education in many disciplines and has not been supplanted in the health care fields.

Threading occupational therapy curricula with relational learning, affective learning, and highly contextualized, active learning ensures that program development evolves in the direction of enhanced teacher-student relationships, attention toward student transformation molded around core values and beliefs, and guided experiential learning in the field. Signature pedagogies can be the plumb line in designing learning experiences, mainly to not lose the core disciplinary tenets. Teacher involvement with students is costly, student transformation takes time and necessitates guided support, and experiential learning involves a village of committed specialists who choose to dedicate efforts in grooming future practitioners. These pedagogies, once demanded, can leverage funding to obtain necessary resources. Implications for occupational therapy education include providing a common language and uniformity across curricula and programs, a reference point for scholarship in teaching and learning, and a springboard for innovation. Scholarship in teaching and learning that exposes the most effective methods for socializing students into professionalism and imparting shared values and beliefs is deficient and requires rigor in discovering best practice approaches (Gupta & Bilics, 2014). Similar to other time-tested educational methods, signature pedagogies will be tested, evolve, and morph into new methods, finding their place in the trajectory of disciplinary teaching and learning.

CONCLUSION

Occupational therapy programs are bound by Accreditation Council for Occupational Therapy Education standards, and a priority requirement is that each program bases its curriculum on its own often individually identified philosophy of teaching and learning. Occupational therapy programs are diverse, so what are the benefits of identifying signature pedagogies for the profession as a whole? The answer lies in the looking, rather than the finding. Programs put forth effort to align with looming changes and challenges, resisting uniformity while conforming to professional standards. Put forward as a continuous and ever-evolving process, identifying signature pedagogies for occupational therapy education can provide a reference point for scholarship in teaching and learning. At its most basic level, discussion and identification of signature pedagogies assist programs in creating curricula that incorporate strategies that work effectively across the profession. With this orientation, a more scientifically guided general uniformity of approach would emerge that could be communicated clearly to occupational therapy faculty. Signature pedagogies, as a guiding principle within each program, may look different (e.g., in the ways that teachers, mentors, or supervisors experience relationship building with students, the designed learning activities that impact and transform student affect, or the locations where students actively engage in the learning process). One size does not fit all; different programs, contexts of programs, and student demographics require tailored approaches. Signature pedagogies can serve as a springboard for innovation for occupational therapy education, revealing a professional identity and guiding the development of those entering the discipline.

Implications for Occupational Therapy Education

Identifying signature pedagogies provides:
- A common foundation and uniformity across curricula and programs,
- A reference point for scholarship in teaching and learning, and
- A springboard for innovation.

Key Reflection Questions

1. If the core signature pedagogies for occupational therapy education are built on relational learning, affective learning, and high contextualized, active engagement, what does this mean for designing learning experiences?
2. What would be implications for the teacher-student relationship of moving occupational therapy education into the virtual environment?
3. Which affective learning strategies are effective in conforming students to the cultural ethos of the profession?
4. Do simulated learning experiences have the same effectiveness on learning as the highly contextualized, active learning experiences in natural settings?

What led you to become an occupational therapy educator?

I began my academic career after serving in Peace Corps Ecuador and working for 13 years in geriatric occupational therapy. Returning to the program where I learned the profession, my goal was to perpetuate the philosophy of health as one of engagement and participation. I am considered a "fast starter," experimenting with new methods of teaching and learning and embracing change as the field of academic occupational therapy evolves.

Patricia Schaber, PhD, OTR/L, FAOTA

I entered the world of academia after 13 years of clinical experience in school-based occupational therapy. I was inspired by the insight gained from my master's degree studies, where the power of theory to connect ideas and usefulness of research to explore them was made evident. As an educator, I remain endlessly fascinated with these as a conduit for teaching, guiding students into making connections between ideas and considered actions, resulting in reflective evidence-based practice.

Catherine Candler, PhD, OTR, BCP

REFERENCES

Allen, I. E., & Seaman, J. (2013). *Changing course: Ten years of tracking online education in the United States*. Babson Park, MA: Babson Survey Research Group.

Bandura, A. (1971). *Social learning theory*. New York, NY: General Learning Press.

Benner, P., Sutphen, M., Leonard, V., & Day, L. (2009). *Educating nurses: A Call for radical transformation*. San Francisco, CA: Jossey-Bass.

Blaschke, L. M. (2012). Heutagogy and lifelong learning: A review of heutagogical practice and self-determined learning. *International Review of Research in Open and Distributed Learning, 13*(1):56-71.

Bloom, B. S. (Ed.). (1956). *Taxonomy of educational objectives: The classification of educational goals. Handbook 1: Cognitive domain*. New York, NY: David McKay.

Cooke, M., Irby, D. M., & O'Brien, B. C. (2010). *Educating physicians: A call for reform of medical school and residency*. San Francisco, CA: Jossey-Bass.

Doherty, R. (2015). Clinical reasoning as signature pedagogy in OT: Teaching and evaluating ways of thinking. Platform session; 2015 AOTA/OTCAS Education Summit Program Guide; October 17-18, 2015.

Fidler, G. (1966). Eleanor Clark Slagle lecture: Learning as a growth process: A conceptual framework for professional education. *American Journal of Occupational Therapy, 20*(1), 1-8.

Foster, C. R., Dahill, L., Golemon, L., & Wang Tolentino, B. (2005). *Educating clergy: Teaching practices and pastoral imagination*. San Francisco, CA: Jossey-Bass.

Gupta, J., & Bilics, A. (2014). Scholarship and research in occupational therapy education. *American Journal of Occupational Therapy, 68*, S87-S92. doi:10.5014/ajot.2014.012880

Hase, S., & Kenyon, C. (2007). Heutagogy: A child of complexity theory. *Complicity: An International Journal of Complexity and Education, 4*(1), 111-118.

Hooper, B. (2006). Beyond active learning: A case study of teaching practices in an occupation-centered curriculum. *American Journal of Occupational Therapy, 60*(5), 551-562.

Hooper, B., King, R., Wood, W., Bilics, A., & Gupta, J. (2013). An international systematic mapping review of educational approaches and teaching methods in occupational therapy. *British Journal of Occupational Therapy, 76*(1), 9-22.

Knowles, M. S. (1968). Andragogy, not pedagogy. *Adult Leadership, 16*(10), 350-352, 386.

Knowles, M. S. (1970). *The modern practice of adult education: Andragogy versus pedagogy*. Oxford, England: Association Press.

Krathwohl, D. R. (2002). A revision of Bloom's taxonomy: An overview. *Theory Into Practice, 41*(4), 212-218. doi:10.1207/s15430421tip4104_2

Krathwohl, D. R., Bloom, B. S., & Masia, B. B. (1956). *Taxonomy of educational objectives: Handbook II: Affective domain*. New York, NY: David McKay Company.

Meyer, A., & Haworth Continuing Features Submission. (1983). The philosophy of occupational therapy. *Occupational Therapy in Mental Health, 2*(3), 79-86.

Mezirow, J. (1997). Transformative learning: Theory to practice. *New Directions for Adult and Continuing Education, 74*, 5-12.

Mezirow, J. (2000). *Learning as transformation.* San Francisco, CA: Jossey-Bass.

Peloquin, S. (2005). 2005 Eleanor Clarke Slagel Lecture—Embracing our ethos, reclaiming our heart. *American Journal of Occupational Therapy, 59*(6), 611-625.

Schaber, P., Marsh, L., & Wilcox, K. (2012). Relational learning and active engagement in occupational therapy professional education. In R. Gurung, N. Chick, & A. Haynie (Eds.), *More signature pedagogies: Approaches to teaching disciplinary habits of mind* (pp. 188–202). Sterling, VA: Stylus Publishing.

Schön, D. A. (1987). *Educating the reflective practitioner: Toward a new design for teaching and learning in the professions.* San Francisco, CA: Jossey-Bass.

Sheppard, S. D., Macatangay, K., Colby, A., & Sullivan, W. M. (2008). *Educating engineers: Designing for the future of the field.* San Francisco, CA: Jossey-Bass.

Shulman, L. S. (2005). Signature pedagogies in the professions. *Daedalus, 134*(3), 52-59.

Sullivan, W. M., Colby, A., Welch Wegner, J., Bond, L., & Shulman, L. S. (2007). *Educating lawyers: Preparation for the profession of law.* San Francisco, CA: Jossey-Bass

5

Bridging the Gap Between Entry-Level Education and the Demands of Clinical Practice

Stacy Smallfield, DrOT, MSOT, OTR/L, BCG, FAOTA
and Lauren E. Milton, OTD, OTR/L

Chapter Objectives

By the end of this chapter, the reader will be able to:

1. Analyze the underlying factors contributing to the divide between entry-level professional education and the realities of clinical practice in occupational therapy.
2. Apply a variety of strategies to narrow the education-practice gap.
3. Conceptualize the intricacies and complexity of the interrelated factors and potential solutions influencing the education-practice gap.

INTRODUCTION

The gap between entry-level occupational therapy professional education and clinical practice can be defined as the perception that knowledge and skills gained in the professional educational program do not translate well into the workplace (Newton, Billett, Jolly, & Ockerby, 2009). Despite extensive academic preparation in knowledge and technical skills required for practice, there is a long-standing and growing body of evidence that occupational therapy students find the transition to clinical practice challenging (Adamson, Hunt, Harris, & Hummel, 1998; Barnitt & Salmond, 2000; Gray et al., 2012; McCombie & Antanavage, 2017; Melman, Ashby, & James, 2016; Morley, Rugg, & Drew, 2007). The purpose of this chapter is to explore the intricacies and challenges of this divide and discuss strategies to bridge the gap.

Taff, S. D., Grajo, L. C., & Hooper, B. R. (Eds.). *Perspectives on Occupational Therapy Education: Past, Present, and Future* (pp. 55-62).
© 2020 Taylor & Francis Group.

Exploring the Divide Between
Occupational Therapy Education and Practice

Although the education-practice gap is not unique to occupational therapy, now more than ever, students are entering an increasingly complex and demanding work environment (Smith & Pilling, 2008). Thriving in this environment requires a combination of knowledge and technical skills and an even wider range of soft skills. To identify or develop strategies to bridge this divide, we need to understand the intricacies of this complex phenomenon. Current literature points to the following influential factors.

Theory-Practice Gap

Kislov (2014) describes two types of knowledge, namely, theoretical knowledge (know that) and procedural knowledge (know how). A student may gain theoretical knowledge but lack the ability to translate this into procedural knowledge, thus creating a gap between education and practice. Students learn the theoretical foundation for occupational therapy practice in an entry-level professional program but may not have many opportunities to apply theoretical knowledge to actual practice.

Soft Skills

A range of soft skills, or a combination of interpersonal skills, emotional intelligence, and character traits, is needed to be successful in clinical practice (Fortune, Ryan, & Adamson, 2013). These include personal agency (the capacity to act independently and make free choices), political adeptness (the ability to not only manage a caseload of clients but also the ability to navigate the complexities of the organization), strategy and adaptability, innovation, stress management, the ability to manage interpersonal conflict, and communication skills (Fortune et al., 2013). Chipchase et al. (2012) identified themes to describe characteristics indicative of student preparedness and noted that three of them—namely, willingness, professionalism, and personal attributes—were seen as more important than knowledge and understanding.

Occupation-Based Practice

Occupation is the core of occupational therapy (American Occupational Therapy Association [AOTA], 2014). However, occupational therapists use a range of interventions in practice, from preparatory to occupation based, to achieve the goal of maximizing occupational performance (AOTA, 2014). Although academic programs emphasize the use of occupation as the primary therapeutic medium, some practice settings, particularly biomedical settings, may have a stronger emphasis on preparatory interventions (Di Tommaso, Isbel, Scarvell, & Wicks, 2016; Wilding & Whiteford, 2007). Workplace culture that differs from educational culture on this core philosophy of the profession may be challenging for new graduates to assimilate (Di Tommaso et al., 2016; Wilding & Whiteford, 2007).

Expectations

Differences in expectations exist between the occupational therapy educator, the student, and the employer. Barnitt and Salmond (2000) found that new graduates expect a gradual transition to the demands of a full caseload, whereas employers no longer have this luxury because of the changing health care environment. For example, health care policies and economics change so rapidly that they may be outdated from the time students learn to the time they use this knowledge in practice. The expectation of educators may be to teach students how to stay up-to-date on topics, whereas employers may expect working knowledge of reimbursement mechanisms, leaving new graduates caught in the middle. Additional qualitative research shows new graduates have high expectations of employers for the quality of supervision they will receive in practice (Morley et al., 2007).

Preparation for Dynamic and Evolving Practice

Students in entry-level occupational therapy education programs prepare for an unknown future (Barnett, 2004). Work environments are increasingly varied, complex, and unpredictable. Preparation for the unknown is difficult. Although educators strive to anticipate the future and vary educational offerings, this is an ongoing, challenging task that may or may not prepare graduates for the demands of current practice (Barnett, 2004; Fortune et al., 2013).

Delays in Knowledge Translation

A significant delay occurs between the discovery of and the implementation of health research into practice. Students learn about, and may contribute to, the latest research efforts in developing effective clinical interventions. It takes years from the time these interventions are first developed to the time they are widespread in clinical practice (Morris, Wooding, & Grant, 2011; Westfall, Mold, & Fagnan, 2007). New graduates may not be equipped to navigate practice issues that arise when working in settings where outdated intervention approaches are used or implement new evidence-based interventions within a complex work environment.

Strategies to Bridge the Gap Between Education and Practice

Research identifies strategies to bridge the gap between education and practice. Although the list is extensive, they are themed here to include purposeful ambiguity, mentorship, experiential learning, collaboration, reflective practice, lifelong learning, and the use of evidence-based practice. These strategies are supported by current research within occupational therapy and related disciplines and are consistent with the core values of occupational therapy education, which include the use of active and diverse learning experiences, lifelong learning, ongoing self-reflection and development of a professional identity, and collaboration (AOTA, 2015). The strategies described later are in addition to clinical competencies (i.e., entry-level knowledge and technical skills needed to apply theory and evidence to the occupational therapy process [AOTA, 2014] across practice settings). Clinical competencies, which are described in Chapter 8, are essential components of professional education and entry to clinical practice. Educational programs can enhance clinical competencies by using strategies described later in this section as well as with a variety of tools introduced within the professional program (e.g., Ikiugu, Smallfield, & Condit, 2009).

Purposeful Ambiguity

The teaching strategy of using purposefully ambiguous experiences includes having students manage questions that do not have concrete answers and situations with no one solution (Fortune et al., 2013). Students are intentionally placed in situations in which the outcome is vague or not yet known, such as in-patient simulations or program development with community agencies, when directives allow students the framework to take risks in decision making and creativity. This promotes problem solving, critical thinking, and decision making and serves to refine soft skills needed to thrive in a complex work environment. Purposeful ambiguity can be facilitated in professional curricula when students are permitted to take the lead, interact with others, influence outcomes, and work in unknown environments to make decisions while considering multiple points of view (Fortune et al., 2013). Program development in which students conceive an idea that requires needs assessment, planning, implementation, and evaluation, along with community interaction, is an example of a purposefully ambiguous experience that can strengthen the ability to enter a new practice setting with confidence.

Mentorship and Supervision

A significant body of literature discusses the use of mentoring or supervision of students and new graduates as a tool for bridging the education-practice gap (McCombie & Antanavage, 2017; Morley et al., 2007; Robertson & Griffiths, 2009; Toal-Sullivan, 2006). Mentorship or supervision is a supportive process through which goals are established and later revisited to determine progress; researchers have found that support in the form of a mentor or supervisor is cited often as a helpful strategy to new graduates in transition to practice (McCombie & Antanavage, 2017; Robertson & Griffiths, 2009). In the educational setting or in clinical practice, a mentoring model is a tool that can be used to support the development of soft skills and personal agency needed to navigate complex work settings.

Experiential Learning

Hands-on learning, such as through simulation or service, enhances the retention of new knowledge and skills by activating multiple senses in the learning experience (Doyle & Zakrajsek, 2013), promoting clinical reasoning and competence in technical and soft skills. Significant learning occurs through simulated experiences with standardized clients, including general preparation for practice (Thomas, Rybski, Apke, Kegelmeyer, & Kloos, 2017) and confidence in skills (Glenn & Gilbert-Hunt, 2012). A deeper exploration of simulated learning can be found in Chapter 8 of this text. Service learning affords students opportunities to immerse themselves in rich learning endeavors, resulting in the development and refinement of personal traits desired by future employers (Flinders, Nicholson, Carlascio, & Gilb, 2013; Levkoe, Brail, & Daniere, 2014). Within health care, recent models for service learning (Flinders, Nicholson, Carlascio, & Gilb, 2013; Otty & Milton, 2016) offer unique frameworks for engaging students in this form of experiential learning.

Collaboration

Opportunities readily exist for collaboration between educational programs and clinical sites in the form of practitioner as lecturer, lab instructor, and adjunct faculty. Practitioners are well suited to serve on external advisory boards to advise academic programs on topics such as curriculum development, admissions, program evaluation, and the overall direction of the program. Student learning activities embedded in coursework offer unique connections between student and practitioner. Anecdotally, one student commented on a semester-long systematic review project that was driven by a question from a practicing occupational therapist by saying, "I was also motivated to produce high-quality work, knowing that the questions came from real clinicians. It made me realize that I will soon be in their shoes, and I want to provide clients with evidence-based treatment."

Reflective Practice

Fitzgerald, Moores, Coleman, and Fleming (2015) describe the use of reflective practice as part of a clinical learning framework for new occupational therapy graduates. Reflective practice occurs when purposeful thought and consideration is given to one's own performance and ability to complete tasks successfully (Parham, 1987). Wilding and Whiteford (2007) describe the use of reflective practice among occupational therapists in acute care settings to resolve the dissonance of occupation-based practice within a biomedical setting, whereas Smith and Pilling (2008) include a reflective component in a program that supports students in the transition to becoming professionals. Reflective practice may include tools such as the National Board for Certification in Occupational Therapy (NBCOT) Entry-Level Self-Assessment Tool (2017), journaling, or discussion with a colleague. Educational programs can incorporate reflection in learning experiences to develop clinical reasoning skills and professional identity.

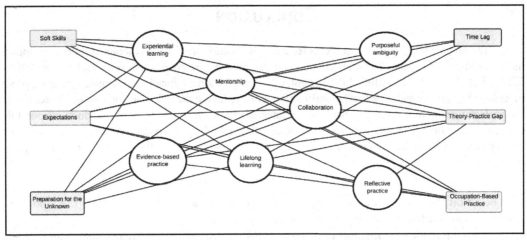

Figure 5-1. A concept map illustrating the bridge between entry-level occupational therapy education and the demands of clinical practice. The strategies to bridge the gap each address multiple factors contributing to the gap.

Lifelong Learning

A conscious and ongoing voluntary effort to pursue knowledge and personal or professional growth, lifelong learning promotes engagement in the professional community. Communities of practice (CoPs) are a vehicle to facilitate lifelong learning. CoPs gained popularity among professional disciplines as an avenue through which those with common interests can informally gather to support each other, learn together, and develop shared resources around a topic of interest (Wenger, 1991). Within occupational therapy, CoPs are gaining momentum as a mechanism for professional growth and development and capacity building (Barry, Kuijer-Siebelink, Nieuwenhuis, & Scherpbier-de Haan, 2017; McLoughlin, Patel, O'Callaghan, & Reeves, 2018; Roberts, 2015).

Evidence-Based Practice

Evidence-based practice is the use of the best available evidence to inform clinical decision making while considering the clinical experience of the practitioner, the unique needs of the client, and the clinical practice setting (Sackett, 1996). It can serve as a bridge between education and practice because through it effective interventions are integrated. Equipping students with the ability to synthesize research to inform practice is a natural bridge across the education-practice gap. Carroll, Herge, Johnson, and Schaaf (2017) designed and implemented a data-driven decision-making process to assist fieldwork students and supervisors in integrating evidence into daily decision making. This model significantly improved student knowledge and skill in the use of evidence in practice.

The Complexity of Interrelated Factors and Strategies of the Education-Practice Gap

Factors influencing the education-practice gap and the strategies to bridge this divide are multiple, complex, and interrelated. The concept map in Figure 5-1 illustrates how factors and strategies are interrelated and how each of the strategies serves to address multiple factors.

CONCLUSION

It is no longer enough to teach students technical skills and hire them as therapists; rather, we must maximize students' capacity to be effective in complex health care environments (Fortune et al., 2013; Liddiard, et al., 2017). Successfully bridging entry-level professional education and clinical practice promotes confidence, competency, and job satisfaction while reducing the risk of losing new graduates from the profession or compromising patient care. Strategies to maximize this transition include purposeful ambiguity, mentorship, experiential learning, collaboration, lifelong learning, reflection, and evidence-based practice. The implementation of these strategies is essential to bridge the education-practice gap.

Implications for Occupational Therapy Education

Based on the latest evidence, occupational therapy educators should consider the following strategies to ease the transition from education to practice:

- Develop models for mentoring students as they transition to practice that reflect on current strengths and areas for development, create a plan for growth, and build confidence.
- Maximize experiential learning opportunities, including the use of simulation experiences, service learning, experiential clinics, and collaborative relationships with practice sites.
- Provide opportunities for students to engage in purposeful ambiguity and lead projects with opportunities to influence the team toward desired outcomes.
- Develop ongoing collaborations with clinical managers and practitioners to develop and teach technical skills as well as soft skills needed to thrive in a complex work environment.

Key Reflection Questions

1. Which of the multiple factors underlying the education-practice gap discussed in this chapter resonate with you when you reflect on your own transition from education to practice? Are there additional factors that you would add to this list?
2. Which soft skills (i.e., professional attributes) are needed most in your work setting? What strategies did you use to develop those skills?
3. Considering your role as student, educator, clinician, or researcher, which strategies can you implement at the personal, organization, or policy level to bridge the education-practice gap?

What led you to become an occupational therapy educator?

Education is in my genes. I was introduced to the profession when my grandmother, a retired elementary school teacher, rehabilitated poststroke. In college, I fell in love with learning and had a hunch I would work in academia one day. Although I value my work with older adult clients, it is rewarding to know that I have an even greater influence on the profession by training future therapists.

Stacy Smallfield, DrOT, MSOT, OTR/L, BCG, FAOTA

My dad, a farmer and a public school educator turned administrator, recognized my need for hands-on learning and took me with him on Saturday mornings to our family farm stand at the city market. I thrived in this real-world context. My desire to pursue a career in health care led me to occupational therapy, and midway through the program, I knew a role as an occupational therapy educator was in my future. Much like the methods my dad used to teach me math, I value engaging students in active, hands-on learning.

Lauren E. Milton, OTD, OTR/L

ACKNOWLEDGMENT

We would like to acknowledge Allison Burns, Kaitlin LaPlant, and Courtney Weber for their assistance with gathering and summarizing the resources used to develop this chapter.

REFERENCES

Adamson, B., Hunt, A., Harris, L., & Hummel, J. (1998). Occupational therapists perceptions of their undergraduate preparation for the workplace. *British Journal of Occupational Therapy, 61*, 173-179.

American Occupational Therapy Association. (2014). Occupational therapy practice framework: Domain and process (3rd ed.). *American Journal of Occupational Therapy, 68*(Suppl. 1), S1-S48. doi:10.5014/ajot.2014.682006

American Occupational Therapy Association. (2015). Philosophy of occupational therapy education. *American Journal of Occupational Therapy, 69*(Suppl. 3), 6913410052. doi:10.5014/ajot.2015.696S17

Barnett, R. (2004). Learning for an unknown future. *Higher Education Research and Development, 23*, 247-261.

Barnitt, R., & Salmond, R. (2000). Fitness for purpose of occupational therapy graduates: Two different perspectives. *British Journal of Occupational Therapy, 63*, 443-448.

Barry, M., Kuijer-Siebelink, W., Nieuwenhuis, L., & Scherpbier-de Haan, N. (2017). Communities of practice: A means to support occupational therapists' continuing professional development. A literature review. *Australian Journal of Occupational Therapy, 64*(2), 185-193. doi:10.1111/1440-1630.12334

Carroll, A., Herge, E. A., Johnson, L., & Schaaf, R. C. (2017). Outcomes of an evidence-based, data driven model fieldwork experience for occupational therapy students. *Journal of Occupational Therapy Education, 1*(1). doi:10.26681/jote.2017.010102

Chipchase, L. S., Buttrum, P. J., Dunwoodie, R., Hill, A. E., Mandrusiak, A., & Moran, M. (2012). Characteristics of student preparedness for clinical learning: Clinical educator perspectives using the Delphi approach. *BMC Medical Education, 12*(1), 1-9. doi:10.1186/1472-6920-12-112

Di Tommaso, A., Isbel, S., Scarvell, J., & Wicks, A. (2016). Occupational therapists' perceptions of occupation in practice: An exploratory study. *Australian Occupational Therapy Journal, 63*(3), 206-213. doi:10.1111/1440-1630.12289

Doyle, T., & Zakrajsek, T. (2013). *The new science of learning: How to learn in harmony with your brain.* Sterling, VA: Stylus.

Fitzgerald, C., Moores, A., Coleman, A., & Fleming, J. (2015). Supporting new graduate professional development: A clinical learning framework. *Australian Occupational Therapy Journal, 62*, 13-20. doi:10.1111/1440-1630.12165

Flinders, B. A., Nicholson, L., Carlascio, A., & Gilb, K. (2013). The partnership model for service learning programs: A step-by-step approach. *American Journal of Health Sciences, 4*(2), 67-77.

Fortune, T., Ryan, S., & Adamson, L. (2013). Transition to practice in supercomplex environments: Are occupational therapy graduates adequately prepared? *Australian Occupational Therapy Journal, 60*, 217-220. doi:10.1111/1440-1630.12010

Glenn, E. K., & Gilbert-Hunt, S. (2012). New graduate occupational therapists experience of showering assessments: A phenomological study. *Australian Occupational Therapy Journal, 59*(3), 188-196. doi:10.1111/j.1440-1630.2012.01000.x

Gray, M., Clark, M., Penman, M., Smith, J., Bell, J., Thomas, Y., & Trevan-Hawke, J. (2012). New graduate occupational therapists feelings of preparedness for practice in Australia and Aotearoa/New Zealand. *Australian Occupational Therapy Journal, 59*, 445-455. doi:10.1111/j.1440-1630.2012.01029.

Ikiugu, M. N., Smallfield, S., & Condit, C. (2009). A framework for combining theoretical conceptual practice models in occupational therapy practice. *Canadian Journal of Occupational Therapy, 76*(3), 162-170.

Kislov, R. (2014). Rethinking capacity building for knowledge mobilization: Developing multilevel capabilities in healthcare organization. *Implementation Science, 9*(166). doi: 10.1186/s13012-014-0166-0

Levkoe, C., Brail, S., & Daniere, A. (2014). Engaged pedagogy and transformative learning in graduate education: A service-learning case study. *Canadian Journal of Higher Education, 44*(3), 68-85.

Liddiard, K., Batten R., Wang, Y., Long, K., Wallis, A., & Brown, C. A. (2017). Job club: A program to assist occupational therapy students' transition to practice. *Education Sciences, 7*(3). doi:10.3390/educsci7030070

McCombie, R. P., & Antanavage, M. E. (2017). Transitioning from occupational therapy student to practicing occupational therapist: First year of employment. *Occupational Therapy in Health Care, 31*(2), 126-142. doi:10.1080/07380577.2017.1307480

McLoughlin, C., Patel, K. D., O'Callaghan, T., & Reeves, S. (2018). The use of virtual communities of practice to improve interprofessional collaboration and education: findings from an integrated review. *Journal of Interprofessional Care, 32*(2), 136-142. doi:10.1080/13561820.2017.1377692

Melman, S., Ashby, S. E., & James, C. (2016). Supervision in practice education and transition to practice: Student and new graduate perceptions. *Internet Journal of Allied Health Sciences and Practice, 14*(3). Retrieved from http://nsuworks.nova.edu/cgi/viewcontent.cgi?article=1589&context=ijahsp

Morley, M., Rugg, S., & Drew, J. (2007). Before preceptorship: New occupational therapists' expectations of practice and experience of supervision. *British Journal of Occupational Therapy, 70*(6), 243-253. doi:10.1177/030802260707000604

Morris, Z. S., Wooding, S., & Grant, J. (2011). The answer is 17 years, what is the question: understanding time lags in translational research. *Journal of the Royal Society of Medicine, 104*, 510-520. doi:10.1258/jrsm.2011.110180

National Board for Certification in Occupational Therapy. (2017). *Self-Assessment.* Retrieved from https://www.nbcot.org/en/Students/Study-Tools/Self-Assessments

Newton, J. M., Billett, S., Jolly, B., & Ockerby, C. M. (2009). Lost in translation: Barriers to learning in health professional clinical education. *Learning in Health and Social Care, 8*(4), 315-327. doi:10.1111/j.1473-6861.2009.00229.x

Otty, R., & Milton, L. (2016). Collaborative structures in a graduate program. In J. Bernstein & B. Flinders (Eds.), *New Directions for Teaching and Learning* (pp. 51-63). San Francisco, CA: Jossey Bass. doi:10.1002/tl.20209

Parham, D. (1987). Toward professionalism: The reflective therapist. *American Journal of Occupational Therapy, 41*(9), 555-561. doi:10.5014/ajot.41.9.555

Roberts, G. I. (2015). Communities of practice: Exploring enablers and barriers with school health clinicians. *Canadian Journal of Occupational Therapy, 82*(5), 294-306. doi:o.1177/0008417415576776

Robertson, L. J., & Griffiths, S. (2009). Graduates' reflections on their preparation for practice. *British Journal of Occupational Therapy, 72*(3), 125-132. doi:10.1177/030802260907200307

Sackett, D. (1996). Evidence-based medicine: What it is and what it isn't. *British Medical Journal, 312*, 71-72.

Smith, R., & Pilling, S. (2008). Supporting the transition from student to professional—a case study in allied health. *Australian Health Review, 32*(1), 134-138.

Thomas, E. M., Rybski, M. F., Apke, T. L., Kegelmeyer, D. A., & Kloos, A. D. (2017). An acute interprofessional simulation experience for occupational and physical therapy students: Key findings from a survey study. *Journal of Interprofessional Care, 31*(3), 317-324. doi:10.1080/13561820.2017.1280006

Toal-Sullivan, D. (2006). New graduates' experiences of learning to practise occupational therapy. *British Journal of Occupational Therapy, 69*(11), 513-524. doi:10.1177/030802260606901105

Wenger, E. (1991). *Communities of practice: Learning, meaning, and identity.* Cambridge, UK: Cambridge University Press.

Westfall, J. M., Mold, J., & Fagnan, L. (2007). Practice-based research—"Blue Highways" on the NIH roadmap. *Journal of the American Medical Association, 297*, 403-406. doi:10.1001/jama.297.4.403

Wilding, C., & Whiteford, G. (2007). Occupation and occupational therapy: Knowledge paradigms and everyday practice. *Australian Occupational Therapy Journal, 54*(3), 185-193. doi:10.1111/j.1440-1630.2006.00621.x

6

Use of Simulation in Occupational Therapy Education

Monica S. Perlmutter, OTD, OTR/L, SCLV, FAOTA
and Susan M. Cleghorn, DrOT, OTR/L, TRS, CAPS, FNAP

Chapter Objectives

By the end of this chapter, the reader will be able to:

1. Distinguish various methods of simulation used in health care education.
2. Recognize the benefits and challenges of simulation.
3. Select appropriate tools for measuring student learning in simulation.
4. Identify student learning gained from simulation experiences.

INTRODUCTION

Occupational therapy educators are challenged to prepare students to manage the complexities of practice and meet increased productivity standards (Knecht-Sabres, Kovic, Wallingford, & St. Amand, 2013). According to a 2014 survey, the majority of U.S. occupational therapy programs incorporate a wide range of simulation learning experiences into their curricula (Bethea, Castillo, & Harvison, 2014). Simulation experiences typically include a case scenario, opportunity to practice skills in a safe environment, and reflection with facilitators and peers (Ozelie, Both, Fricke, & Maddock, 2016). Goals of simulation that were identified by 175 occupational therapy and certified occupational therapy assistant programs included increasing competencies in patient assessment, clinical reasoning, problem solving, communication, intervention, and communication (Bethea et al., 2014). A similar report regarding the use of simulation in Australian occupational therapy programs found that all programs surveyed were using some form of simulation (Rodger, Bennett, Fitzgerald, & Neads, 2010).

Taff, S. D., Grajo, L. C., & Hooper, B. R. (Eds.). *Perspectives on Occupational Therapy Education: Past, Present, and Future* (pp. 63-73).
© 2020 Taylor & Francis Group.

Simulation provides a flexible and low-risk learning opportunity that can be tailored to meet learning objectives, modified to increase or decrease difficulty level, and repeated as needed for skill development (Issenberg, Mcgaghie, Petrusa, Lee Gordon, & Scalese, 2005). The goals of simulation experiences include building occupational therapy student competencies in clinical reasoning, problem solving, decision making (Bethea et al., 2014), goal setting, information gathering, communication, professional behaviors, and intervention (Bennett, Rodger, Fitzgerald, & Gibson, 2017). Support for simulation as a clinical instructional method is demonstrated with the updated 2018 Accreditation Council for Occupational Therapy Education (ACOTE) standards which includes the option for students meeting level 1 fieldwork requirements through participation in simulated environments and with standardized patients (American Occupational Therapy Association, 2018).

A number of systematic reviews reveal that studies regarding the use and efficacy of simulation vary widely in rigor and methodology across health care disciplines (Cook et al., 2011; Issenberg et al., 2005; Mori, Carnahan, & Herold, 2015; Yeung, Dubrowski, & Carnahan, 2013). A recent literature review of simulation use in occupational therapy curricula included 57 articles that were descriptive, used pretest-posttest design, or described student perceptions (Bennett et al., 2017). Simulation methods included written case studies ($n = 22$), standardized patients ($n = 13$), video-based case studies ($n = 15$), role play ($n = 8$), and mannequins or part-task trainers ($n = 4$). Nearly all systemic reviews conclude that more rigorously designed studies that include randomized controlled design and cost-benefit analyses are needed.

Simulation Methods Used in Occupational Therapy Education

A wide range of simulation methods offer students the opportunity to practice clinical skills in a safe environment. Before exploring these methods in more detail, a discussion of simulation fidelity is warranted. *Simulation fidelity* is defined as "the degree to which the simulation mimics reality in terms of equipment, environment and psychological responses" (Shea, 2015, p. 3) and can range from high to low. High-fidelity experiences may involve students interacting with patient educators in a simulated acute hospital suite (Hedge, Neville, & Pickens, 2015). Low-fidelity simulations include written or video-based case studies. Psychological fidelity is the degree that the learner perceives the experience to be authentic (Sharma, Boet, Kitto, & Reeves, 2011). Educators can create more realistic and believable simulations by adding stressors and other emotional components to case scenarios (DeMaria et al., 2010). Additionally, sociological fidelity can be addressed by embedding opportunities for students to collaborate and negotiate with peers and other interprofessional students (Sharma et al., 2011).

Types of Simulation Experiences

Most simulation experiences require a case scenario, which is often provided in written form (Bennett et al., 2017). Written case scenarios are frequently the basis for problem-based learning curricula (Hooper, King, Wood, Bilics, & Gupta, 2013), standardized patient scripts, and other simulation methods. Case updates that reflect changes in medical status, social support, or other realistic "monkey wrenches" can be introduced at key points in the learning experience to provide opportunity for students to pursue multiple lines of reasoning (Poulton, Conradi, Kavia, Round, & Hilton, 2009).

Role-play experiences can be guided by written cases or procedures and are commonly used in occupational therapy curricula (Hooper et al., 2013). The use of a script will help faculty and students to feel more prepared to assume the role of the client (Haddad, 1988). Educators may want to consider using props, adding family members into the mix, and building in psychosocial elements to increase fidelity and complexity.

Videos can be an effective medium for simulation experiences and may be obtained via YouTube and organizations such as the ICE Video Learning Center Library (ICE Learning Center, Inc., n.d.), or faculty can create their own using actual clients (Hall, Marshall, Weaver, Boyle, & Taniguchi, 2011). Tomlin (2005) reported that videos used in combination with drop-down menus with assessment and intervention options were instrumental in evaluating students' decision-making skills as they planned occupational therapy evaluation for a "client" who had a stroke. Occupational therapy–related virtual patient experiences include an interprofessional education experience using VirtualPT and DxR Clinician (DxR DevelopmentGroup, Carbondale, IL) virtual patient software (Shoemaker, Platko, Cleghorn, & Booth, 2014) and software that focuses on home assessment (Sabus, Sabata, & Antonacci, 2011; Sutton, Newberry, & Threapleton, 2016).

Encounters with standardized patients in realistic settings provide students with high-fidelity learning experiences; associated benefits have been reported in the rehabilitation and occupational therapy literature (Lindstrom-Hazel & West-Frasier, 2004; Yeung et al., 2013). Standardized patients are actors or actual clients who are trained to realistically and consistently portray individuals with different medical complaints (Yeung et al., 2013). Standardized patient experiences frequently include post–self-assessment and feedback from faculty and standardized patients regarding clinical and communication skills, although there is limited evidence regarding the best practice of training standardized patients to provide this feedback (Bokken, Linssen, Scherpbier, van der Vleuten, & Rethans, 2009).

BEST PRACTICES IN IMPLEMENTING SIMULATION

The initial step in simulation development is to identify learning objectives that are appropriate for the students' level of knowledge and skill base (Alinier, 2011; Shea, 2015). Alinier (2011) suggests including one to four learning objectives that consider the degree of challenge presented to the students as well as the skill and experience level of faculty involved in the simulation. After learning objectives are identified, case scenario elements can be considered, such as the client's medical and mental health status (Alinier, 2011), occupational performance issues, home environment, social support, and clinical setting (e.g., acute care, outpatient, home health, and school/work setting). In addition, elements of social determinants of health (SDH) can be included when describing client factors in case studies and/or proposed guidelines for case development. SDH serve as a threshold concept that fosters transformative learning and critical thinking and reflects the reality of practice. Examples include ensuring diversity in simulation cases relative to gender identity, economic status and other factors; adding descriptors such as limited access to transportation and work schedule that conflicts with therapy visits; and placing case based client in context of local community (Berg, Philipp & Taff, 2019).

Educators may begin the simulation experience by providing students with a limited amount of case information to facilitate initial thought processes. Then, a comprehensive case can be shared along with occupational therapy evaluation results and reports from other disciplines, if desired. The inclusion of twists and turns such as a medical status change, a sudden plan for discharge, or a challenging family dynamic will promote the authenticity of the experience (Alinier, 2011). Case scenarios may be inspired by faculty experience with actual clients and videos available on YouTube. Occupational therapy textbooks that include collections of case studies may also be useful (Lowenstein & Halloran, 2015; Trickey-Rokenbrod, 2017).

Scripts for standardized patients, faculty, or students playing the part of clients, family members, or other professionals can be written so that roles are portrayed with some consistency. Scripts may include details regarding client appearance and demeanor, props, opening statements about key client concerns, and medical history. Alinier (2011) provides a detailed template for script development.

Faculty will need to train facilitators and standardized patients and rehearse methods of portraying physical, cognitive, and emotional elements of their character. Mock medical records, evaluation results, and documentation may add to the realism of the experience. Ideally, the physical environment where the simulation will occur should be as realistic as possible (Alinier, 2011). Many universities have simulation laboratories that closely mimic acute care hospital or clinic settings.

Students engaged in simulation experiences have the opportunity to take on multiple roles including that of the occupational therapist, family member, and observer (Shea, 2015). Faculty can direct students to play the role of the primary occupational therapist, or students can be paired and interact with the "client" in a tag-team format. Students in observer roles can be assigned the additional responsibility of providing peer feedback after the encounter.

The provision of feedback from faculty, peers, and standardized patients is a critical component of the simulation experience (Issenberg et al., 2005; Zigmont, Kappus, & Sudikoff, 2011). Shea (2015) suggests that although debriefing generally occurs after the simulation experience, real-time feedback from the faculty or students may be beneficial. Additional postsimulation feedback can be provided by faculty, peers, and/or standardized patients to allow students to gain insight into how their communication style, behaviors, and clinical skills influenced their performance (Shea, 2015). Faculty can create guides or related assignments to foster self-appraisal and identification of continued learning needs.

Zigmont et al. (2011, p. 92) assert that "post experience analysis" is the most critical component of the simulation process and provide detailed guidelines for the debriefing process. Their framework is called the 3D model and includes three phases: "defusing, discovering, and deepening." During the initial defusing phase, students are invited to share their immediate reactions to the experience while the faculty member ensures a safe atmosphere and validates student feelings.

The goal of the discovering phase is to foster the students' self-reflection and conceptualization of new information (Zigmont et al., 2011). The facilitator assists the learner with determining strengths and areas for growth. Student, peer, and faculty review of videos of the simulation experience can be used as a basis for self-reflection and the identification of additional leaning needs. During the deepening phase of debriefing, facilitators foster the learners' connection with the simulation experience with practice and, ideally, provide opportunity for additional practice with an actual or standardized patient.

Simulated learning experiences are generally well received by students but present a variety of challenges. Results of a 2014 survey indicate that common hurdles include cost, development, training time, and scheduling conflicts (Bethea et al., 2014). Despite these challenges, the majority of survey respondents (83%, $n = 145$) reported that the simulation experiences were valuable and provided a greater number of positive comments about the benefits vs. the challenges (Bethea et al., 2014; Shoemaker et al., 2014).

IMPACT OF SIMULATION ON STUDENT LEARNING OUTCOMES

The use of simulation for teaching clinical skills and measuring student learning has a long-standing history in medicine, nursing, and pharmacy education (Bradley, Whittington, & Mottram, 2013; Cook et al., 2011; Ray, Wylie, Rowe, Heidel, & Franks, 2012). Student competencies measured in these professions include knowledge of basic science, clinical reasoning and decision making, therapeutic communication, physical and psychosocial assessment, and application of ethical considerations. Tools used to measure these skills include student self-assessment, reflection, survey, questionnaire, video evaluation, pre- and post-tests, and multiple-choice examination. Assessment has been used before and after interaction with standardized patients, mannequins, and virtual cases to measure student competency (Buxton, Phillippi, & Collins, 2015; Harris, Ryan, & Rabuck, 2012; Hoffman et al., 2011; Miles, Mabey, Leggett, & Stansfield, 2014; Raurell-Torredà et al., 2015; Ray et al., 2012).

There is a growing body of evidence supporting the effectiveness of simulation on student learning outcomes in the occupational therapy literature (Bennett et al., 2017; Bethea et al., 2014; Ozelie et al., 2016). Bethea and colleagues (2014) completed a survey of 175 occupational therapy and occupational therapy assistant programs in the United States that identified simulation goals that could impact student learning outcomes, including increasing competencies in patient assessment, clinical reasoning, communication, intervention, and communication. Additional evidence identifies simulation as an effective method for developing student competencies and learning outcomes inclusive of clinical reasoning (Shea, 2015), efficient time use, completeness (Tomlin, 2005), patient evaluation, professional behaviors (Ozelie et al., 2016), self-awareness, confidence, and empathy (Hedge et al., 2015). In addition to development of competencies, student involvement in simulation was found to be positively associated with performance in fieldwork and acute care settings (Bennett et al., 2017; Ozelie et al., 2016).

The majority of student learning in simulation has been measured through student self-report. In a study by Hedge and colleagues (2015), occupational therapy students who engaged in a low-fidelity simulation that included hands-on instruction from patient educators reported a higher level of confidence, awareness of skills, and empathy after the simulation. In addition to self-report, competencies have been measured with the use of didactic and simulation assignment scores. Gibbs, Dietrich, and Dagnan (2017) used pre- and post-test evaluation of occupational therapy students engaged in high-fidelity simulation with mannequins in an intensive care unit environment. Evaluation results included higher levels of confidence, knowledge, and skill after the high-fidelity simulation when working with acute conditions and devices such as heart monitors and intravenous lines. Tomlin (2005) found that higher didactic scores from classroom work combined with simulation experiences predicted higher scores in the areas of completeness of work and the efficient use of time in clinical experiences.

OCCUPATIONAL THERAPY PROGRAM INNOVATIONS

Occupational therapy educators across the country were contacted by the authors and invited to share examples of simulation used in their programs. Table 6-1 includes a few examples that demonstrate how a developmental approach to using simulation in occupational therapy curriculum can scaffold student learning from novice to readiness for Level II fieldwork.

NEW TECHNOLOGIES

Technologies used in simulation have rapidly evolved and become more sophisticated, resulting in more high-fidelity options for health profession educators (Duff, Miller, & Bruce, 2016; Moro, Stromberga, Raikos, & Stirling, 2017). Occupational therapy departments must take into consideration space for equipment, budget constraints, access to technology support, cost of upkeep and upgrading, and scheduling access when shared among other health professions (Bethea et al., 2014; Duff et al., 2016). Table 6-2 outlines examples of technology innovations.

Table 6-1

OCCUPATIONAL THERAPY PROGRAM INNOVATIONS

OCCUPATIONAL THERAPY PROGRAM	SIMULATION EXPERIENCE	STUDENT LEARNING OBJECTIVES	INSTRUCTION
Grand Valley State University Occupational Science & Therapy Department (S. Cleghorn, personal communication, November 1, 2017)	"Baby Lab" with typically developing infants from 1 week to 12 months of age as standardized patients and their caregivers	Research typical developmental milestones and assessment tools. Apply observation and interview skills to gather developmental data. Create a clinical report of developmental findings.	Lecture, discussion, simulation lab, and assignment; students work in pairs to research and create a developmental checklist, interview caregivers, assess infants, and create a report.
University of Mississippi Occupational Therapy Department (P. Rogers & T. Taylor, personal communication, January 8, 2018)	"Integrated Behavioral Health Education" simulation with students from occupational therapy, nursing, social work, and standardized patients	Compare and contrast interprofessional roles in mental health. Demonstrate competency in assessment, intervention, and documentation.	Discussion and simulation lab. Discussion-based instruction roles, responsibilities, training, and techniques among the different professions; students work in interprofessional teams to assess and provide interventions with standardized patients assigned with mental health conditions.
Winston-Salem State University Occupational Therapy Department (D. P. Bethea, personal communication, November 3, 2017)	Assessment lab with use of standardized patient assessment and video with nursing, physical, and occupational therapy students	Demonstrate competencies in goal writing, patient evaluation, clinical reasoning, problem solving, interprofessional collaboration, and patient behavior management.	Simulation lab; students view a video-based case and determine discipline-specific goals individually, develop interdisciplinary goals, and assess the patient.

Table 6-2

TECHNOLOGY INNOVATIONS

TECHNOLOGY DESCRIPTION	SIMULATION METHOD	COST
Anatomage Table (Anatomage, 2018) • Interactive images of realistic, life-size, dissectible, three-dimensional human anatomy. • Used in hospitals, universities, and institutions for education and training of health care professionals and students. • Anatomage (2018) offers software programs including regional and gross anatomy cases and 1000 examples of various pathologies. (R. Chen, personal communication, January 10, 2018)	Virtual reality: three-dimensional, interactive anatomy 	$70,000 to $80,000 per table
ShadowHealth (ShadowHealth, 2018) • Students engage with digital standardized patients. • Uses a conversation engine and interactive three-dimensional environments that mimic real-world verbal exchanges between health professionals/students. • Students are able to ask the virtual patients questions, receive responses, and practice critical thinking skills. • Students practice patient interactions, assessment, intervention, and documentation. (B. Fidrick, personal communication, January 26, 2018)	Virtual reality: virtual patients and clinical environments 	$99 per product per student

continued

Table 6-2 (continued)

TECHNOLOGY INNOVATIONS

TECHNOLOGY DESCRIPTION	SIMULATION METHOD	COST
Sentinal World • Software immerses students in virtual urban and rural communities. • Ten different city and rural environments with 5 to 13 unique citizens, each with original demographics. • Students have 24/7 access to experiences with environments and community members. • Students can complete population health assessments, care planning, disaster preparedness, and case studies. • Software provides a dashboard for faculty to track student hours and activities, curricular mapping tools, and rubrics for grading virtual learning. (Healthcare Learning Innovations, 2018)	Virtual reality: virtual patients and community environments	Cost varies, contact for product estimates
Black Box Theater • Space designed with black walls, a medium to large empty floor, and seating for an audience. • Traditionally used in performance education as an indoor performance area for participants to practice engaging in uniquely created sets or environments. • A canvas for creating unique environments, such as responding to a disaster, practicing a surgical technique, or practicing skills in a simulated medical environment. • The space is constructed similar to black box theaters with plain black walls, open floor spaces, medical equipment, cameras used for recording student experiences, projectors, and software to create desired sounds, smells, and images. (K. Branch, personal communication, January 23, 2017)	Virtual reality: adaptable space/ able to create use based on need	$2,000 and $125,000 depending on equipment needed

Implications for Occupational Therapy Education

- Simulation prepares students for working in challenging health care environments by addressing skills related to clinical reasoning; problem solving; and communication, assessment, and intervention.
- A wide range of simulation experiences provide flexible opportunities for students to engage with complex case scenarios in low-risk environments.
- Simulation requires training, equipment, supplies, and support from the educational institution.
- Cost, training, technology support, and scheduling access must be considered before adopting new technologies.
- More rigorously designed research on the efficacy of simulation in occupational therapy education is needed to determine best practice.

Key Reflection Questions

1. How might you use simulation in your courses? What student learning outcomes will you target?
2. What challenges might your department encounter when planning and implementing simulation?
3. What tools will you consider for measuring student learning with simulation?
4. How can you contribute to the evidence about simulation in occupational therapy education?

What led you to become an occupational therapy educator?

My love of teaching began at an early age when I coerced my younger brothers to be my students while we played "school." Early experiences as a teaching assistant during my undergraduate occupational therapy program, clinical instructor for Level I and II students, and kinesiology lab instructor sparked my interest in education. Teaching allows me to combine my love of interacting with people of all ages, personalities, and backgrounds with my love for learning. Watching students develop critical thinking and problem-solving skills and gain confidence is extremely rewarding.

Monica S. Perlmutter, OTD, OTR/L, SCLV, FAOTA

My occupational therapy mentor and friend Denise Meier encouraged me to try my hand at teaching by asking that I develop a school-based occupational therapy module for Grand Valley State University early in my career as a therapist. I was hooked after the first day of instructing and leapt at the opportunity to become a full-time occupational therapy educator 7 years later. After 10 years of teaching, I still feel there is so much learn about adult education. What I do know is that occupational therapy education can transform students' thinking about people, communities, health care, and the world. I enjoy creating learning opportunities that require students to think outside of the box in their view of health, wellness, and the role of occupational therapist.

Susan M. Cleghorn, DrOT, OTR/L, TRS, CAPS, FNAP

REFERENCES

Alinier, G. (2011). Developing high-fidelity health care simulation scenarios: A guide for educators and professionals. *Simulation & Gaming, 42*(1), 9-26. doi:10.1177/1046878109355683

American Journal of Occupational Therapy. (2018) Accreditation council for occupational therapy education (ACOTE) standards and interpretive guide. *American Journal of Occupational Therapy, 72* (Suppl. 2), 1-54. doi: 10.5014/ajot.2018.72S217

Anatomage. (2018, January 3). Retrieved from http://www.anatomage.com/anatomage-medical/

Bennett, S., Rodger, S., Fitzgerald, C., & Gibson, L. (2017). Simulation in occupational therapy curricula: A literature review. *Australian Occupational Therapy Journal, 64*, 314-327. doi:10.1111/1440-1630.12372

Bethea, D. P., Castillo, D. C., & Harvison, N. (2014). Use of simulation in occupational therapy education: Way of the future? *American Journal of Occupational Therapy, 68*, S32-S39. doi:10.5014/ajot.2014.012716

Berg, C., Philipp, R., & Taff, S. D. (2019). Critical thinking and transformational learning: Using case studies as narrative frameworks for threshold concepts. *Journal of Occupational Therapy Education, 3*(3), 13.

Bokken, L., Linssen, T., Scherpbier, A., van der Vleuten, C., & Rethans, J. J. (2009). Feedback by simulated patients in undergraduate medical education: A systematic review of the literature. *Medical Education, 43*(3), 202-210. doi:10.1111/j.1365-2923.2008.03268.x

Bradley, G., Whittington, S., & Mottram, P. (2013). Enhancing occupational therapy education through simulation. *British Journal of Occupational Therapy, 76*(1), 43-46.

Buxton, M., Phillippi, J. C., & Collins, M. R. (2015). Simulation: A new approach to teaching ethics. *Journal of Midwifery Women's Health, 60*(1), 70-74. doi:10.1111/jmwh.12185

Cook, D. A., Hatala, R., Brydges, R., Zendejas, B., Szostek, J. H., Wang, A. T., … Hamstra, S. J. (2011). Technology-enhanced simulation for health professions education: A systematic review and meta-analysis. *Journal of the American Medical Association, 306*(9), 978-988. doi:10.1001/jama.2011.1234

DeMaria, S., Jr., Bryson, E., Mooney, T., Silverstein, J., Reich, D., & Bodian, C. (2010). Adding emotional stressors to training in simulated cardiopulmonary arrest enhances participant performance. *Medical Education, 44*(10), 1006-1015. doi:10.1111/j.1365-2923.2010.03775.x

Duff, E., Miller, L., & Bruce, J. (2016). Online virtual simulation and diagnostic reasoning: A scoping review. *Clinical Simulation in Nursing, 12*(9), 377-384. doi:10.1016/j.ecns.2016.04.001.

Gibbs, D. M., Dietrich, M., & Dagnan, E. (2017). Using high fidelity simulation to impact occupational therapy student knowledge, comfort, and confidence in acute care. *Open Journal of Occupational Therapy, 5*(1), 10. doi:10.15453/2168-6408.1225

Haddad, A. M. (1988). Teaching ethical analysis in occupational therapy. *American Journal of Occupational Therapy, 42*, 300-304. doi:10.5014/ajot.42.5.300

Hall, P., Marshall, D., Weaver, L., Boyle, A., & Taniguchi, A. (2011). A method to enhance student teams in palliative care: piloting the McMaster-Ottawa team observed structured clinical encounter. *Journal of Palliative Medicine, 14*(6), 744-750.

Harris, D. M., Ryan, K., & Rabuck, C. (2012). Using a high-fidelity patient simulator with first-year medical students to facilitate learning of cardiovascular function curves. *Advances in Physiology Education, 36*(3), 213-219. doi:10.1152/advan.00058.2012

Healthcare Learning Innovations. (2018, January 3). Retrieved from https://healthcarelearninginnovations.com/

Hedge, N., Neville, M. A., & Pickens, N. D. (2015). How patient educators teach students: Giving a face to a story. *Open Journal of Occupational Therapy, 3*(1), 4. doi:10.15453/2168-6408.1143

Hoffman, K., Dempsey, J., Levett-Jones, T., Noble, D., Hickey, N., Jeong, S., … Norton, C. (2011). The design and implementation of an Interactive Computerised Decision Support Framework (ICDSF) as a strategy to improve nursing students' clinical reasoning skills. *Nurse Education Today, 31*(6), 587-594. doi:10.1016/j.nedt.2010.10.012

Hooper, B., King, R., Wood, W., Bilics, A., & Gupta, J. (2013). An international systematic mapping review of educational approaches and teaching methods in occupational therapy. *British Journal of Occupational Therapy, 76*, 9-22. doi:10.4276/030802213X13576469254612

ICE Learning Center, Inc. (n.d.). Retrieved from https://www.icelearningcenter.com/

Issenberg, S. B., Mcgaghie, W. C., Petrusa, E. R., Lee Gordon, D., & Scalese, R. J. (2005). Features and uses of high-fidelity medical simulations that lead to effective learning: A BEME systematic review. *Medical Teacher, 27*(1), 10-28. doi:10.1080/01421590500046924

Knecht-Sabres L. J., Kovic, M., Wallingford, M., & St. Amand, L. E. (2013). Preparing occupational therapy students for the complexities of clinical practice. *Open Journal of Occupational Therapy, 1*(3), 4. doi:10.15453/2168-6408.1047

Lindstrom-Hazel, D., & West-Frasier, J. (2004). Preparing students to hit the ground running with problem-based learning standardized simulations. *American Journal of Occupational Therapy, 58*(2), 236-239. doi:10.5014/ajot.58.2.236

Lowenstein, N., & Halloran, P. (2015). *Case studies through the health care continuum.* Thorofare, NJ: SLACK Incorporated.

Miles, L. W., Mabey, L., Leggett, S., & Stansfield, K. (2014). Teaching communication and therapeutic relationship skills to baccalaureate nursing students: A peer mentorship simulation approach. *Journal of Psychosocial Nursing and Mental Health Services, 52*(10), 34-41. doi:10.3928/02793695-20140829-01

Mori, B., Carnahan, H., & Herold, J. (2015). Use of simulation learning experiences in physical therapy entry-to-practice curricula: a systematic review. *Physiotherapy Canada, 67*(2), 194-202. doi:10.3138/ptc.2014-40E

Moro, C., Stromberga, Z., Raikos, A., & Stirling, A. (2017). The effectiveness of virtual and augmented reality in health sciences and medical anatomy. *American Sciences Education, 10*(6), 549-559. doi:10.1002/ase.1696

Ozelie, R., Both, C., Fricke, E., & Maddock, C. (2016). High-fidelity simulation in occupational therapy curriculum: Impact on level II fieldwork performance. *Open Journal of Occupational Therapy, 4*(4), 9. doi:10.15453/2168-6408.1242

Poulton, T., Conradi, E., Kavia, S., Round, J., & Hilton, S. (2009). The replacement of 'paper' cases by interactive online virtual patients in problem-based learning. *Medical Teacher, 31*(8), 752-758. doi:10.1080/01421590903141082

Raurell-Torredà, M., Olivet-Pujol, J., Romero-Collado, À., Malagon-Aguilera, M. C., Patiño-asó, J., & Baltasar-Bagué, A. (2015). Case-based learning and simulation: Useful tools to enhance nurses' education? Nonrandomized controlled trial. *Journal of Nursing Scholarship, 47*(1), 34-42. doi:10.1111/jnu.12113

Ray, S. M., Wylie, D. R., Rowe, A. S., Heidel, E., & Franks, A. S. (2012). Pharmacy student knowledge retention after completing either a simulated or written patient case. *American Journal Pharmaceutical Education, 76*(5), 86. doi:10.5688/ajpe76586

Rodger, S., Bennett, S., Fitzgerald, C. & Neads, P. (2010). Use of simulated learning activities in occupational therapy curriculum. Queensland: University of Queensland. Retrieved from https://web.archive.org/web/20160328031147/http://hwa.gov.au/sites/default/files/simulated-learning-in-occupational-therapy-curricula-201108.pdf

Sabus, C., Sabata, D., & Antonacci, D. (2011). Use of a virtual environment to facilitate instruction of an interprofessional home assessment. *Journal of Allied Health, 40*(4), 199-205. Retrieved from http://www.ingentaconnect.com/content/asahp/jah/2011/00000040/00000004/art00008 VR/computer based patients

ShadowHealth. (2018). Retrieved from www.ShadowHealth.com

Sharma, S., Boet, S., Kitto, S., & Reeves, S. (2011). Interprofessional simulated learning: The need for 'sociological fidelity'. *Journal of Interprofessional Care, 25*(2), 81-83. doi:10.3109/13561820.2011.556514

Shea, C. K. (2015). High-fidelity simulation: A tool for occupational therapy education. *Open Journal of Occupational Therapy, 3*(4), 8. doi:10.15453/2168-6408.1155

Shoemaker, M. J., Platko, C. M., Cleghorn, S. M., & Booth, A. (2014). Virtual patient care: An interprofessional education approach for physician assistant, physical therapy, and occupational therapy students. *Journal of Interprofessional Care, 28*(4), 365-367. doi:10.3109/13561820.2014.891978

Sutton, G., Newberry, K., & Threapleton, K. (2016). Evaluating unity created teaching simulations within occupational therapy. *Journal of Assistive Technologies, 10*(3), 162-170. doi:10.1108/JAT-11-2015-0030

Tomlin, G. (2005). The use of interactive video client simulation scores to predict clinical performance of occupational therapy students. *American Journal of Occupational therapy, 59*(1), 50-56. doi:10.5014/ajot.59.1.50

Trickey-Rokenbrod, D. (2017). *Occupational therapy in action: A library of case studies.* Philadelphia, PA: Wolters-Kluwer.

Yeung, E., Dubrowski, A., & Carnahan, H. (2013). Simulation-augmented education in the rehabilitation professions: A scoping review. *International Journal of Therapy and Rehabilitation, 20*(5), 228-236. doi:10.12968/ijtr.2013.20.5.228

Zigmont, J. J., Kappus, L. J., & Sudikoff, S. N. (2011). The 3D model of debriefing: defusing, discovering, and deepening. *Seminars in Perinatology, 35*(2), 52-58. doi:10.1053/j.semperi.2011.01.003

7

Measuring Educational Outcomes in Occupational Therapy
Course- and Curriculum-Level Examples

Lenin C. Grajo, PhD, EdM, OTR/L and Sharon A. Gutman, PhD, OTR, FAOTA

Chapter Objectives

By the end of this chapter, the reader will be able to:

1. Describe outcomes of occupational therapy education based on evolving official professional documents.
2. Describe some examples of measuring course-level and curricular outcomes in occupational therapy education.
3. Describe how properly designed rubrics and test blueprints can aid in effective measurement of course-level learning outcomes.
4. Reflect on opportunities and challenges to effectively measure educational outcomes.

OUTCOMES OF HIGHER EDUCATION AND OCCUPATIONAL THERAPY EDUCATION

Assessment is the process of appraising knowledge, skills, beliefs, and attitudes acquired as the result of learning through coursework (Barkley & Major, 2016). A variety of educational outcomes exist for higher education. For example, Fink (2013) highlighted the following six categories of outcomes related to significant learning: (1) learning how to learn or learning to inquire and construct knowledge and becoming self-directed and intentional learners; (2) caring or becoming passionate about a topic or subject; (3) human dimension or learning about self (e.g., leadership, cultural competence, and ethics); (4) integration or connecting multiple domains of knowledge; (5) application or learning critical thinking, creativity, and performance skills; and (6) foundational knowledge or learning concepts and facts in an area of study. Fink's outcomes for significant learning encompass broader outcomes for higher education such as enabling (a) active, engaging, diverse, and inclusive

Taff, S. D., Grajo, L. C., & Hooper, B. R. (Eds.). *Perspectives on Occupational Therapy Education: Past, Present, and Future* (pp. 75-93). © 2020 Taylor & Francis Group.

learning within and beyond the classroom environment; (b) a collaborative process that builds on learners' prior knowledge and experience; (c) professional judgment, evaluation, and self-reflection; and (d) lifelong learning.

Many of the outcomes for higher education are mirrored in the educational documents of occupational therapy. The revised "Philosophy of Occupational Therapy Education" (American Occupational Therapy Association, 2018) asserts that the goal of occupational therapy education is to prepare practitioners to address the occupational needs of individuals, groups, communities, and populations. Current accreditation standards (Accreditation Council for Occupational Therapy Education [ACOTE], 2018) assert that the goal of occupational therapy education is to prepare graduates who are generalists, theory guided, evidence based, and occupation centered; who are holistic, ethical, and committed to lifelong learning; and who are collaborative and actively involved in professional development, leadership, and advocacy. Students demonstrate achievement of these educational outcomes by passing the certification examination of the National Board for Certification in Occupational Therapy (NBCOT). The NBCOT (2019) certification examination evaluates outcomes with regard to students' abilities to (a) acquire information about factors that influence clients' occupational performance, (b) formulate conclusions about client needs and priorities to develop and monitor intervention plans, (c) select and evaluate the effectiveness of client-centered interventions, and (d) manage and direct occupational therapy services to promote quality practice. How occupational therapy programs interpret ACOTE standards and prepare students to master NBCOT certification competencies varies depending on the nature and goals of their institutions and how curricular- and course-level outcomes are defined.

Therefore, multiple educational outcomes exist for higher education and for occupational therapy, making assessment of learning quite challenging. In this chapter, we (a) provide examples of occupational therapy curricular and course-level goals and (b) describe how these educational goals can be measured.

Measuring Outcomes

In this section, we examine occupational therapy education research for examples of course- and curricular-level outcomes. At the course level, we highlight examples of how student learning objectives and skill competencies are addressed and measured. At the curricular level, we highlight examples of how outcomes of teaching-learning strategies are addressed and measured based on how they contribute to program-, department-, or university-level objectives. Whether at the course or curricular level, it is critical that the measurement of educational outcomes be aligned with course or curriculum level objectives and the most current version of the ACOTE (2018) standards.

Hooper et al. (2015) stated that occupation is the focus of occupational therapy education, and its degree of explicitness must be continually reassessed. Hooper and colleagues added that the profession's distinct knowledge base lies in how the curriculum and all courses are organized to intersect with the concept of occupation. In this section, we briefly introduce six teaching-learning strategies used in educational programs and the highlighted outcomes of these strategies. Specifically, we discuss outcomes in relation to (1) occupation-centered education, (2) interprofessional collaboration, (3) evidence-based practice (EBP) in the curriculum, (4) integration of service learning, (5) skill attainment through the use of simulation, and (6) clinical competency through fieldwork education. This section is followed by a summary table (Table 7-1) with examples of measuring educational outcomes at the course and curriculum levels. This list is not meant to be exhaustive but rather an overview of different examples of measuring educational outcomes.

Occupation-Centered Education

Because occupation is central to the profession's core values and serves as a guiding principle in both education and practice, it is critical that educators assess occupation as a learning outcome. Several studies examined how and to what degree occupation is presented at curricular and

Table 7-1

TEACHING-LEARNING STRATEGIES AND METHODS OF MEASURING RESEARCH AND TEACHING OUTCOMES

TEACHING-LEARNING STRATEGY	EXAMPLES OF METHODS TO MEASURE COURSE-LEVEL LEARNING OUTCOMES	EXAMPLES OF METHODS TO MEASURE CURRICULAR LEARNING OUTCOMES
Occupation as central theme	Qualitative analysis of case discussions and practical examinations on the use of occupation during clinical and critical reasoning activities in problem-based learning and clinical courses. Use of structured assessments (e.g., the Occupation-Centered Intervention Assessment [Jewell & Pickens, 2017]) to analyze whether therapeutic interventions are occupation centered during fieldwork experiences. Occupation analysis, reflective assignments, case studies, and case simulation examinations with critical questions on the use of occupation in clinical decision making embedded within courses.	Analysis of educational artifacts across courses within the program and identifying which courses are strong at or have opportunities to strengthen occupation as a central theme. Use of a curriculum matrix mapping out how each course within the curriculum addresses occupation and completing a strengths-weaknesses-opportunities-threats analysis to revise curriculum.
Interprofessional collaboration	Use of structured assessments to measure the effects of interprofessional education strategies on student sense of clinical competence (e.g., Ascent to Competence Scale [Berg-Poppe, Karges, Nissen, Deutsch, & Webster, 2017]) and readiness to engage in interprofessional collaboration (e.g., Readiness for Interdisciplinary Education Perception Scale [Parsell & Bligh, 1999] and Interdisciplinary Education Scale [Baughan, Macfarlane, Dentry, & Mendoza, 2014]). Use of case studies and reflective assignments expanding on the understanding of and appreciation for interprofessional health care team roles and the impact on client service provision.	Programmatic assessments of transfer of interprofessional learning in a clinical setting (Institute of Medicine, 2015) of a program through surveys and focus groups of various stakeholders (advisory board, alumni, fieldwork educators, and employers).

continued

Table 7-1 (continued)

TEACHING-LEARNING STRATEGIES AND METHODS OF MEASURING RESEARCH AND TEACHING OUTCOMES

TEACHING-LEARNING STRATEGY	EXAMPLES OF METHODS TO MEASURE COURSE-LEVEL LEARNING OUTCOMES	EXAMPLES OF METHODS TO MEASURE CURRICULAR LEARNING OUTCOMES
Service learning	Qualitative analysis of reflective assignments and field notes on the professional development of students during service activities (Lau, 2016). Qualitative analysis on the impacts of service learning on student perspectives on disability (Gitlow & Flecky, 2005). Qualitative measurement of the perceived effects on student cultural competence as a result of international service learning activities (Lawson & Olson, 2017).	Structured measurement through quantitative analysis (e.g., number of contact hours of service in the community) of program and university impacts as well as assessment of financial impacts, enhancements in infrastructure and health service provision, and changes in community morale on communities served.
Evidence-based practice	Use of case studies, development of critically appraised topic articles, and quantitative and qualitative assessment of student participation in scholarship activities that includes the development of research proposals and the completion and presentation of research projects.	Use of a structured assessment in measuring effects of curricular changes in the delivery of EBP instruction across cohorts of students (Benevides, Vause-Earland, & Walsh, 2015). Curriculum evaluation and analysis of effects of horizontal integration of courses on EBP (Cohn, Coster, & Kramer, 2014).
Simulation activity	Use of a comprehensive practical examination using patient simulations and reflective case videos on readiness of students for fieldwork (Giles, Carson, Breland, Coker-Bolt, & Bowman, 2014).	Programmatic comparison of students' fieldwork performance based on the introduction of client simulation activities in the curriculum (Tomlin, 2005; Ozelie, Both, Fricke, & Maddock, 2016). Qualitative analysis of the integration of various courses that offered high-fidelity simulations and impacts on student learning (Shea, 2015).

continued

Table 7-1 (continued)

TEACHING-LEARNING STRATEGIES AND METHODS OF MEASURING RESEARCH AND TEACHING OUTCOMES

TEACHING-LEARNING STRATEGY	EXAMPLES OF METHODS TO MEASURE COURSE-LEVEL LEARNING OUTCOMES	EXAMPLES OF METHODS TO MEASURE CURRICULAR LEARNING OUTCOMES
Fieldwork experiences	Qualitative analysis of perceptions of self-efficacy after fieldwork (Andonian, 2017). Use of structured assessments (e.g., Goal Attainment Scaling) as a measure of student learning during fieldwork (Chapleau & Harrison, 2015). Comparison of perceived personal and professional skills as a result of traditional vs. community-based fieldwork (Gat & Ratzon, 2014).	Programmatic analysis of fieldwork reports and correlation analysis with NBCOT passing (Novalis, Cyranowksi, & Dolhi, 2017). Analysis of the relationship of program admissions process with fieldwork performance of students (Bathje, Ozelie, & Deavila, 2014).

instructional levels (Hooper, Krishnagiri, Price, Taff, & Bilics, 2018; Krishnagiri, Hooper, Price, Taff, & Bilics, 2017; Price, Hooper, Krishnagiri, Taff, & Bilics, 2017; for more details, see Chapter 12). This body of literature found that many occupational therapy programs taught occupation through threads that were revisited throughout the curriculum and through theoretical models. The teaching of occupation ranged from explicit (i.e., visible and integrated into curricular materials) to implicit (i.e., partially or not visible), with many educators reporting that other topics vied for prominence and created a situation in which the core theme of occupation as a learning outcome was lost.

Interprofessional Collaboration

Interprofessional education appears frequently in the literature. Interprofessional education refers to learning activities in which students from various health professions collaborate to promote greater understanding of each profession's role as well as mutual respect and interprofessional communication skills (Rose et al., 2009; Shoemaker et al., 2011). The majority of these studies have found that the opportunity for students from varying professions (including occupational therapy) to work together on specific clinical learning activities promotes the following outcomes: increased skills competence, enhanced sense of practice autonomy, and the desire to work cooperatively for the patient's highest good. Students have indicated that interprofessional education facilitates outcomes related to their ability to describe and advocate for occupational therapy services. Barriers to interprofessional education have been noted as labor-intensive planning, cost, and curricular scheduling.

Service Learning

Service learning has also been extensively examined in occupational therapy education and can be defined as a learning strategy in which embedded community service combined with expert instruction and student reflection is undertaken to promote clinical skills, global civic responsibility, and ways to assist the community with their health-related needs (Gitlow & Flecky, 2005). Service learning, along with community involvement and social justice activities, has been embedded in curricular and university-wide outcomes of many institutions. Service learning methods are related to outcomes that measured students' direct exposure to people from other cultures residing in communities with insufficient resources to meet health care needs and students' clinical skills during the provision of needed services (Gitlow & Flecky, 2005; Lau, 2016). Studies have also suggested that service learning promoted outcomes of respect for diversity, cultural competency, and consciousness and helped students apply course content through real-life experiences. Researchers have further demonstrated that the use of virtual technologies provided students with service learning opportunities facilitating outcomes related to global perspectives of human occupation and intercultural competence, without the cost and time requirements of traditional embedded service learning experiences (Aldrich & Grajo, 2017; Cabatan & Grajo, 2017).

Instruction Related to Evidence-Based Practice Outcomes

Occupational therapy scholarship has examined how students and practitioners develop EBP skills. EBP is the method through which clinical practice decisions are made by weighing available evidence including empirical research, a practitioner's clinical judgment, and the patient's health care goals (Davidoff, Haynes, Sackett, & Smith, 1995). Several studies investigated teaching EBP to students through direct engagement in research activities, intervention courses, and fieldwork (Baarends, Van der Klink, & Thomas, 2017; Benevides et al., 2015; Moyers, Finch Guthrie, Swan, & Sathe, 2014). These studies collectively found that although such methods increased students' value of and skills in EBP, participants did not generally report engaging in EBP in fieldwork or in their first year of practice. Participants reported that barriers to EBP included time restraints, high productivity demands, and lack of administrative support and access to research databases.

	FORMATIVE ASSESSMENT	SUMMATIVE ASSESSMENT
Table 7-2 FORMATIVE AND SUMMATIVE ASSESSMENTS		
PRIMARY PURPOSE *(Bennett, 2011)*	Assessment for learning; part of the teaching process	Assessment of learning; part of the assessment of curricular and programmatic effectiveness
REFERENCE (POINT OF COMPARISON) *(Harlen & James, 1997)*	Often ipsative (monitoring the progress of the individual); can be but not purely criterion referenced	Criterion referenced (progression of learning against a public criteria)
NEED FOR VALIDITY AND RELIABILITY *(Harlen & James, 1997)*	Validity and usefulness are more important than reliability	Requires methods that determine reliability without compromising validity

Simulation

The use of simulation experiences to enhance clinical skills of students has increased in recent years. Simulation is the immersion of students in situations that mirror real-life clinical situations without the risk of patient harm (Sørensen et al., 2017). Several recent studies have found that simulation experiences using trained actors presenting with specific clinical conditions, mock clinical settings with authentic medical equipment, clinical scenarios and vignettes, patient simulator mannequins, and digital videos for postperformance reflection can effectively increase learning outcomes related to complex practice skills that could otherwise involve patient injury or harm if performed incorrectly (Baird, Raina, Rogers, O'Donnell, & Holm, 2015; Baird et al., 2015; Cahill, 2015).

Fieldwork Education

Another line of scholarship involves assessing outcomes from fieldwork education. One study found that students perceived their learning to be facilitated by fieldwork supervisors who were approachable, had realistic expectations of student performance, and created a supportive learning environment (Grenier, 2015). A second study found that students placed in nontraditional fieldwork settings without a full-time, on-site occupational therapist reported higher outcomes in perceived competence and advocacy skills (Gat & Ratzon, 2014).

Measuring Course-Specific Outcomes: Developing Learning Assessment Techniques

Occupational therapy educators must ensure that course outcomes contribute to overall curricular and programmatic goals through an iterative assessment process. Learning assessments have often been categorized in the literature as either formative or summative. A summary of differences between formative and summative assessments is provided in Table 7-2. Various learning activities (e.g., written assignments, examinations, quizzes, and case studies) can be used as formative and summative assessments to measure specific learning outcomes. Educators can also use these specific learning outcomes to assess how the specific learning activities may contribute toward the overall course-level outcomes and curricular outcomes.

Specific learning outcomes must align with course- and curriculum-level outcomes. Educators must explicitly identify how targeted assignments or learning activities contribute toward course-level objectives and the bigger program, department, or institution objectives. Learning activities and course-level or institution-level objectives must also be aligned with the ACOTE standards for accreditation. For example, a reflection assignment after developing a community-based program for a fieldwork activity in an underserved community may serve as a way to measure the course-level objective of "develop occupational justice-promoting programs within the context of community-based occupational therapy service provision." This course-level objective can be aligned to the curriculum-level objective of "identify specific ways that occupation-centered education is a central theme in the curriculum" and a university-level objective of "increasing participation and service in underserved communities." The course-level, curriculum-level, and institution-level objective can then be aligned with one of the ACOTE B standards on Community and Primary Care Programs (Standard B.4.27: Evaluate access to community resources, and design community or primary care programs to support occupational performance for persons, groups, and populations.)

One way of measuring alignment between course and curricular outcomes is through the development of learning assessment techniques (LATs). According to Barkley and Major (2016), LATs have a three-part, interconnected structure: (1) the identification of significant learning goals, (2) the implementation of learning activities, and (3) the analysis and report of outcomes. Although there are several methods for developing LATs, this section focuses on two specific methods to measure and align specific learning activities with course-level outcomes: (1) rubrics and (2) blueprints for test construction.

Using Rubrics to Measure Course Outcomes

In a review of higher education literature, Panadero and Jonsson (2013) described several ways in which the summative and formative use of rubrics can improve student performance by increasing transparency, reducing anxiety, aiding the feedback process, improving student self-efficacy, and supporting student self-regulation. According to the authors, well-constructed rubrics can (a) enhance the communication of clear course expectations and elucidate how expectations will impact grades (thereby enhancing transparency and reducing anxiety), (b) be used to help students understand the scoring of specific assignments and areas for needed improvement (feedback), and (c) help students to self-monitor performance and assess their learning (student self-efficacy and self-regulation). Panadero and Jonsson (2013) also emphasized the value of embedding facilitated discussions into course instruction regarding student performance and grade rationale based on rubric criteria.

Stevens and Levi (2013) suggested that effective rubrics contain four elements: (1) assignment description, (2) grading scale, (3) assignment dimensions, and (4) dimension descriptors.

1. Assignment descriptions are the actual written directions for an assignment and can include written reports, oral presentations, skill demonstration, and classroom behavioral expectations (i.e., professional behaviors and class participation) and learning objectives for the assignment.

2. Grading scales depict the quality of student performance on a given assignment and can be represented as gradations of (a) mastery levels (e.g., emerging to competent), (b) quality levels (e.g., low to high), and (c) completion levels (e.g., incomplete to complete).

3. Assignment dimensions are criteria that articulate how each aspect of an assignment is to be completed.

4. Dimension descriptors describe levels of performance based on the expected assignment dimensions and grading scale. Dimension descriptors should elucidate performance-level criteria from low to high but, at the very least, must indicate the criteria for the highest performance level.

Educator Resource A and B at the end of this chapter show two examples of rubrics with different scale gradations and dimension descriptors.

Using Blueprints for Test Construction

Written tests are common methods used by occupational therapy educators as summative assessments of course-level outcomes. Therefore, quality examination construction is critical for assessing learning outcomes. Many test constructors often struggle to cover as much content as possible in written tests. In a seminal article, Nunally (1978) proposed that one mechanism for ensuring content validity of written examinations is to create a test blueprint. A blueprint generates a relationship between the subject matter delivered through instruction and the items that appear on the test (Bridge, Musial, Frank, Roe, & Sawilowsky, 2003). A test blueprint has the following three components that can be physically placed within columns or panels:

- Panel 1 lists specific course learning objectives or topics.
- Panel 2 lists both the (a) total number of test items and the (b) number of test items for each learning objective or topic.
- Panel 3 lists the course mastery domain. It is typical for written examinations to use the cognitive domain of the revision to Bloom's learning taxonomy when describing mastery domains (Anderson & Krathwohl, 2001). For each course topic or learning objective, the test constructor must explicate the level or cognitive domain that was used to achieve mastery. The test constructor then assigns a number of test items to each cognitive domain.

Educator Resource C provides an example of a test blueprint for an introduction to occupational therapy theory class. In panel 1, the educator listed five topics to be covered in the written examination. The test constructor wished to allot a total of 60 points for the examination and distributed these based on the depth and amount of information covered per topic (10-15 points). The educator then identified the cognitive domains that were targeted in each course topic. For example, when discussing the model of human occupation (MOHO), the instructor facilitated learning that covered a variety of lower- and higher-order thinking skills (recall, comprehension, application, and analysis). The test constructor then distributed the allotted 15 points for this topic. Based on this test blueprint, the educator then formulated three questions that measured the recall of constructs related to MOHO, three questions that measured the comprehension of MOHO constructs, three questions that measured the ability to apply MOHO concepts, and six questions that measured the ability to analyze the use of MOHO in practice.

CONCLUSION

Occupational therapy education must encompass an explicit articulation and alignment of ways to measure course- and curricular-level objectives. Curricular and course objective alignment requires strategic and intentional coordination of methods to measure student learning outcomes. This process can be an arduous task, and program directors and occupational therapy educators must use effective educational measurement methods to both (a) align the curriculum with institutional goals and accreditation standards and (b) produce graduates that successfully pass the National Certification Examination.

Implications for Occupational Therapy Education

- Simulation prepares students for working in challenging health care environments by addressing skills related to clinical reasoning; problem solving; and communication, assessment, and intervention.
- Occupational therapy curricula should (a) focus on occupation as a central tenet; (b) be aligned with course content so that courses support curricular, programmatic, institutional, and accreditation objectives; and (c) strive to facilitate student learning opportunities beyond the classroom through interprofessional education, EBP, service learning, and fieldwork.
- Educators should adopt LATs through the construction of rubrics and test blueprints. Rubrics should contain assignment descriptions, grading scales, assignment dimensions, and dimension descriptors. Test blueprints should distribute test items based on the relationship between course objectives, test item number, and course mastery domains.

Key Reflection Questions

1. How do your course topics and course assessment practices provide evidence for your curriculum and institutional goals?
2. What factors facilitate and/or hinder development of rubrics and/or test blueprints for course use?
3. What supports do educators need to ensure the development and use of effective formative and summative assessments?

What led you to become an occupational therapy educator?

My first recollections of pretend play at the age of 5 were memories of me and four to six other playmates in a pretend classroom setting. With a pointer stick in hand and chalk, I would write and draw and talk about various children's stories and ask my "students" questions about these stories. Some 12 years later, the passion for teaching became stronger as I carefully observed professors, who later became mentors, in occupational therapy school. I just knew that I am passionate about sharing, discussing, and dissecting information and facilitating learning. I have been very grateful to have amazing mentors from the Philippines, St. Louis, and New York who continue to inspire my teaching today.

Lenin C. Grajo, PhD, EdM, OTR/L

Just the facts please. As an educator for 25 years, I've recognized that students have a variety of blended learning styles and capacities (some identified in the literature, others not readily described)—much like the patients I've treated. I've also realized that most students learn best when complex information is broken down into simpler categories and is clearly organized, when course and assignment expectations are clear and simply conveyed, when instructional methods are delivered through a variety of modalities, and when the learning environment is supportive and recognizes that mistakes are part of the learning process. When a colleague of mine first began teaching, a mentor advised her to simplify her lectures by stating, "Just give it to me A, B, C so that I understand it." This has been my educational motto.

Sharon A. Gutman, PhD, OTR, FAOTA

REFERENCES

Accreditation Council for Occupational Therapy Education. (2018). 2018 ACOTE standards and interpretive guide. Retrieved from https://www.aota.org/~/media/Corporate/Files/EducationCareers/Accredit/StandardsReview/2018-ACOTE-Standards-Interpretive-Guide.pdf

Aldrich, R. M., & Grajo, L. C. (2017). International educational interactions and students' critical consciousness: A pilot study. *American Journal of Occupational Therapy, 71*, 7105230020. doi:10.5014/ajot.2017.026724

American Occupational Therapy Association. (2018). Philosophy of occupational therapy education. *American Journal of Occupational Therapy, 72*(Suppl. 2), 7212410070. doi:10.5014/ajot.2018.72S201

Anderson, L. W., & Krathwohl, D. R. (2001). *A taxonomy for learning, teaching, and assessing: A revision of Bloom's taxonomy of educational objectives.* New York, NY: Longman.

Andonian, L. (2017). Occupational therapy students' self-efficacy, experience of supervision, and perception of meaningfulness of level II fieldwork. *Open Journal of Occupational Therapy, 5*(2), 7. doi:10.15453/2168-6408.1220

Baarends, E., Van der Klink, M., & Thomas, A. (2017). An exploratory study on the teaching of evidence-based decision making. *Open Journal of Occupational Therapy, 5*(3), 8. doi:10.15453/2168-6408.1292

Baird, J. M., Raina, K. D., Rogers, J. C., O'Donnell, J., & Holm, M. B. (2015). Wheelchair transfer simulations to enhance procedural skills and clinical reasoning. *American Journal of Occupational Therapy, 69*(Suppl. 2), 6912185020. doi:10.5014/ajot.2015.018697

Baird, J. M., Raina, K. D., Rogers, J. C., O'Donnell, J., Terhorst, L., & Holm, M. B. (2015). Simulation strategies to teach patient transfers: Self-efficacy by strategy. *American Journal of Occupational Therapy, 69*(Suppl. 2), 6912185030. doi:10.5014/ajot.2015.018705

Barkley, E., & Major, C. (2016). *Learning assessment techniques: A handbook for college faculty.* San Francisco, CA: Jossey-Bass.

Bathje, M., Ozelie, R., & Deavila, E. (2014). The relationship between admission criteria and fieldwork performance in a masters-level OT program: Implications for admissions. *Open Journal of Occupational Therapy, 2*(3), 6. doi:10.15453/2168-6408.1110

Baughan, B., MacFarlane, C., Dentry, T., & Mendoza, G. (2014). The interdisciplinary education perception scale (IEPS): which factor structure? *Education in Medicine Journal, 6*(3), e67-e71. doi: 10.5959/eimj.v6i3.259

Bennett, R. E. (2011). Formative assessment: A critical review. *Assessment in Education: Principles, Policy & Practice, 18*(1), 5-25. doi:10.1080/0969594X.2010.513678

Benevides, T. W., Vause-Earland, T., & Walsh, R. (2015). Impact of a curricular change on perceived knowledge, skills, and use of evidence in occupational therapy practice: A cohort study. *American Journal of Occupational Therapy, 69*(Suppl. 2), 6912185010. doi:10.5014/ajot.2015.018416

Berg-Poppe, P. J., Karges, J. R., Nissen, R., Deutsch, S., & Webster, K. (2017). Relationship between occupational and physical therapist students' belongingness and perceived competence in the clinic using the ascent to competence scale. *Journal of Occupational Therapy Education, 1*(3). doi:10.26681/jote.2017.010303

Bridge, P., Musial, J., Frank, R., Roe, T., & Sawilowsky, S. (2003). Measurement practices: Methods for developing content-valid student examinations. *Medical Teacher, 25*(4), 414-421. doi:10.1080/0142159031000100337

Cabatan, M. C. C., & Grajo, L. C. (2017). Centennial topics—internationalization in an occupational therapy curriculum: A Philippine–American pilot collaboration. *American Journal of Occupational Therapy, 71*, 7106165010. doi:10.5014/ajot.2017.024653

Cahill, S. M. (2015). Perspectives on the use of standardized parents to teach collaboration to graduate occupational therapy students. *American Journal of Occupational Therapy, 69*(Suppl. 2), 6912185040. doi:10.5014/ajot.2015.017103

Chapleau, A., & Harrison, J. (2015). Fieldwork I program evaluation of student learning using goal attainment scaling. *American Journal of Occupational Therapy, 69*(Suppl. 2), 6912185060. doi:10.5014/ajot.2015.018325

Cohn, E. S., Coster, W. J., & Kramer, J. M. (2014). Conference proceedings—Facilitated learning model to teach habits of evidence-based reasoning across an integrated master of science in occupational therapy curriculum. *American Journal of Occupational Therapy, 68*, S73-S82. doi:10.5014/ajot.2014.685S05

Davidoff, F., Haynes, B., Sackett, D., & Smith, R. (1995). Evidence based medicine. *British Medical Journal, 310*(6987), 1085-1086. Retrieved from https://www.ncbi.nlm.nih.gov/pmc/articles/PMC2549494/pdf/bmj00590-0009.pdf

Fink, L. D. (2013). *Creating significant learning experiences: An integrated approach to designing college courses.* San Francisco, CA: Jossey-Bass.

Gat, S., & Ratzon, N. Z. (2014). Comparison of occupational therapy students' perceived skills after traditional and non-traditional fieldwork. *American Journal of Occupational Therapy, 68*, e47-e54. doi:10.5014/ajot.2014.007732

Giles, A. K., Carson, N. E., Breland, H. L., Coker-Bolt, P., & Bowman, P. J. (2014). Conference proceedings—Use of simulated patients and reflective video analysis to assess occupational therapy students' preparedness for fieldwork. *American Journal of Occupational Therapy, 68*, S57-S66. doi:10.5014/ajot.2014.685S03

Gitlow, L., & Flecky, K. (2005). Integrating disability studies concepts into occupational therapy education using service learning. *American Journal of Occupational Therapy, 59*, 546-553. doi:10.5014/ajot.59.5.546

Grenier, M. L. (2015). Facilitators and barriers to learning in occupational therapy fieldwork education: Student perspectives. *American Journal of Occupational Therapy, 69*(Suppl. 2), 6912185070. doi:10.5014/ajot.2015.015180

Harlen, W., & James, M. (1997) Assessment and learning: Differences and relationships between formative and summative assessment. *Assessment in Education: Principles, Policy & Practice, 4*(3), 365-379. doi:10.1080/0969594970040304

Hooper, B., Krishnagiri, S., Price, P., Taff, S. D., & Bilics, A. (2018). Curriculum-level strategies that U.S. occupational therapy programs use to address occupation: A qualitative study. *American Journal of Occupational Therapy, 72*, 7201205040. doi:10.5014/ajot.2018.024190

Hooper, B., Mitcham, M. D., Taff, S. D., Price, P., Krishnagiri, S., & Bilics, A. (2015). The issue is—energizing occupation as the center of teaching and learning. *American Journal of Occupational Therapy, 69*(Suppl. 2), 6912360010. doi:10.5014/ajot.2015.018242

Institute of Medicine. (2015). *Measuring the impact of interprofessional education on collaborative practice and patient outcomes.* Washington, DC: The National Academies Press.

Jewell, V. & Pickens, N. (2017). Psychometric evaluation of the occupation-centered intervention assessment. *OTJR: Occupation, Participation and Health, 37*(2), 82-88. doi:10.1177/1539449216688619.

Krishnagiri, S., Hooper, B., Price, P., Taff, S. D., & Bilics, A. (2017). Explicit or hidden? Exploring how occupation is taught in occupational therapy curricula in the United States. *American Journal of Occupational Therapy, 71*, 7102230020. doi:10.5014/ajot.2017.024174

Lawson, J., & Olson, M. (2017) International service learning: Occupational therapists' perceptions of their experiences in Guatemala. *Open Journal of Occupational Therapy, 5*(1), 11. doi.org/10.15453/2168-6408.1260

Lau, C. (2016). Impact of a child-based health promotion service-learning project on the growth of occupational therapy students. *American Journal of Occupational Therapy, 70*, 7005180030. doi:10.5014/ajot.2016.021527

Moyers, P. A., Finch Guthrie, P. L., Swan, A. R., & Sathe, L. A. (2014). Interprofessional evidence-based clinical scholar program: Learning to work together. *American Journal of Occupational Therapy, 68*, S23-S31. doi:10.5014/ajot.2014.012609

National Board for Certification in Occupational Therapy. (2019). Certification renewal handbook. Retrieved from https://www.nbcot.org/-/media/NBCOT/PDFs/Renewal_Handbook.ashx?la=en

Novalis, S., Cyranowski, J., & Dolhi, C. (2017) Passing the NBCOT examination: Preadmission, academic, and fieldwork factors. *Open Journal of Occupational Therapy, 5*(4), 9. doi:10.15453/2168-6408.1341

Nunally, J. (1978) *Psychometric theory.* New York, NY: McGraw Hill.

Ozelie, R., Both, C., Fricke, E., & Maddock, C. (2016). High-fidelity simulation in occupational therapy curriculum: Impact on level II fieldwork performance. *Open Journal of Occupational Therapy, 4*(4), 9. doi:10.15453/2168-6408.1242

Panadero, E., & Jonsson, A. (2013). The use of scoring rubrics for formative assessment purposes revisited: A review. *Educational Research Review, 9*, 129-144. doi:10.1016/j.edurev.2013.01.002

Parsell, G., & Bligh, J. (1999). The development of a questionnaire to assess the readiness of health care students for interprofessional learning (RIPLS). *Medical Education, 33*(2), 95-100. doi: https://doi.org/10.1046/j.1365-2923.1999.00298.x

Price, P., Hooper, B., Krishnagiri, S., Taff, S. D., & Bilics, A. (2017). A way of seeing: How occupation is portrayed to students when taught as a concept beyond its use in therapy. *American Journal of Occupational Therapy, 71*, 7104230010. doi:10.5014/ajot.2017.024182

Rose, M. A., Smith, K., Veloski, J. J., Lyons, K. J., Umland, E., & Arenson, C. A. (2009). Attitudes of students in medicine, nursing, occupational therapy, and physical therapy toward interprofessional education. *Journal of Allied Health, 38*(4), 196-200. Retrieved from http://www.ingentaconnect.com/content/asahp/jah/2009/00000038/00000004/art00003

Shea, C. (2015). High-fidelity simulation: A tool for occupational therapy education. *Open Journal of Occupational Therapy, 3*(4), 8. doi:10.15453/2168-6408.1155

Shoemaker, M. J., Beasley, J., Cooper, M., Perkins, R., Smith, J., & Swank, C. (2011). A method for providing high-volume interprofessional simulation encounters in physical and occupational therapy education programs. *Journal of Allied Health, 40*(1), 15E-21E. Retrieved from http://www.ingentaconnect.com/content/asahp/jah/2011/00000040/00000001/art00012

Sørensen, J. L., Østergaard, D., LeBlanc, V., Ottesen, B., Konge, L., Dieckmann, P., & Van der Vleuten, C. (2017). Design of simulation-based medical education and advantages and disadvantages of in situ simulation versus off-site simulation. *BMC Medical Education, 17*(1), 20. doi:10.1186/s12909-016-0838-3

Stevens, D., & Levi, A. (2013). *Introduction to rubrics: An assessment tool to save grading time, convey effective feedback, and promote student learning* (2nd ed). Sterling, VA: Stylus.

Tomlin, G. (2005). The use of interactive video client simulation scores to predict clinical performance of occupational therapy students. *American Journal of Occupational Therapy, 59*, 50-56.

Appendix

Rubric Example 1. Rubric that describes the highest-level competency expected for each dimension.

Assignment 1 (assignment description): You will write a 10-page literature synthesis that will evaluate the trustworthiness, accuracy, and rigor of conducted experimental-type and quantitative studies and synthesize critical findings from experimental-type and quantitative research on a preselected topic.

EDUCATOR RESOURCE A

PAPER SECTION (DIMENSIONS)	EXPECTED COMPETENCY (DIMENSION DESCRIPTOR)	EXCEEDS EXPECTATIONS (SCALE GRADATION)	MEETS EXPECTATIONS (SCALE GRADATION)	BELOW EXPECTATIONS (SCALE GRADATION)
A. Introduction (20 points)	Clearly articulated description of choice of topic, relevance to their future practice of interest, and methods of selecting and gathering literature (including search engines used, examples of key words used to gather literature, any assistance from librarians, etc.).			
B. Summary of studies (20 points)	Provides an overview of the 8 to 10 studies used for analysis. Methodically presents a summary of studies using visual or text descriptions (table or descriptive). Develops qualifiers in the summary (e.g., all studies used convenience sampling as sampling method of choice) that provides evidence that all studies were synthesized and analyzed.			

continued

(continued)

EDUCATOR RESOURCE A

PAPER SECTION (DIMENSIONS)	EXPECTED COMPETENCY (DIMENSION DESCRIPTOR)	EXCEEDS EXPECTATIONS (SCALE GRADATION)	MEETS EXPECTATIONS (SCALE GRADATION)	BELOW EXPECTATIONS (SCALE GRADATION)
C. Analysis of rigor (20 points)	Provides evidence of thoughtful analysis of the rigor of all 8 to 10 studies based on information gathered from annotated bibliography and research checklists. Describes strengths and weaknesses of the studies based on annotations.			
D. Findings (30 points)	Provides a succinct presentation of what is available evidence related to the topic of choice. Describes what is available in the occupational therapy body of knowledge. Findings are presented as objective findings with no personal judgment of research members.			
E. Discussion and implications (30 points)	Describes what is available in occupational therapy literature without making sweeping statements of generalizability of findings. Provides at least two to three statements or bullet points on implications of findings on occupational therapy practice.			

continued

(continued)

Educator Resource A

PAPER SECTION (DIMENSIONS)	EXPECTED COMPETENCY (DIMENSION DESCRIPTOR)	EXCEEDS EXPECTATIONS (SCALE GRADATION)	MEETS EXPECTATIONS (SCALE GRADATION)	BELOW EXPECTATIONS (SCALE GRADATION)
F. References and use of APA format (15 points)	Provides a succinct presentation of what is available evidence related to the topic of choice. Describes what is available in the occupational therapy body of knowledge. Findings are presented as objective findings with no personal judgment of research members.			
G. Grammar and writing style (15 points)	Free of syntactical and grammatical errors. Sentences flow smoothly. Thoughts are presented cogently and coherently.			
TOTAL (150 points)				

Abbreviation: APA, American Psychological Association.

Rubric Example 2. Rubric that describes the competency expected for each dimension gradated with the scale. Assignment (assignment description): Given a theoretical case study, you will apply concepts of an occupation-based theory, list clinical questions that will guide in clinical and professional reasoning, and identify one occupational role that will be addressed as part of intervention.

EDUCATOR RESOURCE B

CRITERIA (DIMENSIONS)	EXCEEDS EXPECTATIONS (SCALE)	MEETS EXPECTATIONS (SCALE)	BELOW EXPECTATIONS (SCALE)
Application of theory concepts (15 points)	• Learner shows clear understanding and ability to apply major constructs of chosen theory. • Learner is able to provide clear rationales and definitions of the chosen constructs as applicable in the case. • There is evidence of clear scientific clinical reasoning and grasp of occupational therapy theories based on clear articulation of examples cited from theoretical case.	• One to two questionable or unclear applications of constructs of chosen theory. • Learner provides some clear rationales/definitions of constructs. Some definitions of constructs need further expansion/clarification. • There is evidence of emerging scientific clinical reasoning and grasp of theories based on articulation of examples cited from case.	• Several questionable applications of constructs of theory. • Rationales and definitions of theoretical constructs need clarity and further explanation. • There is some evidence of scientific clinical reasoning but not strongly related to theoretical concepts.
Clinical questions (15 points)	• Learner lists a set of questions that demonstrate thorough understanding of the case and the theory being applied. • Learner lists questions that pertain to occupational performance and participation of the client.	• One to two questions listed are unclear as to how they apply to the theory chosen.	• Clinical questions listed do not strongly relate to theoretical concepts. • Questions listed adhere to a biomedical perspective rather than an occupational perspective.

continued

(continued)

EDUCATOR RESOURCE B

CRITERIA (DIMENSIONS)	EXCEEDS EXPECTATIONS (SCALE)	MEETS EXPECTATIONS (SCALE)	BELOW EXPECTATIONS (SCALE)
Clinical questions (15 points)	• The questions contribute to formation of an occupational profile (strengths and weaknesses of the client in terms of occupational performance and participation).	• Learner lists questions related to occupational performance of client. One to two questions appear to be using a medical model approach and are primarily concerned with enhancement of client skills without direction connection to occupation.	
Occupational role (15 points)	• Learner identifies one important occupational role from the case. • Learner uses constructs and concepts from the theory to describe how occupational role will be addressed. • Learner identifies general intervention approaches, guided by the theory, to address occupational role.	• Learner identifies one important role from the case. • One to two constructs from the theory needed clarification as to how they apply with addressing occupational role. • One to two intervention approaches do not directly relate to chosen theory or need further clarification as to how they relate to chosen theory.	• Learner does not identify an occupational role. • Manner of addressing occupational role does not reflect theoretical perspectives. • Intervention approaches listed do not reflect theoretical perspectives.

continued

(continued)

EDUCATOR RESOURCE B

CRITERIA (DIMENSIONS)	EXCEEDS EXPECTATIONS (SCALE)	MEETS EXPECTATIONS (SCALE)	BELOW EXPECTATIONS (SCALE)
Grammar and format (5 points)	• Learner uses correct grammar and punctuation and complete and simple sentences to articulate thoughts. • Learner uses correct APA 6th edition in-text citation (as needed) and referencing format.	• Two to three errors in grammar and punctuation. • Two to three errors in APA 6th edition in-text citation and referencing.	• Multiple grammatical and punctuation errors. • Multiple APA formatting errors.
TOTAL (50 points)			

Abbreviation: APA, American Psychological Association.

Educator Resource C: Sample Test Blueprint for an Introduction to Occupational Therapy Theory Course

LEARNING OBJECTIVE OR COURSE TOPIC (PANEL 1)	% OR n OF ITEMS FOR THE TEST (PANEL 2)	COGNITIVE DOMAIN BASED ON BLOOM'S TAXONOMY AND % OR n OF TEST ITEMS TO BE DEVELOPED MEASURING THAT COGNITIVE DOMAIN (PANEL 3)					
		Recall	Comprehend	Apply	Analyze	Evaluate	Create
Model of human occupation	15	3	3	3	6	0	0
Occupational adaptation theory	15	3	2	5	5	0	0
Person-environment-occupation model	10	0	3	3	4	0	0
Person-environment-occupation-performance model	10	0	3	3	4	0	0
Ecology of human performance	10	0	1	5	4	0	0
Total test items	60 points	6	12	19	23	0	0

Recent Developments in Educational Research and Evaluation

A Vision for the Future of Occupational Therapy Education Research

Hirokazu Yoshikawa, PhD

Chapter Objectives

By the end of this chapter, the reader will be able to:

1. Identify recent advances in educational research methods, including causal impact evaluation, implementation science, and research on scaling of programs and policies.
2. Relate these approaches to the future growth of occupational therapy education research.

INTRODUCTION

Education research in occupational therapy has been described as "early stage," meaning its methods, interventions, and assessments are descriptive and rely heavily on student perceptions to establish outcomes (Hooper, King, Wood, Bilics, & Gupta, 2013). Therefore, examining recent developments in educational research methods may be relevant for maturing occupational therapy education research. In this chapter, I discuss recent advances in several areas of educational research and evaluation including (1) causal impact evaluation; (2) implementation science, particularly using mixed qualitative/quantitative methods; and (3) research on expansion and scaling of interventions. For each area, examples are presented that illustrate exemplary research to improve teaching, learning, and/or mental health outcomes. The examples included can help the reader envision just how robust occupational therapy education research can become. A concluding section will draw implications for occupational therapy education research.

Taff, S. D., Grajo, L. C., & Hooper, B. R. (Eds.). *Perspectives on Occupational Therapy Education: Past, Present, and Future* (pp. 95-101).

CAUSAL IMPACT EVALUATION: ADVANCES IN
QUASIEXPERIMENTAL METHODS

Educational research has undergone a shift from largely descriptive research to extensive use of causal impact evaluation methods. This shift occurred first through the application of experimental methods in fields ranging from agriculture to medicine and later extended to social sector programs (Michalopoulos, 2005). Despite extensive use of experiments in specific areas of education dating back to the 1950s and 1960s (e.g., preschool education), the use of randomized controlled trials did not really become common practice until the 1990s. One of the pioneering educational experiments was the Tennessee STAR study in which the state of Tennessee funded a study randomly assigning a cohort of over 10,000 kindergarteners to different class sizes and then followed them through third grade (Schanzenbach, 2006).

Quasiexperimental methods or controlled studies in which random assignment is not conducted have advanced considerably in recent years as well. In cases in which random assignment is not feasible or is difficult, quasiexperimental designs may be a good scientific solution. In education and in related areas like policy evaluation, several have proven useful and attracted the attention of methodologists.

First, regression discontinuity is one of the strongest quasiexperimental designs (Cook, Campbell, & Shadish, 2002). It relies on the fact that those eligible vs not eligible to avail themselves of a policy or program are distinguished by a cutoff value on a forcing variable. For example, many public prekindergarten programs in the United States offer enrollment only for those older than a given birthday cutoff. This allows for comparison at the cutoff of children who were vs were not eligible for preschool in a given year, thus enabling a causal impact evaluation of the effect of 1 year of preschool. This method was applied in an influential evaluation of the Tulsa prekindergarten program (Gormley, Gayer, Phillips, & Dawson, 2005) and, subsequently, to a variety of other state or city prekindergarten programs (Wong, Cook, Barnett, & Jung, 2008). It has also been applied to evaluations of remedial education (Jacob & Lefgren, 2004) based on the fact that access to remedial education is often based on a test score cutoff.

Studies in which eligibility is based on the cutoff on a skills-based assessment may be relevant to occupational therapy education research. For example, consider the pool of applicants admitted and not admitted to an occupational therapy program based on an applicant score cutoff. Those just above and below the cutoff can be considered equal in expectation of outcomes, with the difference in outcomes an estimate of the impact of being admitted to the program.

The regression discontinuity design has been creatively applied to important policy evaluations with implications for equity and inclusion. For example, the strongest causal impact evaluation of the Obama administration's national effort to provide relief from deportation for unauthorized youth, the Deferred Action for Childhood Arrivals (DACA) program, used this technique. Hainmueller and colleagues (2017) assessed the impact of DACA on children's mental health by using a complete state-level Medicaid data set to track rates of diagnoses of disorders in children whose mothers were on either side of the strict eligibility cutoff of age of eligibility at the point that DACA went into effect. Reductions of roughly half in the rates of anxiety disorders were observed after the passage of DACA, a causal impact (Hainmueller et al., 2017).

Second, the econometric technique of synthetic control analysis has been widely disseminated and used in policy analysis (Abadie, Diamond, & Hainmueller, 2010). This analysis is useful when the effects of policy change affect all people in a given jurisdiction but no other jurisdictions in a state or country. In this approach, a single unit's preintervention characteristics are used to weigh the outcomes in that unit relative to a combined set of other unit's preintervention characteristics that are similar in profile to those of the single unit. Recently, outcomes from a single state that experienced a particular policy change can be compared with those from a weighted combination of the other 49 states based on preexisting measured characteristics in that single state. For example, the approach was used to estimate the effects on firearm suicide rates of two state laws requiring a permit to purchase a handgun, one in Connecticut establishing such a law and one in Missouri repealing such a law. The study showed that the Connecticut law's passage brought about a 15.4% reduction in firearm suicide rates in that state relative to a weighted combination of states similar on prepassage characteristics. The researchers showed that the Missouri repeal of its permit to purchase law resulted in a 16.1% increase in firearm suicide rates in that state (Crifasi, Meyers, Vernick, & Webster, 2015). This method could be applied to situations in which a policy affecting occupational therapy outcomes occurs in different states or jurisdictions at different times.

Third, advances in propensity score matching help match individuals in intervention and comparison groups when the random assignment of individuals is not possible. Individuals are matched on a weighted set of preexisting observed characteristics that predict membership in the intervention group. It allows comparison of the groups in their balance on observed preexisting characteristics. However, it cannot balance on unobserved characteristics. This approach is now widely used in educational program evaluation and in many other fields (e.g., medicine and public health; D'Agostino, 1998). One study improved on the noncausal literature linking teacher-child interaction quality to student achievement by applying a multilevel propensity score model at the student and teacher level. Characteristics of students and teachers in the interaction drove selection processes into different levels of teacher-child interaction quality. In a dual propensity score model, observed selection factors in both students and teachers were used to estimate propensity for different levels of teacher-child interaction quality. Causal associations of teacher-child interaction quality with later student achievement were estimated, showing significant associations with math achievement (McCormick, O'Connor, Cappella, & McClowry, 2013).

The use of these quasiexperimental approaches still seems rare in occupational therapy education despite calls for their use (Hooper et al., 2013; Kielhofner, Hammel, Finlayson, Helfrich, & Taylor, 2004). However, Watkins and colleagues (2014) used propensity score methods in practice-based research to assess the effects of physical and occupational therapy on children's motor skills.

IMPLEMENTATION SCIENCE

Advances in implementation science have deepened the understanding of the "how" in educational program evaluation. Implementation science refers to the research field that studies quality of dissemination, educational program provision, and experiences of intended beneficiaries with the intent to provide evidence to inform program improvement. Research in this area answers the following questions: How do participants experience educational programs or services? Does variation in implementing the program matter for educational and other outcomes? Do impacts of education programs vary depending on the quality of implementation?

Education programs can be implemented with great intentions and even good conceptualization, but, with low quality of or great variation in implementation, the hoped-for outcomes are often not achieved. A recent policy failure in global education occurred during the years of the Millennium Development Goals and their education counterpart, the Education for All goals. These explicitly established universal access to primary education as a goal for all countries by 2015. Substantial progress was made toward education access in many countries with the lowest access levels previously (particularly in regions such as sub-Saharan Africa or the poorest countries in Asia). However, research generally showed that learning levels (as measured by national assessments of basic literacy or numeracy skills) did not improve in most of these countries. The answer to this puzzle was that investments in the quality of education (e.g., teaching, pedagogy, qualifications, learning materials, content of curricula, and family engagement) were not made in the push toward greater access.

Durlak and DuPre (2008) put forward an influential multidimension model for measuring the quality of implementation of educational programs. First, fidelity examines the adherence of implementation to the intended program model. Fidelity may be measured by aspects such as whether the content of a program's curriculum or session sequence is reflected in implementation. Second, dosage measures the actual duration, frequency, and mode of contact with the target population relative to what was intended in the design of a program. Third, implementation is studied based on the quality of the services provided. This can include (for human services programs) the quality of provider-client interaction, structural features of quality such as basic safety or qualifications of providers, and specific areas of implementation regarding content (e.g., core clinical or therapeutic areas of content in occupational therapy programs and responsiveness to other concerns raised by clients). Fourth, implementation research is concerned with participant responsiveness or engagement often characterized by rate or level of take-up or utilization of services and experiences with services. Responsiveness is influenced by the cultural match or mismatch between services and the diversity of the target population. Fifth, program differentiation or uniqueness from other programs is measured through a traditional literature review of a general program approach to understand the novelty and innovation of the program at hand. Sixth, a description of the nature and amount of services received by the control or comparison conditions is critical to understanding the effects of the program (i.e., relative to what related services the control or comparison group has used). Seventh, program reach or coverage measures the percent of intended population who participated. Finally, features related to adaptation of the original program can also be measured as features of implementation. All of these topics are relevant to research on occupational therapy education, such as examining the quality of implementation of entry-level master's and doctorate training programs.

When implementation research accompanies impact evaluation, the results can be more effectively translated into improvements in teaching and learning. For example, a recent set of studies on a large-scale professional development program for public preschool teachers to improve language and literacy instruction in Chile used several kinds of implementation research put forth by Durlak and DuPre (2008). The intervention involved both didactic workshops and in-person biweekly coaching of teachers by trained coaches across a 2-year curriculum with 12 modules. Basic dosage analyses showed that the large majority of intended sessions of both workshops and coaching were provided. Minute-by-minute coding of classroom videotapes indicated that although a randomized controlled trial of this program significantly increased minutes of targeted language instruction and reduced nontargeted language instruction, the overall number of minutes in the targeted instruction was still low in the intervention group at the end of the experiment (Mendive, Weiland, Yoshikawa, & Snow, 2016). The quality of coaching was assessed by surveys of both coaches and teachers; satisfaction and reported coverage of topics were high. These studies have informed practice and policy in early childhood education in the Latin American region. Cross-country learning processes are enhanced when empirical publications of various kinds (e.g., experimental, quasiexperimental, case study descriptions, and mixed method) are disseminated that open up the "black box" of implementation to reveal specific practices that can be adapted and implemented in other contexts.

RESEARCH ON SCALE

A challenge in education, including occupational therapy education, is that of scale. Two processes of research on scale have been noted in the literature (Yoshikawa, Wuermli, Raikes, Kim, & Kabay, 2018): "small to bigger" and "big to better." This method is concerned with how successful programs' quality and impacts are maintained when they go through expansion and scaling processes, such as expansion from a pilot demonstration program to a growing number of additional sites. This question is addressed through evidence on "small to bigger" forms of scale, when an initial implementation serving a relatively smaller number of beneficiaries gradually expands to reach more and more of the target population. In contrast, the "big to better" form of scale involves educational or service systems that are already at large scale but may require attention to quality improvement or maximization of benefits to the target population. This form of scale is characterized by reform efforts such as a state's educational system seeking to improve quality provision or to more effectively assure learning of at-risk students.

Research on scaling of educational interventions is still nascent. There is more extensive conceptualization and measurement of scale interventions in health. However, some examples can be drawn. One addresses the massive challenge of targeting educational interventions in public schools in India to the skill level of individual children. The typical elementary school classroom in India may have skill levels that cover a range of five or six grades (Muralidharan, Singh, & Ganimian, in press). As a response, the education nongovernmental organization Pratham implemented in one state in India an approach that grouped students by skill level in providing remedial support (an approach they termed "teaching at the right level"). By assessing student learning levels and then matching interventions to those levels, improvement in achievement and learning were observed (Banerjee et al., 2016).

Research on "big to better" is even more challenging because assessing the functioning of a system at scale, such as a national mental health, health, or educational system, is often only done at the level of outcomes or basic features, such as numbers of beneficiaries reached. For example, understanding the bottlenecks or barriers in systems functioning at a national scale requires detailed examination of administrative structures and bureaucracies, an area that is often outside the expertise of evaluation scientists. However, some recent examples illustrate this form of research. In India, the challenges of reforming the educational system make the systems of other countries seem literally puny. The administrative structure reaches from the individual school level up to block and district levels. A typical district may be responsible for hundreds of thousands of government schools (the size of an entire nation's schooling system in other contexts). One recent ethnographic study examined the specific roles, responsibilities, daily constraints, and incentives affecting the work duties of all education staff at the block and district level offices in one state (Aiyar & Bhattacharya, 2016). Both in-depth interviews and time-use studies (conducted through a series of half-day visits to block and district staff) showed that block-level staff focused almost entirely on conveying higher-level directives to lower-level staff rather than on using data from lower levels to inform higher-level decision making. The directionality of governance was thus entirely top-down, and moreover did not stretch down to school management stakeholders such as parents. This study illustrates that the nature of "vertical" relationships in a system (i.e., what occurs across administrative levels higher up and lower down in a system relative to a single level) may be essential to understanding why large-scale systems do not function effectively to meet their goals (in this case to improve learning of all students in the public education system). Similarly, analysis of "horizontal" relationships may also be useful at different levels of scale.

A challenge in the implementation of services at a national scale is that of cultural appropriateness and sensitivity of services. For example, national quality standards for education do not generally allow a process through which marginalized communities can contribute to notions of quality through their own culturally specific lenses. A process is encouraged of community-wide discussions of quality standards and their implementation so that multiple stakeholders can express their knowledge, experiences, and needs. A recent case study of the Modalidad Propia in the Kamentsa community of Colombia in Putumayo indicated success in adapting the notion of interdisciplinary teams covering nutrition, psychosocial support, education, and health for young children (Ponguta, et al., 2019). This community incorporated local healing leaders as well as elders in health, nutrition, and support to fulfill the roles typically filled in urban settings by a health and nutrition expert and a mental health practitioner. In addition, the Kamentsa based their curriculum on understanding the land, mountain, sky, and other aspects of the natural context of their community and language.

The utility and use of research on scale, whether the "small to bigger" or "big to better" kind, has rarely been encouraged systematically. One exception is the Brookings Institution's new "real-time scaling lab" initiative in education research and practice. This initiative follows Brookings' multicase study of examples of successful scaling of educational interventions, Millions Learning (Robinson, Winthrop, & McGivney, 2016). In the scaling lab approach, partnerships are assembled between research, policy leaders, and practitioners to apply learnings about the scaling process to ongoing implementation science. As initiatives go to scale, they produce evidence for the process. Several efforts across the United States and other countries are included in this scaling lab initiative (Robinson & Curtiss, 2018).

Conclusion and Implications for Occupational Therapy

In this chapter, I have described three areas of innovation and development in educational research related to causal impact evaluation, implementation science, and scaling of educational programs and policies. I summarize lessons from each of these three areas and indicate a few further crosscutting areas of research that may be useful to occupational therapy education.

First, innovations in causal impact evaluation stretch far beyond innovations in experimental research to a variety of quasiexperimental methods described in this chapter (i.e., regression discontinuity, synthetic control, and propensity score matching designs). These may be useful in achieving stronger causal inference in linking occupational therapy education to outcomes. Second, the rapidly expanding field of implementation science in education (as well as mental health and health) may also be of use to researchers in occupational therapy education. The use of mixed methods studies has been particularly rich. Finally, multimethod research on scale may help delineate the larger systems and conditions for successful implementation of occupational therapy education for diverse populations. For example, research on processes to incorporate the voices and autonomy of diverse communities may facilitate cross-country or cross-context learning regarding inclusive practices and policies.

However, by necessity, I have left out several other research approaches in education that have been influential in informing practice and policy. These include the potential of longitudinal studies to inform processes of implementation and their impact on human development and learning across the life span; the role of qualitative research in improving education interventions, whether alone or in combination with quantitative methods; and studies of the costs as well as benefits of occupational therapy education, to name a few. Some of these have been discussed regarding their relevance to occupational therapy research in general (e.g., Clarke, 2009; Graff et al., 2008) but have not yet been discussed widely regarding their relevance to occupational therapy education research.

In sum, the communication of advances in research methods across areas of professional practice is rare because disciplinary and professional boundaries are often impermeable. However, initiating two-way dialogue, not only between research and educational practice but also among research practice models across professional sectors such as occupational therapy and education, may be fruitful in building toward our common goals of maximizing human potential for all.

Key Reflection Questions

1. How could applying recent advances in causal impact evaluation, implementation science, and research on scaling interventions be useful to occupational therapy education research and practice?

2. How might the assumptions of the educational vs occupational therapy sectors regarding practice or research be different or similar? What are implications for how researchers and practitioners conduct their work?

3. In what ways do the methods in this chapter fit with your own research or practice experiences, goals, and future directions?

Acknowledgments

Supported in part by funding from the NYU Abu Dhabi Research Institute to the Global TIES for Children Center.

REFERENCES

Abadie, A., Diamond, A., & Hainmueller, J. (2010). Synthetic control methods for comparative case studies: Estimating the effect of California's tobacco control program. *Journal of the American statistical Association, 105*(490), 493-505.

Aiyar, Y., & Bhattacharya, S. (2016). The post office paradox. Economic & Political Weekly, 51(11), 61.

Banerjee, A., Banerji, R., Berry, J., Duflo, E., Kannan, H., Mukherji, S., ... Walton, M. (2016). *From proof of concept to scalable policies: Challenges and solutions, with an application (NBER working paper w22931)*. Cambridge, MA: National Bureau of Economic Research.

Clarke, C. (2009). An introduction to interpretative phenomenological analysis: A useful approach for occupational therapy research. *British Journal of Occupational Therapy, 72*(1), 37-39.

Cook, T. D., Campbell, D. T., & Shadish, W. (2002). *Experimental and quasi-experimental designs for generalized causal inference.* Boston, MA: Houghton Mifflin.

Crifasi, C. K., Meyers, J. S., Vernick, J. S., & Webster, D. W. (2015). Effects of changes in permit-to-purchase handgun laws in Connecticut and Missouri on suicide rates. *Preventive Medicine, 79*, 43-49.

D'Agostino, R. B. (1998). Propensity score methods for bias reduction in the comparison of a treatment to a non-randomized control group. *Statistics in Medicine, 17*(19), 2265-2281.

Durlak, J. A., & DuPre, E. P. (2008). Implementation matters: A review of research on the influence of implementation on program outcomes and the factors affecting implementation. *American Journal of Community Psychology, 41*, 327.

Gormley W. T. Jr., Gayer, T., Phillips, D., & Dawson, B. (2005). The effects of universal pre-K on cognitive development. *Developmental Psychology, 41*(6), 872.

Graff, M. J., Adang, E. M., Vernooij-Dassen, M. J., Dekker, J., Jönsson, L., Thijssen, M., ... Rikkert, M. G. O. (2008). Community occupational therapy for older patients with dementia and their care givers: cost effectiveness study. *BMJ, 336*(7636), 134-138.

Hainmueller, J., Lawrence, D., Martén, L., Black, B., Figueroa, L., Hotard, M., ... Laitin, D. D. (2017). Protecting unauthorized immigrant mothers improves their children's mental health. *Science, 357*(6355), 1041-1044.

Hooper, B., King, R., Wood, W., Bilics, A., & Gupta, J. (2013). An international systematic mapping review of educational approaches and teaching methods in occupational therapy. *British Journal of Occupational Therapy, 76*(1), 9-22.

Jacob, B. A., & Lefgren, L. (2004). Remedial education and student achievement: A regression-discontinuity analysis. *Review of Economics and Statistics, 86*(1), 226-244.

Kielhofner, G., Hammel, J., Finlayson, M., Helfrich, C., & Taylor, R. R. (2004). Documenting outcomes of occupational therapy: The Center for Outcomes Research and Education. *American Journal of Occupational Therapy, 58*(1), 15-23.

McCormick, M. P., O'Connor, E. E., Cappella, E., & McClowry, S. G. (2013). Teacher–child relationships and academic achievement: A multilevel propensity score model approach. *Journal of School Psychology, 51*(5), 611-624.

Mendive, S., Weiland, C., Yoshikawa, H., & Snow, C. E. (2016). Opening the black box: Intervention fidelity in a randomized trial of a preschool teacher professional development program in Chile. *Journal of Educational Psychology, 108*, 135-145.

Michalopoulos, M. (2005). Precedents and prospects for randomized experiments. In H. Bloom (Ed.), *Learning more from social experiments* (pp. 1-36). New York, NY: Russell Sage Foundation.

Muralidharan, K., Singh, A., & Ganimian, A. J. (in press). Disrupting education? Experimental evidence on technology-aided instruction in India. *American Economic Review.*

Ponguta, L. A., Maldonado-Carreño, C., Kagan, S. L., Yoshikawa, H., Nieto, A. M., Aragón, C. A., ... & Guerrero, P. A. (2019). Adaptation and Application of the Measuring Early Learning Quality and Outcomes (MELQO) Framework to Early Childhood Education Settings in Colombia. Zeitschrift für Psychologie.

Robinson, J. P., & Curtiss, M. (2018). *Millions Learning real-time scaling labs: Designing a adaptive learning process to support large-scale change in education.* Washington, DC: Brookings Institution, Center for Universal Education.

Robinson, J., Winthrop, R., & McGivney, E. (2016). Millions learning: Scaling up quality learning in developing countries. Brookings Institution. Retrieved from https://www. brookings.edu/wp-content/uploads/2016/04/FINAL-Millions-Learning-Report.pdf

Schanzenbach, D. W. (2006). What have researchers learned from Project STAR? *Brookings Papers on Education Policy, 9*, 205-228.

Watkins, S., Jonsson-Funk, M., Brookhart, M. A., Rosenberg, S. A., O'Shea, T. M., & Daniels, J. (2014). Preschool motor skills following physical and occupational therapy services among non-disabled very low birth weight children. *Maternal and Child Health Journal, 18*(4), 821-828.

Wong, V. C., Cook, T. D., Barnett, W. S., & Jung, K. (2008). An effectiveness-based evaluation of five state pre-kindergarten programs. *Journal of Policy Analysis and Management, 27*(1), 122-154.

Yoshikawa, H., Wuermli, A. J., Raikes, A., Kim, S., & Kabay, S. B. (2018). Achieving high quality early childhood development program and policies at national scale: Directions for research in global contexts. *Social Policy Report of the Society for Research in Child Development, 31*(1), 1-36.

9

Supporting Diversity and Inclusion in Occupational Therapy Education

Yolanda Suarez-Balcazar, PhD; Jaime P. Muñoz, PhD, OTR/L, FAOTA;
and Amy R. Early, OTD, OTR/L

Chapter Objectives

By the end of this chapter, the reader will be able to:

1. Explain the importance of diversity and inclusion in occupational therapy education.
2. Articulate what it means to create a diverse and inclusive educational environment.
3. Identify strategies for supporting diversity and inclusion.

INTRODUCTION

The American Occupational Therapy Association's (AOTA's) Centennial Vision (2007) articulated a commitment to a diverse workforce, supporting diversity and inclusion within the occupational therapy community and meeting the needs of diverse populations. Yet, in her farewell address as AOTA president, Clark (2013) acknowledged that the diversity components of the Centennial Vision had not been addressed as well as other priorities. She argued for the necessity of diversity and that diversity would make occupational therapy an even more vibrant profession. In a compelling story of a clinical encounter, Clark's farewell address illustrated the devastating impact cultural misunderstandings can have on the effectiveness of occupational therapy interventions. Similarly, the following AOTA president, Stoffel (2016), suggested in her presidential farewell address that the profession of occupational therapy could do more to foster systematic change in our professional culture, policies, and practices to achieve diversity and inclusion. A takeaway message from these recent leaders is that to truly transform our profession, we need to honor inclusivity and diversity. Notably, AOTA's Vision 2025 (2017) retains the pillars of inclusion and diversity, includes accessibility as a core tenet of the vision statement, and specifically targets the delivery of culturally responsive services.

Despite recognizing the need for and actively working to achieve a more diverse and inclusive profession and the corresponding benefits, occupational therapy remains primarily female (90.9%)

Taff, S. D., Grajo, L. C., & Hooper, B. R. (Eds.). *Perspectives on*
Occupational Therapy Education: Past, Present, and Future (pp. 103-115).
© 2020 Taylor & Francis Group.

and mostly White, reported at 87% in 2012 and then at 83.8% in 2015 (U.S. Department of Health and Human Services [USDHHS], 2014, 2017). In their workforce analysis of health professions data from 2011 to 2015, the USDHHS reports the racial demographics of 32 different U.S. health occupations. Only three professions, chiropractors (86.7% White), speech-language pathologists (86.1%), and advanced practice registered nurses (84%), were less ethnically/racially diverse than occupational therapists (USDHHS, 2017). Similar demographics for race are noted among faculty (Table 9-1).

The data in Table 9-1 indicate that occupational therapy is primarily composed of White individuals, although the United States has experienced rapid demographic changes in the past 40 years. In 2011, more births were recorded to minorities than to nonminorities for the first time in the nation's history (Cohn, 2016). The Asian population increased by 6% during the past 10 years, and analysts predict that the Latino population will increase from 18% of the U.S. population in 2017 to 24% in 2065 (Flores, 2017). However, there is incontrovertible evidence that low-income and low-literacy populations (Paasche-Orlow & Wolf, 2007), racial and ethnic minorities (Thompson, Molina, Viswanath, Warnecke, & Prelip, 2016), people with disabilities (Krahn, Walker, & Correa-De-Araujo, 2015), and the lesbian, gay, bisexual, transgender, and queer (or questioning) (LGBTQ) community (Hafeez, Zeshan, Tahir, Jahan, & Naveed, 2017) continue to experience disparities in health, participation, and rehabilitation outcomes (Ben-Moshe & Magaña, 2014). Therefore, a sharpened focus on the social determinants of health, population trends, and established evidence of health care disparities for diverse populations also contribute to the rationale for building diversity and inclusion in health professions. Indeed, there is ample evidence that diversity in the health care workforce can improve health care access, lead to better health outcomes, and foster effective patient-provider relationships marked by increased patient engagement in treatment and enhanced willingness to ask questions, express concerns, and communicate preferences related to treatment options (Cooper & Powe, 2004; Cooper-Patrick et al., 1999; Evans, Colburn, Stith, & Smedley, 2001).

For decades, scholars internationally have given voice to the need for diversity and inclusion within occupational therapy (Abreu & Peloquin, 2004; Beagan, 2015; Black, 2002; Grady, 1995; Muñoz, 2007; Suarez-Balcazar et al., 2009; Taff & Blash, 2017; Taylor, 2007). We must continue to address diversity, sensitivity, and cultural competency through strengthening our commitment to enact sustained, system-focused efforts that can transform our profession's diversity and inclusivity. This chapter defines diversity and inclusion, provides strategies for supporting diversity and inclusion in occupational therapy education, and highlights the benefits of these strategies for occupational therapy students and their future clients.

DEFINITION AND MODELS THAT PROMOTE DIVERSITY AND INCLUSION

Diversity and inclusion are complex, intrinsically related terms, yet diversity does not necessarily indicate inclusion. For the purpose of this chapter, we use the following definition put forward by the Society for Community Research and Action (SCRA) of the American Psychological Association:

The concept of diversity encompasses acceptance and respect for the full range of human characteristics in their sociocultural, historical, and cultural contexts, as well as understanding that each individual, family, community and societal group has uniqueness that make them different from others. The concept of diversity does not mean equality, inclusion, or pluralism; although these concepts are interrelated. (SCRA, 2018b)

From this definition, the term *diversity* should include the key components of "acceptance" and "respect" and should allow for variance and uniqueness. Diversity can occur at the surface level (i.e., physical and observable attributes), such as age, race, language, sex, and disability (Harrison, Price, & Bell, 1998), or diversity may exist on a deeper level and include unobservable traits such as religious

Table 9-1

RACIAL DEMOGRAPHICS IN OCCUPATIONAL THERAPY

	WHITE	BLACK	ASIAN	HISPANIC/ LATINO	OTHER
FACULTY	88.6%	3.9%	4.3%	2.1%	Not reported
PRACTITIONERS	85.3%	3.1%	4.4%	3.2%	Not reported
OCCUPATIONAL THERAPY DOCTORATE STUDENTS	85%	3%	7%	3%	5%
MSOT STUDENTS	80%	5%	7%	7%	8%
OCCUPATIONAL THERAPY ASSISTANT STUDENTS	74%	11%	5%	13%	8%

Abbreviation: MSOT, master of science in occupational therapy.
Adapted from American Occupational Therapy Association. (2018). *Academic programs annual data report: Academic year 2017-2018.* Retrieved from https://www.aota.org/~/media/Corporate/Files/EducationCareers/Educators/2017-2018-Annual-Data-Report.pdf.

affiliation, immigration status, sexual orientation, past trauma, ethnicity, and sometimes disability, to name a few (Harrison, Price, & Bell, 1998).

However, as the definition provided previously specifies, the concept of diversity does not necessitate inclusion. Scholars argue that definitions of diversity must acknowledge the pervasive discrimination certain individuals experience (e.g., people of color, people with disabilities, and members of the LGBTQ community; Betancur & Herring, 2013). Therefore, we define inclusion as instances in which these diverse groups have a voice that is recognized as unique and valuable (Shore et al., 2011). An inclusive environment involves diverse individuals as "insiders" empowered to engage fully in decision making, collaboration, and core activities to contribute in meaningful ways while receiving respect from peers and colleagues for their contributions (Shore et al., 2011; Taff & Blash, 2017).

Recently, Taff and Blash (2017) audited the profession's efforts to address diversity and inclusion. Citing Plaut (2002), these scholars reviewed four models used to address diversity and inclusion. These included the sameness model, which decategorizes individuals and views people as essentially similar; the common identity model, which minimizes differences through emphasizing shared group values and goals; the value-added model, which acknowledges differences and posits these differences benefit the organization; and the mutual accommodation model, which seeks to ensure an organizational climate where all members feel valued and connected. Taff and Blash (2017) proposed that occupational therapy use the mutual accommodations model as follows: "Building a culture of mutual accommodation requires a more explicit focus on doing, stepping outside comfort zones, and making systemic changes in policy and procedures" (p. 78). Such an approach would necessitate that educational programs identify actions, define policies and procedures, and reinforce habits of accountability focused on diversity and inclusivity.

Effectively fostering diversity and inclusion in a work or school environment can lead to significant benefits for those involved. For example, an inclusive workplace is correlated with increased job satisfaction, decreased turnover rates, and greater psychological well-being (Shore et al., 2011). Diverse teams frequently display increased creativity, innovation, and productivity compared with homogenous groups (Roberge & van Dick, 2010). In the academic setting, these benefits may affect

Table 9-2

STRATEGIES FOR RECRUITING AND RETAINING A DIVERSE STUDENT APPLICANT POOL

- Attend career fair days at local universities that attract a diverse student body.
- Host information sessions at various times, including evenings/late afternoons and/or Saturdays, to accommodate undergraduates who work.
- Add a statement on the department's website about commitments to diversity and inclusion, including commitment to ethnic, LGBTQ, racial, and ability diversity.
- Start a pre–occupational therapy club. In public institutions, this club typically attracts diverse students.
- Develop holistic admissions criteria attending to other potential qualifications of students aside from GPA, GRE, and prerequisites (e.g., work, volunteer and leadership experiences, experience in dealing with adversity, and other unique qualifications).
- Post visual symbols around the department of your commitment to diversity, safety, and inclusion, such as the pride flag or disability pride logo.
- Highlight academic and financial supports at your institution; when possible, waive application fees, provide specific scholarships, and target students from underrepresented groups or resource-scarce backgrounds for graduate assistant positions.
- Ensure a supportive environment and invite and mentor diverse students in scholarly, leadership, and professional socialization opportunities.
- Develop a strong commitment to community engagement; provide students with opportunities to conduct community practice and volunteer at these organizations.

Abbreviations: GPA, grade point average; GRE, graduate record examinations.

graduation rates, career choice satisfaction, classroom participation, subject matter engagement, and student social and emotional health, as well as decreased student burnout, leading to better educated and more innovative future practitioners.

However, settings lacking appropriate inclusion and diversity promotion tactics risk increased conflict, decreased communication and cohesiveness between group members, increased turnover and poor organizational commitment, and resulted in detrimental cognitive, emotional, physical, and behavioral health (Roberge & van Dick, 2010; Shore et al., 2011). Thus, it is essential for occupational therapy educators and program directors to understand and implement strategies that foster diversity and inclusion within their academic programs and the profession as a whole (Muñoz, 2007; Taff & Blash, 2017).

STRATEGIES FOR SUPPORTING DIVERSITY AND INCLUSION IN OCCUPATIONAL THERAPY EDUCATION

Enhancing diversity in occupational therapy education must begin with recruiting a diverse faculty and student body (Table 9-2).

During the application process, it is important to consider applicants holistically. Recent articles have demonstrated the limited usefulness of Graduate Record Examinations (GRE) scores to predict graduate school success markers, including the number of presentations/publications, likelihood of graduation, and certification examination pass rates for both PhD and clinical/professional programs (Moneta-Koehler, Brown, Petrie, Evans, & Chalkley, 2017; Moore et al., 2019). Although grade point average is widely used as a criterion and is indeed a strong indicator of academic success, other indicators, including letters of recommendation and nonobjective application components, should be requested to avoid overemphasizing learned performance in traditional academic settings (Moneta-Koehler et al., 2017). Embracing a holistic admissions process that focuses on the whole student adds richness to the class, the learning environment, and the profession (Association of American Medical Colleges, n.d.). Students from diverse backgrounds bring unique qualifications, life experiences, and attributes to the cohort that might otherwise be overlooked in a numbers-focused admissions process. Given the current call for holistic admissions in the health professions (Artinian et al., 2017), institutions of higher education are beginning to adopt strategies that ensure a diverse class of students. Here we highlight the holistic model of the Department of Occupational Therapy at the University of Illinois at Chicago.

The University of Illinois at Chicago embraces a holistic admissions process that recognizes a broad spectrum of human experiences, including volunteerism, leadership roles, work experience, community service, personal experience with disability, overcoming adversity, and being a first-generation college student, among other experiences. Consequently, during the past few years, between 35% and 41% of enrolled students were from diverse ethnic and racial backgrounds (Black, Latino/Hispanic, and Asian/Pacific Islander). We also know that the overall diversity has increased as well, yet this is harder to calculate because students do not necessarily disclose their gender preference, disability, and/or other indicators of diversity. Numerous students cite diversity of the student body as a strength of the program. Positive experiences of diversity and inclusion within academic programs come as a result of intentional prioritization of diversity and careful implementation of strategies aimed at fostering inclusive environments (Table 9-3). For example, at the University of Illinois at Chicago, class learning experiences draw on diverse perspectives to enrich learning (e.g., students give presentations on living and studying with a disability, post on discussion boards about religious discrimination on fieldwork, and thoughtfully discuss cultural humility and personal experiences as diverse individuals interacting with health care professionals).

Sue (2016) offers the following guidelines for hosting conversations on diversity and inclusion: set respectful and inclusive norms, connect the discussion to class learning objectives, invite multiple perspectives, incorporate writing and self-reflection, help students connect the topic to their personal experiences, connect class dynamics to larger social dynamics, evaluate the experience of engaging topics of diversity, and encourage community service opportunities (see SCRA, 2018a).

Sue (2016) also cautions against unsuccessful strategies, suggesting not to allow race, disability, and other difficult topics to brew in silence; to remain passive during difficult verbal exchanges with students and/or colleagues; to cut off dialogue; or to fail to provide a safe space to discuss issues of diversity. Although students and faculty may experience varying levels of discomfort when discussing diversity and inclusion, ignoring these topics creates hostility, deters a rich educational experience, and neglects preparing future occupational therapy practitioners to engage with diversity effectively.

At the University of Illinois at Chicago, occupational therapy students have the opportunity to gain a certificate in health and diversity to expand their knowledge and skills for working with diverse populations. Participating students partner with community organizations in underserved areas to complete a 45-hour service learning experience. Increased community engagement provides additional learning opportunities that support learning diversity and inclusion within the context of occupational scholarship and practice (Hammel et al., 2015; Suarez-Balcazar, Mirza, & Witchger-Hansen, 2015). Health and diversity fellows complete a project for their community site that meets the needs of the agency or the participants. Past examples include tutoring formerly incarcerated youth and adults, designing group protocols to promote healthy eating for Latino adults with intellectual

Table 9-3

STRATEGIES FOR SUPPORTING DIVERSITY AND INCLUSION IN OCCUPATIONAL THERAPY EDUCATION

- Be intentional about diversity and inclusion by setting specific goals and talking about them openly during faculty meetings and with students.
- Work with your institution to ensure that diversity and inclusion are also embraced at the institutional level, addressing different levels of the academic system.
- Embed diversity and inclusion topics throughout the curriculum (e.g., working with people with disabilities; individuals from diverse ethnic, racial, and LGBTQ backgrounds; social determinants of health; social justice and equity; power and privilege; health care disparities; racism; and bias). Add conversations about diversity to your professional development lectures/seminars throughout the program of study.
- Define explicit strategic actions in departmental plans related to diversity and inclusion and, when possible, spread accountability across faculty.
- Create a diversity and inclusion committee within the department and assign clear, measurable goals and expectations for this committee.
- Sponsor ongoing conversations about diversity and inclusion with students; ensure a safe space to talk about these issues and bring experts or consultants as needed.
- Bring experts from the disability resource center to speak to faculty about accommodations for students with disabilities.
- Hire a diverse faculty and staff.
- Invite speakers from diverse backgrounds and highlight their strengths during class presentations and encourage SOTA and other student groups to do the same; create a position in student government for diversity and inclusion.
- Use community-engaged learning and target communities and populations where students learn side by side with diverse populations.
- Use inclusive language such as "partner" or "spouse" instead of gendered language, and establish inclusive norms such as asking students and guests their preferred pronouns.
- Represent clients from diverse backgrounds in curriculum case studies. Accordingly, discuss the deeper issues that diversity brings to the case (e.g., inclusion, bias, diverse conceptions about occupation, values, independence, cultural nuances, and cultural adaptations).
- Connect students with multicultural occupational therapy networking groups (see Resources).
- Create opportunity for all students to provide feedback and contribute to class structure and group processes (Thomas & Heath, 2014).
- Provide students with a safe space to have their own student-sponsored conversations about diversity.
- Foster strong collective identity between students (Roberge & van Dick, 2010).

Abbreviation: SOTA, Student Occupational Therapy Association.

disabilities, creating sensory spaces to promote self-regulation for minority children attending an after-school program, and developing an ongoing group program to facilitate attainment of gross and fine motor milestones for an organization serving children with Down syndrome. Students achieve several learning outcomes through this experience, including gaining an understanding of the population they are working with, identifying and applying culturally relevant strategies for delivering occupation-based activities, and communicating with diverse populations. Students also complete a reflection report illustrating the specific materials, protocols, or resources developed for the agency and/or participants and how the experience will influence their future practice.

Most, if not all, student participants are immersed in settings and amongst populations previously unfamiliar to them. These experiences challenge students' preconceived notions about diverse populations and place them in humbling situations where instead of providing assistance or training to community members as they initially expected, the community members teach the students important truths about disability, parenting, inclusion, systemic injustice, and much more. Students pursuing the certificate also participate in seminars examining discrimination, health disparities, social justice, working with limited English proficiency clients, social determinants of health, cultural relevant practice, community-based participatory research and community-engaged research, and inclusion and participation. The university offers several elective courses on the above topics as well. Scholars indicate that exposure to these didactic and experiential encounters enhances knowledge, attitudes/perceptions, and skills toward diversity and inclusion (Calzada & Suarez-Balcazar, 2014; Suarez-Balcazar et al., 2009; Witchger Hansen et al., 2007).

Occupational therapy departments can also foster inclusive and diverse environments through the formation of a collective group identity as "future occupational therapists." Diversity research indicates individuals from varied backgrounds work most cohesively and productively when a uniting group identity supersedes perceptions of differences (Roberge & van Dick, 2010). Group members focus on shared interests, group status, and goals while maintaining their diverse perspectives and experiences within the group (Roberge & van Dick, 2010). Formation of the collective identity as "future occupational therapists" should begin on day 1 and extend the length of the program. Strategies may include group discussions on students' reasons for entering the profession and the occupational therapy values they connect with, interstudent collaboration on assignments and study guides via electronic sharing methods, avoidance of competitive program cultures such as identifying the top student or grade point average/rank sharing, and initiation of class social events. Additionally, faculty may remind students of their shared values and ethics as future therapists and the importance of treating classmates as future colleagues.

Finally, occupational therapy programs must consider the impact of faculty teaching strategies on the learning environment. Thomas and Heath (2014) describe several principles to promote inclusive teaching in higher education focused on supporting students from lower socioeconomic status backgrounds. These strategies include setting clear expectations for the class in jargon-free language, getting to know students, providing additional materials to students as needed to scaffold their learning, reflecting on one's own teaching strategies, and offering flexibility and choice in teaching and assessment methods (Thomas & Heath, 2014).

Offering flexibility and choice parallels the principles of universal design for learning, which advocates for eliminating barriers to participation in educational activities and learning environments by providing multiple means of interacting with the material (ACCESS Project, 2011). Occupational therapy programs must provide the following options: study materials should be available in both paper and electronic format; PDF files should contain real text so students can search for key ideas or use text-to-speech software to read files aloud; all videos shown in class and for homework should include captioning; classroom environments should allow for students to stand, sit, and use learning aids as needed; and teaching methods should incorporate visual, auditory, and kinesthetic learning styles when presenting information (ACCESS Project, 2011). These principles foster inclusion in the classroom and place the burden of student success on the curriculum so students with diverse abilities can engage in the learning process. By ensuring these options are available, occupational therapy programs can reduce barriers to education and promote participation for students with diverse abilities and learning styles.

PREPARING STUDENTS FOR WORKING WITH DIVERSE POPULATIONS

Several strategies can help prepare occupational therapy students to work with diverse populations. One such strategy is building students' awareness of cognitive shortcuts. Cognitive shortcuts serve as heuristics and are used for decision making based on the information available to the individual (Smedley, Stith, & Nelson, 2003). Cognitive shortcuts can easily transform into stereotypes, a common practice among health professionals due to practice constraints such as limited time with clients, high turnover, and decentralization of the health care system (Smedley et al., 2003). These cognitive shortcuts cause us to group individuals according to their more salient characteristics—having a visual disability, speaking with an accent, being racially or ethnically different from the therapist, or being openly gay or lesbian. Developing a habit of self-reflection and acknowledgment of one's own assumptions and biases is an optimal strategy for eliminating these shortcuts. Thus, having open conversations with students about stereotypes and biases will help them establish habits of self-reflection early in their careers and prepare them to serve a diverse client base.

Second, as culturally responsive individuals who embrace social justice, diversity, and inclusion, we need to stand against racism, homophobia, sexism, ableism, and other forms of-ism whenever and wherever we see it. Students need to learn to advocate for the rights of all clients and research participants to be who they are and to fulfill their occupational needs in meaningful ways according to their desires or those of their families regardless of their cultural background. Advocacy can be taught throughout the curriculum and through professional development seminars and workshops such as a virtual Hill Day (Barker & Fisher, 2018). Third, we also need to study and conceptualize diversity and inclusion from a broader perspective within the field of occupational therapy; diversity and inclusion are complex concepts intertwined with culture and cultural relevance (addressed in Chapter 33), discrimination, social justice, and equity. It is our shared responsibility to build a better society, aspire to become better professionals and scholars, and care for the well-being of all, regardless of their race, culture, abilities, gender preference, religion, sexual orientation, or other diverse characteristics. Promoting diverse and inclusive occupational therapy programs is an important first step on the road to a better profession and a better society. Fourth, occupational therapy programs need to be intentional in addressing diversity and inclusion within their mission statements, the values and principles they embrace, and their program curriculum. Fifth, occupational therapy programs can benefit from evaluating their own progress toward diversity and inclusion, reflecting on strategies that work and do not work within their own cultural context and institutional environment, creating checks and balances. identifying accountability measures, and setting clear goals to move forward. Finally, involve students in the process of embracing diversity and inclusion. Students can be part of a faculty/student diversity and inclusion committee or student recruitment and diversity affairs committee, provide ongoing input, and spearhead diversity events and conversations with faculty support, as needed. In all, occupational therapy programs need to make an intentional commitment to address diversity and inclusion to better prepare students for working with diverse clients and to prepare a diverse workforce.

Implications for Occupational Therapy Education

The authors offer the following suggestions in the spirit of enhancing diversity and inclusion within occupational therapy education:

- Intentionally recruit and train a diverse workforce of future occupational therapists.
- Prepare all occupational therapy practitioners and scholars to address health and participation disparities among diverse groups.
- Integrate conversations on diversity and inclusion throughout the curriculum.
- Provide students opportunities for community-engaged scholarship and practice.
- Foster diverse and inclusive educational environments and teaching and learning approaches.
- Offer required and elective courses on health disparities, global health, social justice, culturally responsive occupational therapy, gender issues, occupational therapy practice with refugees and immigrants, community partnerships, power structures within health care, disability issues, ethics, and more.
- Integrate race, culture, disparities, and social justice across the curriculum.
- Examine documents and department-level structures that reflect commitment to diversity and inclusion in curriculum philosophy, strategic plan, hiring, mentoring, and systems for addressing reports of discrimination or bias.

What led you to become an occupational therapy educator?

I was raised as the 5th child in a family of 12 kids and when we were little, we often played school. A couple of us were the teachers and the rest of my siblings the students. At an early age, I strongly advocated for playing the role of the teacher. Besides, my older siblings and I were often charged with crafting activities to help entertain my younger siblings. As an adolescent, my parents took all of us kids to volunteer as teacher aids at a school for poor children in the outskirts of Bogota, Colombia. Since then, I knew well that I wanted to become an educator and also study psychology. I saw this path as a way to help others and foster critical thinking in my students. I was heavily influenced by Paulo Freire, a Brazilian educator, who criticized the traditional banking notion of education and I firmly agree with him that education is a way to achieve real democratic empowerment. Now, I synergize my roles as an educator and researcher and in my journey I am equally transformed by my students and the community research partners from whom I learn a lot.

Yolanda Suarez-Balcazar, PhD

I have never really thought about the origins of my identity as a teacher. I am from a very large family; a family of artists, healers and people whose craft is in their hands. I suppose in one way or another I was always being shown and told how to do something and our family culture expected me to pay it forward and teach the next person the lessons I learned. My mother tells stories of how, as a child, my lessons were often making my chores seem like a game and teaching my younger siblings and cousins how to do my work, do it right, and think it was fun. I was invited to guest lecture in a colleague's classroom and shortly afterwards a stroke of serendipity found me teaching my own course; an then another. For years I kept one foot in the clinic and another in the classroom, then transitioned completely to academia. The people I treated, my students, and my academic colleagues have taught me all of the most important lessons about how to perfect my craft as an educator.

Jaime P. Muñoz, PhD, OTR/L, FAOTA

REFERENCES

Abreu, B. C., & Peloquin, S. M. (2004). The issue is: Embracing diversity within our profession. *American Journal of Occupational Therapy, 58*(3), 353-359.

ACCESS Project. (2011). *Universal design for learning: A concise introduction.* Retrieved from http://accessproject.colostate.edu/udl/modules/udl_introduction/udl_concise_ intro.pdf

American Occupational Therapy Association. (2007). AOTA's Centennial Vision and executive summary. *American Journal of Occupational Therapy, 61*(6), 613-614. doi:10.5014/ajot.61.6.613

American Occupational Therapy Association. (2017). Vision 2025. *American Journal of Occupational Therapy, 71*, 37103420010. doi:10.5014/ajot.2017.713002

American Occupational Therapy Association. (2018). *Academic programs annual data report: Academic year 2017-2018.* Retrieved from https://www.aota.org/~/media/Corporate/Files/EducationCareers/Educators/2017-2018-Annual-Data-Report.pdf

Artinian, N. T., Drees, B. M., Glazer, G., Harris, K., Kaufman, L. S., Lopez, N., ... Michaels, J. (2017). Holistic admissions in the health professions: Strategies for leaders. *College and University, 92*(2), 65-68. Retrieved from https://www.ncbi.nlm.nih.gov/pmc/articles/PMC5708588/pdf/nihms915516.pdf

Association of American Medical Colleges. (n.d.). Holistic admissions. Retrieved from https://www.aamc.org/initiatives/holisticreview/about/

Barker, N. C. S., & Fisher, G. (2018). Take a stand with technology: Advocating for the profession with virtual hill days. *OT Practice, 23*(16), 18-20. doi:10.7138/otp.2018.2316.cr

Beagan, B. L. (2015). Approaches to culture and diversity: A critical synthesis of occupational therapy literature. *Canadian Journal of Occupational Therapy, 82*(5) 272-282. doi: 10.1177/0008417414567530

Ben-Moshe, L., & Magaña, S. (2014). An introduction to race, gender, and disability: Intersectionality, disability studies, and families of color. *Women, Gender, and Families of Color, 2*(2), 105-114. Retrieved from http://www.jstor.org/stable/10.5406/womgenfamcol.2.2.0105

Betancur, J. J., & Herring, C. (2013). *Reinventing race, reinventing racism.* Chicago, IL: Haymarket Books.

Black, R. M. (2002). Occupational therapy's dance with diversity. *American Journal of Occupational Therapy, 56*(2) 140-148. doi:10:5014/ajot.56.2.140

Calzada, E., & Suarez-Balcazar, Y. (2014). *Enhancing cultural competence in social service agencies: A promising approach to serving diverse children and families.* The Office of Planning, Research, and Evaluation. Retrieved from https://www.acf.hhs.gov/sites/default/files/opre/brief_enhancing_cultural_competence_final_022114.pdf

Clark, F. (2013). As viewed from above: Connectivity and diversity in fulfilling occupational therapy's Centennial Vision (Farewell Presidential Address). *American Journal of Occupational Therapy, 67*, 624-632. doi:10.5014/ajot.2013.676003

Cohn, D. (2016, June 23). *It's official: Minority babies are the majority among the nation's infants, but only just.* Pew Research Center. Retrieved from http://www.pewresearch.org/fact-tank/2016/06/23/its-official-minority-babies-are-the-majority-among-the-nations-infants-but-only-just/

Cooper, L. A., & Powe, N. R. (2004, July 1). *Disparities in patient experiences, health care processes, and outcomes: The role of patient-provider racial, ethnic, and language concordance.* The Commonwealth Fund. Retrieved from https://www.commonwealth fund.org/sites/default/files/documents/___media_files_publications_fund_report_2004_jul_disparities_in_patient_experiences__health_care_processes__and_outcomes__the_role_of_patient_provide_cooper_disparities_in_patient_experiences_753_pdf.pdf

Cooper-Patrick, L., Gallo, J. J., Gonzales, J. J., Vu, H. T., Powe, N. R., Nelson, C., & Ford, D. E. (1999). Race, gender, and partnership in the patient-physician relationship. *Journal of the American Medical Association, 282*(6), 583-589. doi:10.1001/jama.282.6.583

Evans, C. H., Colburn, L., Stith, A. Y., & Smedley, B. D. (2001). *The right thing to do, the smart thing to do: Enhancing diversity in health professions.* Washington, DC: National Academies Press.

Flores, A. (2017, September 18). *How the U.S. Hispanic population is changing.* Pew Research Center. Retrieved from https://www.pewresearch.org/fact-tank/2017/09/18/how-the-u-s-hispanic-population-is-changing/

Grady, A. P. (1995). Building inclusive community: A challenge for occupational therapy. *American Journal of Occupational Therapy, 49*, 300-310. doi:10.5014/ajot.49.4.300

Hafeez, H., Zeshan, M., Tahir, M. A., Jahan, N., & Naveed, S. (2017). Health care disparities among lesbian, gay, bisexual, and transgender youth: A literature review. *Cureus, 9*(4), 1-7. doi:10.7759/cureus.1184

Hammel, J., Magasi, S., Mirza, M., Fischer, H., Preissner, K., Peterson, E., & Suarez Balcazar, Y. (2015). A scholarship of practice revisited: Creating community-engaged occupational therapy practitioners, educators, and scholars. *Occupational Therapy and Health Care, 29*(4), 352-369.

Harrison, D. A., Price, K. H., & Bell, M. P. (1998). Beyond relational demography: Time and the effects of surface- and deep-level diversity on work group cohesion. *Academy of Management Journal, 41*, 96-107. Retrieved from https://www.jstor.org/stable/256901

Krahn, G. L., Walker, D. K., & Correa-De-Araujo, R. (2015). Persons with disabilities as an unrecognized health disparity population. *American Journal of Public Health, 105*(S2), S198-S206. doi:10.2105/AJPH.2014.302182

Moneta-Koehler, L., Brown, A. M., Petrie, K. A., Evans, B. J., & Chalkley, R. (2017). The limitations of the GRE in predicting success in biomedical graduate school. *PLoS One, 12*(1), e0166742. doi:10.1371/journal.pone.0166742

Moore, S., Clark, C., Haught, A., Hinde, B., Reckner, D., Robinson, J., ... Horsempa, J. (2019). Factors associated with academic performance in physician assistant graduate programs and national certification examination scores. A literature review. *Health Professions Education, 5*(2), 103-110. doi:10.1016/j.hpe.2018.06.003

Muñoz, J. P. (2007). Culturally responsive caring in occupational therapy. *Occupational Therapy International, 14*(4), 256-280. doi:10.1002/oti.238

Paasche-Orlow, M. K., & Wolf, M. S. (2007). The causal pathways linking health literacy to health outcomes. *American Journal of Health Behavior, 31*(Suppl. 1), S19-S26. doi:10.5555/ajhb.2007.31.supp.S19

Plaut, V. (2002). Cultural models of diversity in America: The psychology of difference and inclusion. In R. A. Shweder, M. Minow, & H. R. Markus (Eds.), *Engaging cultural differences: The multicultural challenge in liberal democracies* (pp. 365-395). New York, NY: Russell Sage Foundation.

Roberge, M. É., & van Dick, R. (2010). Recognizing the benefits of diversity: When and how does diversity increase group performance? *Human Resource Management Review, 20*, 295-308. doi:10.1016/j.hrmr.2009.09.002

Shore, L. M., Randel, A. E., Chung, B. G., Dean, M. A., Ehrhart, K. H., & Singh, G. (2011). Inclusion and diversity in work groups: A review and model for future research. *Journal of Management, 37*(4), 1262-1289. doi:10.1177/0149206310385943

Smedley, B., Stith, A., & Nelson, A. (2003). *Unequal treatment: Confronting racial and ethnic disparities in health care.* Washington, DC: The National Academies Press.

Society for Community Research and Action. (2018a). *Conversations about diversity.* Retrieved from http://www.scra27.org/resources/webinars/diversity-conversations/

Society for Community Research and Action. (2018b). *Who we are.* Retrieved from http://www.scra27.org/who-we-are/

Stoffel, V. (2016). Coming home to family: Now is the time! (Farewell Presidential Address). *American Journal of Occupational Therapy, 70*, 7006120010. doi:10.5014/ajot.2016.706003

Suarez-Balcazar, Y., Mirza, P. M., & Witchger-Hansen, A.M. (2015). Unpacking university-community partnerships to advance Scholarship of Practice. *Occupational Therapy in Health Care, 29*(4),370-382. doi: 10.3/09/07380577.2015.1037945

Suarez-Balcazar, Y., Rodawoski, J., Balcazar, F. E., Taylor-Ritzler, T., Portillo, N., Barwacz, D., & Willis, C. (2009). Perceived levels of cultural competence among occupational therapists. *American Journal of Occupational Therapy, 63*(4), 498-505. doi:10.5014/ajot.63.4.498

Sue, D. W. (2016). *Race talk and the conspiracy of silence: Understanding and facilitating difficult dialogue on race.* Philadelphia, PA: John Wiley & Sons.

Taff, S. D., & Blash, D. (2017). Diversity and inclusion in occupational therapy: Where we are, where we must go. *Occupational Therapy in Health Care, 31*(1), 72-83. doi:10.1080/07380577.2016.1270479

Taylor, M. C. (2007). The Cason Memorial Lecture 2007: Diversity amongst occupational therapists—rhetoric or reality? *British Journal of Occupational Therapy, 20*(7), 276-283.

Thomas, L., & Heath, J. (2014). Institutional wide implementation of key advice for socially inclusive teaching in higher education. A practice report. *International Journal of the First Year in Higher Education, 5*(1), 123-133. doi:10.5204/intjfyhe.v5i1.206

Thompson, B., Molina, Y., Viswanath, K., Warnecke, R., & Prelip, M. L. (2016). Strategies to empower communities to reduce health disparities. *Health Affairs, 35*(8), 1424-1428. doi:10.1377/hlthaff.2015.1364

U.S. Department of Health and Human Services. (2014). *Sex, race, and ethnic diversity of U.S. health occupations (2010-2012).* Rockville, MD: Health Resources and Services Administration.

U.S. Department of Health and Human Services. (2017). *Sex, race, and ethnic diversity of U.S. health occupations (2011-2015).* Rockville, MD: Health Resources and Services Administration.

Witchger Hansen, A., Muñoz, J., Crist, P. A., Gupta, J., Ideishi, R., Primeau, L. A., & Tupé, D. (2007) Service learning: Meaningful, community-centered professional skill development for occupational therapy students. *Occupational Therapy In Health Care, 21*(1-2), 25-49. doi:10.1080/J003v21n01_03

RESOURCES

Association of American Colleges and Universities. Retrieved from https://www.aacu.org/resources/diversity-equity-and-inclusive-excellence

Banks, J. A. (2006). *Cultural diversity and education: Foundations, curriculum, and teaching* (5th ed.). Boston, MA: Pearson Education.

Banks, J. A. (2010). Approaches to multicultural curriculum reform. In J. A. Banks & C. A. McGee Banks (Eds.), *Multicultural education: Issues and perspectives* (7th ed., pp. 233-256). New York, NY: John Wiley & Sons.

Diversity in the curriculum. Retrieved from http://asjmc.org/resources/diversity_booklet/5_curriculum.pdf

Stoll, L.C. (2013). Race and gender in the classroom: Teachers, privilege, and enduring social inequities. Lanham, MD: Lexington Books.

Journal of Best Practices in Health Professions Diversity: Research, Education and Policy. https://www.uncpress.org/journals/journal-of-best-practices-in-health-professions-diversity/

Teaching tolerance. Educating for a diverse democracy. Retrieved from https://www.tolerance.org/

University of Nebraska. A model for infusing cultural diversity concepts across the curriculum. Retrieved from https://digitalcommons.unl.edu/cgi/viewcontent.cgi?referer=https://search.yahoo.com/&httpsredir=1&article=1196&context=podimproveacad

Appendix

STUDENT AND PROFESSIONAL ORGANIZATIONS PROMOTING DIVERSITY WITHIN OCCUPATIONAL THERAPY

ORGANIZATION	MISSION/VISION	LINK
BrOT	"To ensure the realization of the AOTA centennial vision, by creating a widely recognized, diverse and powerful profession … Our goal will be met by gaining the support of current students and professionals while promoting gender and cultural diversity throughout occupational therapy programs across the country."	http://www.brotmovement.com/
Coalition of Occupational Therapy Advocates for Diversity (COTAD)	"Increasing diversity within the occupational therapy workforce by empowering occupational therapy practitioners, educators, and students to enhance cultural humility and promote diversity and inclusion."	https://www.cotad.org/
Multicultural, Diversity, and Inclusion Network (MDI)	A network of independent groups of various diverse identities and affiliations based on race/ ethnicity, disability, sexual orientation, and religious affiliation that collectively support the increase of diversity and inclusion in occupational therapy.	https://www.aota.org/Practice/Manage/Multicultural/Cultural-Competency-Tool-Kit.aspx Asian/Pacific Heritage Occupational Therapy Association; National Black Occupational Therapy Caucus; Network for Lesbian, Gay, Bisexual, and Transgender Concerns in Occupational Therapy; Network of Occupational Therapy Practitioners With Disabilities and Their Supporters; Occupational Therapy Network for Native Americans; Orthodox Jewish Occupational Therapy Chavrusa; and Terapia Ocupacional para Diversidad, Oportunidad, y Solidaridad (TODOS) Network of Hispanic Practitioners

10

The Principles of Occupation-Centered Education

Barbara R. Hooper, PhD, OTR/L, FAOTA;
Sheama Krishnagiri, PhD, OTR/L, FAOTA; and Pollie Price, PhD, OTR/L, FAOTA

Chapter Objectives

By the end of this chapter, the reader will be able to:

1. Broaden the definition of occupation-centered curriculum to occupation-centered education and justify the broader definition.
2. Describe six principles of occupation-centered education.
3. Connect the principles of occupation-centered education to well-established and evidence-based principles of learning from the field of education.
4. Implement each principle in curricula, teaching, and learning.

INTRODUCTION

Occupational therapy educators have used the term *occupation-centered curriculum* since the end of the 20th century (Wood et al., 2000; Yerxa, 1998). The term generally refers to breaking open the concept of occupation and configuring from its elements a central organizing framework for an entire curriculum (Yerxa, 1998). Knowledge of occupation can be broken into three parts: subconcepts of occupation, associated reasoning processes, and the impact learning occupation has on professional identity. These elements then become themes or threads that are infused into and across all courses in a curriculum, becoming the organizing framework. For example, Wood and colleagues (2000) broke occupation into the subconcepts of "nature of occupation," "view of the person as an occupational being" (p. 367), "occupation as a medium of change" (p. 590), and these became crosscutting curricular threads. Additionally, certain reasoning processes help students engage with the concept of occupation and create therapy based on it. For example, Yerxa (1998) noted that "occupational therapist thinking emphasizes not the diagnosis and treatment of pathology but the development of skill that enables persons to achieve their purposes and connect with the routines of their culture" (p. 368). Similarly, Fortune and Kennedy-Jones (2014) stated that "thinking in an occupational way

Taff, S. D., Grajo, L. C., & Hooper, B. R. (Eds.). *Perspectives on Occupational Therapy Education: Past, Present, and Future* (pp. 117-127).
© 2020 Taylor & Francis Group.

should underpin most of what students learn throughout the curriculum" (p. 297). These authors and others promote systems thinking, thinking that considers the dynamic transactions of things, as a fit for engaging the complexity of occupation. Finally, knowledge of occupation can be analyzed from the vantage point of how it impacts professional identity formation, who students will become as a result of learning about occupation, and its requisite thinking processes. For example, Wood et al. (2000) added the thread of "occupational therapists as scholars and change agents in systems," reflecting who they hoped students would become through the curriculum (p. 590).

In sum, the term *occupation-centered curriculum* has been understood as creating an organizing framework based on occupation, specifically breaking occupation into subconcepts, associated reasoning processes, and students' possible identities. The framework then serves as a basis for selecting, deselecting, organizing, and teaching content in a curriculum. Each course makes contributions to student understandings of the framework's threads.

However, an occupation-centered curriculum extends beyond this macrodesign for the curriculum to include the microlearning students do each day (i.e., an occupation-centered curriculum encompasses how each course is conceptualized, each class session is structured, each learning activity is designed, and learning is assessed). Rather than introductory courses alone, occupation-centered education requires students to relate all courses and topics to occupation-related threads. Hence, in this chapter, we broaden the term occupation-centered curriculum to *occupation-centered education* to denote all teaching and learning activities and assessment strategies within a curriculum (Hooper, Krishnagiri, Price, Taff, & Bilics, 2018). Given the span of time since the concept of occupation-centered education was introduced, there are now sufficient seminal works and subsequent scholarship to distill key principles of occupation-centered education, which we next identify and discuss.

PRINCIPLES OF OCCUPATION-CENTERED EDUCATION MAPPED TO LEARNING PRINCIPLES

The following principles for occupation-centered education were extracted from seminal and current publications. However, the principles identified are valuable for designing learning only to the degree that they manifest established, evidence-based principles of learning from education. Therefore, we validate extracted principles of occupation-centered education by mapping them to best principles of learning (see Principles 1-6 below). We also illustrate each principle with examples drawn from a study of how occupational therapy programs in the United States address occupation (Hooper et al., 2018; Krishnagiri, Hooper, Price, Taff, & Bilics, 2017; Price, Hooper, Krishnagiri, Taff, & Bilics, 2017).

Principle 1: All Learning Is Linked to The Big Idea(s) of Occupational Therapy

We define this principle as designing all learning—from macrocurriculum designs to microlearning tasks—in such a way that students cannot escape, except by making explicit links among the topic of the day, occupation, and associated reasoning processes. As educators are well aware, most curricula and courses in occupational therapy are filled, if not overfilled, with a plethora of topics—all the things faculty and accreditors believe students need to know to succeed on fieldwork and as therapists. However, without explicit expectations that students link these topics to the big ideas of occupational therapy, students can feel inundated by the sheer number of topics they must read about, show competence in, and be assessed on (Whiteford & Wilcock, 2001). Thus, scholars have recommended that curricula and individual courses be designed to help students link their learning to the big ideas of the field. Big ideas are also referred to as core disciplinary knowledge and a field's core subject (Hooper, Greene, & Sample, 2014). The big ideas for occupational therapy have been identified as occupation (Hooper et al., 2015; Mitcham, 2014; Yerxa, 1998; Wood et al., 2000), occupation and its relation to health and well-being (Fortune & Kennedy-Jones, 2014), and a five-concept constellation of "purposeful and meaningful occupation, client centered practice, the inseparable nature of theory and practice, integrated reasoning (thinking critically, reflecting), and professional identity" (Rodger & Turpin, 2011, p. 547). Knowledge that supports occupation, such as neuroscience, is taught in direct relation to these big ideas, not as stand-alone topics (Whiteford & Wilcock, 2001).

The principle that all learning is linked to the big idea(s) of occupational therapy reflects long-established principles of learning in education. In *Idea-Based Learning: A Course Design Process to Promote Conceptual Understanding*, Hansen (2012) explains that "unless big overarching ideas that hold the content together are provided, the course [curriculum] could appear as one long string of disconnected content bits" (p. 5). Connecting learning to a field's big ideas directly influences students' knowledge transfer, what Schell (2018) defined as the ability to apply knowledge learned in one context to multiple contexts. In other words, **learners are able to transfer knowledge and apply it flexibly when they learn topics in direct relation to the logic, the core disciplinary knowledge, and the macroperspective of a field or discipline** (Bruner, 1960; Paul, 1995).

Similarly, in *How People Learn: Brain, Mind, Experience, and School*, Bransford and the National Research Council (2000) summarized that **learning must be driven by general principles over isolated content areas.** Learners are more likely to transfer learning to multiple contexts if the topics they learn are grounded in core disciplinary concepts and if they have opportunity to use those concepts to solve problems in multiple situations. Thus, Mitcham's (2014) edict to "think and link" was aligned with a central understanding in learning science—**learners must have opportunities to relate topics to the overarching ideas of their discipline** (e.g., Bruner, 1960; Paul, 1995; Wiggins & McTighe, 2011). This is related to another learning principle: learning involves quality over quantity, deep understanding of key concepts over superficial breadth and quantity of content (Wiggins & McTighe, 2011).

In sum, linking topics to occupation and its dynamic in health is more likely to promote learning and transfer than learning isolated topics such as kinesiology, activity analysis, standardized assessments, or preparatory methods. Even so, Hooper and colleagues (2014) found that connections in occupational therapy classrooms were commonly made across topics, say from research to practice, but not consistently back to the big idea of the field, occupation.

Principle 2: Students Learn Occupation as a Concept Unto Itself Apart From Therapy

We define this principle as students becoming steeped in knowledge of occupation as it transacts with factors ranging from the intrapersonal, interpersonal, institutional, community, geopolitical, cultural, and global. Yerxa (1998) proposed a set of concepts that students should understand about occupation apart from therapy, including the human need and drive for occupation and humans as open systems acting in tandem with the environment through occupation over the life span. Students should understand how occupation connects people to communities, relates to health and development, and holds culturally situated meanings. Additionally, students need deep understandings of occupation as a "medium of transformation" (Wood et al., 2000).

Price et al. (2017) found that some occupational therapy curricula in the United States, despite being overfilled with numerous topics and standards, teach occupation as a concept apart from practice. Their study framed learning occupation as a concept unto itself as "learning occupation as a way of seeing self, others and the profession" (Price et al., 2017, p. 3). In learning to see self, students analyzed and reflected on their own occupations' contributions to identity, meaning, values, interests, capacities, and health. Students reflected on how occupation shaped their development and how growing up in a certain family, community, and culture shaped some occupational opportunities and limited others. For example, one assignment required students to take up an occupation they had always wanted to learn. They wrote a paper about their experiences, with attention paid to the impact the occupation had on their roles, identities, skills and capacities, social connections, esteem, and competence, among others. Students presented their experience to peers, highlighting occupation as a medium for transformation.

Other examples included having students attend community cultural events and conduct in-depth interviews with people from backgrounds different from their own. Students processed the experiences by writing about how occupations at the events were shaped in, for, and with the culture and about how interviewees' backgrounds shaped their occupational opportunities, values, beliefs, identity, and habitual ways of being in the world. Learning was assessed against rubrics with criteria for how well students understood the meaning and centrality of occupation in life. In these examples, students learned occupation not as an abstract concept or a therapeutic application but as one with which they and others have rich lifelong experiences.

Learning occupation through one's experiences relates to several key learning principles in education. First, **all learning is filtered through prior knowledge and experience; therefore, like the previous examples, new learning must be intentionally tied to students' former experience** (Bransford & National Research Council, 2000; Bybee et al., 2006; Wiggins & McTighe, 2011). Best practices in education involves engaging students' prior knowledge and experience. However, Bransford and the National Research Council (2000) added the following warning: if prior knowledge and meaning perspectives are inadequate or contradictory with new knowledge, students may develop understandings that are very different from those the instructor intended, and we add very different from the core disciplinary knowledge of occupational therapy (Hooper, 2010). In sum, tapping, evaluating, and revising prior knowledge and experience, such as experiences with occupation, enhances learning.

There is a second learning principle related to learning occupation apart from therapy: **learning is sparked by emotion and motivation** (Bybee et al., 2006). When students see how they and others have developed into the people they are with the capacities they have because of their culturally situated occupations, they can develop value, motivation, and commitment for the content. This can be achieved when students tell and elicit stories. Taff et al. (2018) and Frank (2016) highlighted the importance of stories in becoming passionate about occupation's transformative power.

Principle 3: Students Learn Occupation as a Tool for Practice

Having developed deep understandings of why occupation is a transforming agent, students translate that understanding into interventions that optimize occupational participation (Molineux, 2010). Wood et al. (2000) suggested that as students grasp why change occurs through occupation, they can hone a "complex of proficiencies" (p. 592) for enabling occupation, such as systematic observations of occupation, assessment of occupational performance, simultaneous attention to the biomedical condition and the life worlds of clients, and interventions that target clients' optimal participation. Students learn to use occupation as assessment, intervention, and outcome of therapy, what some refer to as *occupation-based practice* (Fisher, 2014).

The process of occupation-based practice begins with understanding clients' histories, identities, and meanings shaped by and expressed through occupation. Then, therapists consider how those occupations interact with clients' daily life contexts. Therapists then observe performance for the "extent of any observable disruption … their performance skills and environmental opportunities" that support performance (Hocking, 2001, p. 465). Therapists next consider impairments as they transact with the "wider occupational perspective" established through the process thus far (Molineux, 2004, p. 11). Pierce (1999) suggested further that learning to use occupation therapeutically is supported by learning about top-down assessment, client-centered practice, occupation as an end and means, and "skills for creative design of powerful therapeutic occupations" (p. 3).

Krishnagiri et al. (2017) found that sometimes, despite different intentions, occupation was minimally present when students learned interventions. For example, students analyzed an area or type of occupation from the Occupational Therapy Practice Framework (American Occupational Therapy Association, 2014) by its required motor, sensory, emotional, cognitive, and communication requirements; students related levels of spinal cord injury to functional implications for performing activities of daily living; and they used purposeful activity to remediate functional deficits such as putting dishes away to address shoulder range of motion or simulated impairments while doing activities of daily living. In these instances, it seemed that learning occupation was "jumped over" and equated with learning activity analysis, functional deficits, types of occupation, and types of intervention.

The principle, learning occupation as a tool for practice, relates to three learning principles from education, namely, that **learning requires practice in authentic performances and situations** (Young, 1993; Fink, 2013); **knowledge is distributed across the student, instructor, tool, and context** (Brown, Collins, & Duguid, 1989); and **learning requires intentional knowledge transfer.** Learning situations must have certain ingredients to meet the criteria of authenticity. One, the learning situation's meaning is clear (i.e., it should be clear to students why they are engaged in a learning activity). Two, the activity will require students to transfer learning (i.e., students apply both the content and the thinking process they learned in one situation to novel situations). To aid knowledge transfer, educators may add prompts like the following: (a) What principles, skills, and tools related to enabling occupation did you use in this experience? (b) Identify three contexts where you have previously used the same principles, skills, and tools; and (c) Identify one additional practice situation (setting or population) where the principles, skills, and tools used in this experience would apply and how. Three, authentic activities will facilitate taking multiple perspectives; for example, students may first simply identify occupations occurring in a situation and then look a second time at the same situation for how the environment shapes the identified occupations, a third examination may focus on examining justice issues associated with the situation, and so on. Finally, during and after an authentic experience, students will reflect on how they used the core knowledge of the profession. Therefore, authentic practice experiences include the actual performance plus linking the performance to the core of occupation as a medium of change plus transferring the performance and what was learned to other contexts.

In the following example, students performed a set of skills, linked the skills to the profession's big ideas, and transferred their learning to another context. Students conducted an interview, created an occupational profile, identified disruptions to the interviewee's meaningful occupations, linked the disruptions to wellness risks, developed three wellness goals, and created interventions using occupation for obtaining optimal wellness. Interventions targeted clients' environmental factors, occupational demands, habits and routines, performance skills, and client factors. Students explained how the interventions related to enabling wellness through occupation. Learning was assessed based on how well the occupational profile drove the rest of the process and how well students linked occupation and wellness. In class, students related their learning to another experience, one they had on fieldwork.

Principle 4: Students Learn Occupational Science and Other Interdisciplinary Sciences That Illumine Occupation

This principle refers to prioritizing basic and applied sciences that study and elaborate the nature and impacts of occupation. Kristensen and Petersen (2016) argued that if the core disciplinary knowledge driving occupational therapy relates to occupation as a health agent, then the sciences that unpack those concepts and their transactions should be the foundational sciences in learning. The authors further proposed that the rationale, evidence, and principles for therapy are primarily located in occupational science, positioning occupational science as paramount for curricula. This argument is not hegemonic because occupational science is in part a science of synthesis (Yerxa, 1998) (i.e., a science of extracting knowledge pertaining to occupation from psychology, biology, philosophy, human development, neuroscience, physiology, theology, anthropology, and many others). Wood et al. (2000) noted that occupational science also generates new knowledge focused on "occupational behavior across the lifespan, in diverse cultural contexts, and with persons with and without disabling conditions" (p. 591). Therefore, occupational science has been elaborating the big ideas of the field for decades. The science generates this knowledge using four levels of research (Pierce, 2014): basic descriptions of the nature and dynamics of occupations, relational research integrating concepts of occupation with concepts of other disciplines, predictive research, and prescriptive intervention research.

Teaching the knowledge development process of occupational science is what Hooper, Krishnagiri, Taff, Price, and Bilics (2016) referred to as "teaching the science itself" (p. 526). Teaching the science itself refers to teaching the discipline's central phenomenon of interest, how concepts and research generated by the science relate to the discipline's central phenomenon, the types of questions the science explores, how its knowledge is so far organized, the tensions and debates within the discipline, the language of the science, and how the science is disseminated. However, rather than teaching the science itself, programs often teach the products of the science in relation to occupational therapy practice. Products of the science are "the concepts and research findings the science has generated" (p. 526). A few examples of these concepts include occupational justice, co-occupations, occupational deprivation, and lifestyle redesign. Therefore, occupational science concepts have been positively appropriated by curricula and infused into courses focused on occupational therapy yet sometimes apart from the context of the science. In one example, the concept occupational justice was introduced in a foundations course without students being exposed to the origins of the concept; the concept of co-occupation, another important occupational science concept, was embedded in pediatric content devoid of the research context in which the term was identified. Thus, Pierce (1999) concluded that teaching occupational science is challenging due to limited opportunities for educators to learn about the science, prevailing curriculum structures emphasizing disability, and too few resources outside of the *Journal of Occupational Science* such as textbooks although these have increased in recent years (e.g., Pierce, 2014; Whiteford & Hocking, 2011).

This principle is related to Principle 1: **learning is maximized when students continuously make connections to the big ideas of their field.** Occupational science generates knowledge from an occupational view of humans and daily life. Therefore, studying the science gives students opportunity to develop an occupational perspective. Such study also provides opportunity to construct identities as future scholars (i.e., as students interact through publications with the occupational therapists who became scientists of occupation, they can envision themselves doing similarly). Finally, studying the science that created some of the concepts behind practice provides knowledge by which to justify and advocate for those services.

Principle 5: Students Learn Through Collaborative, Participatory Pedagogies

This principle is defined as active learning. Alongside creating innovative authentic experiences, occupational therapy educators are masters at actively engaging students (Schaber, 2014). Because of our professional perspective and beliefs about doing, it is as if actively engaging students is part of our educational DNA. However, the familiarity with active learning may interfere with recalling the fullness of its meaning. According to the *Greenwood Dictionary of Education* (Collins & O'Brien, 2011), active learning is defined as follows:

> The process of having students engage in some activity that forces them to reflect upon ideas and how they are using those ideas. Requiring students to regularly assess their own degree of understanding and skill at handling concepts or problems in a particular discipline. (p. 6)

At the heart of active learning lies the education principle that **learning is shaped by context and is actively coconstructed with the context** (Wenger, 2009). Thus, the authentic performances students engage in, whether a case study or video or community experience, naturally elicit active engagement and, in turn, based on how the activities are set up, shape the nature of student engagement and what is learned. Therefore, as educators, we design authentic performance opportunities and also carefully craft what students do with those performances. Weimer (2011) suggested that educators design authentic activities to promote interaction with information, reflection, and confront students "with their knowledge and skill level."

One dimension of the learning-shaping context includes students' own culturally inherited assumptions and experiences. Thus, as noted in Principle 2, knowledge construction is guided by students' existing perspectives and past experiences. Learning scholars suggest that unless there is an explicit challenge imposed to prior knowledge by specific prompts, learners will make a learning experience fit what they know rather than change what they know based on an experience. Consequently, if context shapes learning and if students learn topics and skills in a context that does not include occupation, then the likelihood is low that students learn the relevance of the topic or skill to occupation. In sum, **the context of learning, including the prompts and criteria for an activity and its assessment, will shape what is learned and what knowledge students construct.** For example, occupational therapy students sometimes engage with people in homeless shelters. While taking a pediatrics course, they may focus on the children in the shelter. The context, including students' prior experience and learning, their emotional responses, and the instructions they receive about what to do will shape their learning. For example, they may, because of the structure of the course, focus on the sensory impairments and developmental delays of the children. But if the prompts change, they can additionally address occupational opportunities the shelter provides for the children and their mothers to be meaningfully occupied during their stay there. If the learning context prompts them, students can also explore the occupational injustices the families may face. In other words, as the learning context changes, such as prompts provided, the emphases of learning shift.

It strikes us that this learning principle—**learning is shaped by context and actively coconstructed with the context**—offers an opportunity for reinforcing students' knowledge about occupation. In other words, if students can come to see their learning as an occupation and if they can illumine how their learning is shaped by context (e.g., their values and beliefs, the institution, profession, instructor, vision and mission of the curriculum, interaction with peers), they can then be asked to generalize that experience to reinforce the general principle that occupation is shaped by context. Like active learning, then, the education principle here that **learning is a transaction with context** is grounded in the heart of occupational therapy's belief that occupation is a transaction with context (Dickie, Cutchin, & Humphry, 2006; Law et al., 1996).

Principle 6: Knowledge and Skills Are Assessed Through Educative Strategies

Like learning design, assessing how well students link their learning to human occupation requires (a) authentic tasks that specifically require students to generate those relationships, (b) clear criteria of what it looks like when they do make a quality connection to occupation, and (c) opportunity for students to assess their own and others' work based on the stated criteria. Together, these components constitute an educative learning assessment strategy (Fink, 2013).

Educational theory and research suggest that **learning is enhanced through educative assessment, which requires students to use knowledge as they will in future practice.** Educative assessment is often contrasted with auditive assessment, which assesses knowledge covered in the past unit of a course (Wiggins, 1998). The classic two examinations and a final is an auditive assessment strategy, the purpose of which is to audit learning and determine grades (Fink, 2013). Educative assessment involves selecting tasks that are authentic to how students will use knowledge in the future.

As noted, occupational therapy educators are masterful at creating authentic tasks. We structure assignments requiring students to interview others, write goals, observe others, and work in teams, all of which they will have to do in practice. However, these assessments sometimes omit the additional elements of robust educative assessment, such as explicit criteria and self-assessment. Price et al. (in press) found that occupational therapy assignments often omitted clear criteria and standards for performance, particularly related to what students should do with the experience in relation to occupation. When included, criteria often specify instructions about the tasks students should complete but not the conceptual understandings they should develop and exhibit. Self-assessment is often present in assessments in the form of asking students to reflect on the experience generally or on how they performed a task such as interviewing or teaching. Seldom, however, are students asked to evaluate the learning and thinking strategies pertaining to occupation that they used during and after the experience.

Take, for example, the previously described learning activity in the homeless shelter. To clarify what students should do with the experience in relation to occupation, faculty may provide prompts such as "What are the central occupational problems in this situation?" and "What is possible to change in this setting that would have a positive impact on the daily routines of those seeking shelter?" The self-assessment component may be addressed by reflecting on the key knowledge domains that were required to create occupation-based intervention and students' strengths and growth areas in each domain.

Learning assessment is generally one of the underdeveloped lines of scholarship in occupational therapy education (Hooper, King, Wood, Bilics, & Gupta, 2013), and assessment specific to how well students link learning experiences to occupation may be even further undeveloped (Price et al., 2017). This is evident in that the key seminal pieces on occupation-centered education barely addressed assessment (Pierce, 1999; Wood et al., 2000; Yerxa, 1998). They addressed the types of learning activities needed for students to explore the depths of occupation but not how to assess if students master those depths.

CONCLUSION

In this chapter, we distilled principles that can guide the design and implementation of occupation-centered education. However, such principles must also be validated against discoveries in education science on how people learn. Thus, each principle was matched to findings in learning science. The result is a robust guide and rationale for occupation-centered education. Implementing these principles will require study and reflection on occupation and its place in the curriculum. Implementing these principles all the way from the macrodesign of the curriculum down to the microprocesses of the classroom is at once challenging and exhilarating.

Implications for Occupational Therapy Education

- Educators can use the principles of occupation-centered education to guide curriculum and instructional design and assessment.
- Educators can justify occupation-centered education as grounded in established learning principles from education that are known to assist students in creating disciplinary knowledge, reasoning, and identity.

Key Reflection Questions

1. Which principles are most evident in your curriculum and in your own courses and teaching processes?
2. Which principles could be strengthened, and how?
3. Identify one change you would like to make related to the principles of occupation-centered education. What impact might such a change have on you as an educator and on student learning?
4. To what degree are students required to link all learning to occupation and to what degree are they assessed on how well they make such links?

What led you to become an occupational therapy educator?

I was an educator of sorts from a very young age. On the farm I grew up on was an old abandoned schoolhouse, complete with classrooms, desks, and chalkboards. I taught imaginary students and reluctant neighbors. As I got older, I taught Sunday school classes and flag corps routines and neuroanatomy reviews. When later given an opportunity to fill in for an occupational therapy faculty sabbatical, it was a natural fit. I was a naive practitioner-educator intent on setting students on a better learning course than they were getting from the academics. I've learned a great deal since then.

Barbara R. Hooper, PhD, OTR/L, FAOTA

My family and friends noted that I was good at explaining things from a very young age. After I became an occupational therapist and further refined my skills of breaking things down and teaching clients, I realized that I liked teaching. My doctoral training in occupational science expanded my perspective on occupation and its power. I felt compelled to share what I knew, a powerful way of knowing, doing, and being, and so moved into academia. I am thrilled that I can do research in occupational science and teach students and colleagues about the power of occupation.

Sheama Krishnagiri, PhD, OTR/L, FAOTA

I was not a natural teacher. Operating from a right brain imbued with passion, ambition, and a sense of justice, I became an occupational therapist. As a new grad, I always knew I wanted to do research, write, and teach, and studying occupational science fueled my passion and conviction for occupational therapy even more. I transitioned to teaching while in my doctoral studies, which challenged me to move from big picture thinking to a more linear and sequential process. Through learning how to more effectively teach, I have become better able to convey the therapeutic process of occupational therapy. Engaging in educational research has expanded my knowledge about best practices in course design.

Pollie Price, PhD, OTR/L, FAOTA

REFERENCES

American Occupational Therapy Association. (2014). Occupational therapy practice framework: domain and process (3rd edition). *American Journal of Occupational Therapy, 68*(Suppl. 1), S1-S48. doi:10.5014/ajot.2014.682006.

Bransford, J., & National Research Council (2000). *How people learn: Brain, mind, experience, and school* (Expanded ed.). Washington, DC: National Academy Press.

Brown, J. S., Collins, A., & Duguid, P. (1989). Situated cognition and the culture of learning. *Educational Researcher, 18*(1), 32-42.

Bruner, J. S. (1960). *The process of education: A searching discussion of school education opening new paths to learning and teaching.* New York, NY: Vintage Books.

Bybee, R. W., Taylor, J. A., Gardner, A., Van Scotter, P., Powell, J. C., Westbrook, A., & Landes, N. (2006). *The BSCS 5E instructional model: Origins and effectiveness* (pp. 88-98). Colorado Springs, CO: BSCS.

Collins, J. W., & O'Brien, N. P. (2011). *The Greenwood dictionary of education.* Santa Barbara, CA: ABC-CLIO.

Dickie, V., Cutchin, M. P., & Humphry, R. (2006). Occupation as transactional experience: A critique of individualism in occupational science. *Journal of Occupational Science, 13*(1), 83-93.

Fink, L. D. (2013). *Creating significant learning experiences: An integrated approach to designing college courses.* Philadelphia, PA: John Wiley & Sons.

Fisher, A. G. (2014). Occupation-centered, occupation-based, occupation-focused: Same, same or different? *Scandinavian Journal of Occupational Therapy, 21*(Suppl. 1), 96-107.

Fortune, T., & Kennedy-Jones, M. (2014). Occupation and its relationship with health and wellbeing: The threshold concept for occupational therapy. *Australian Occupational Therapy Journal, 61*(5), 293-298.

Frank, G. (2016). Collective occupations and social transformation: a mad hot curriculum. In D. Sakellariou & N. Pollard (Eds.), *Occupational therapy without borders: Integrating justice with practice* (2nd ed., pp. 596-602). Edinburgh, UK: Elsevier/Churchill Livingston.

Hansen, E. J. (2012). *Idea-based learning: A course design process to promote conceptual understanding.* Sterling, VA: Stylus Publishing, LLC.

Hocking, C. (2001). Implementing occupation-based assessment. *American Journal of Occupational Therapy, 55*(4), 463.

Hooper, B. (2010). On arriving at the destination of the centennial vision: Navigational landmarks to guide occupational therapy education. *Occupational Therapy in Health Care, 24*(1), 97-106.

Hooper, B., Greene, D., & Sample, P. L. (2014). Exploring features of integrative teaching through a microanalysis of connection-making processes in a health sciences curriculum. *Advances in Health Sciences Education, 19*(4), 469-495.

Hooper, B., King, R., Wood, W., Bilics, A., & Gupta, J. (2013). An international systematic mapping review of educational approaches and teaching methods in occupational therapy. *British Journal of Occupational Therapy, 76*(1), 9-22.

Hooper, B., Krishnagiri, S., Price, P., Taff, S. D., & Bilics, A. (2018). Curriculum-level strategies that U.S. occupational therapy programs use to address occupation: A qualitative study. *American Journal of Occupational Therapy, 72*, 7201205040. doi:10.5014/ajot.2018.024190

Hooper, B., Krishnagiri, S., Taff, S., Price, P., & Bilics, A. (2016). Teaching knowledge generated through occupational science and teaching the science itself. *Journal of Occupational Science, 24*(4), 525-531. doi:1080/14427591.2016.1238405

Hooper, B., Mitcham, M. D., Taff, S. D., Price, P., Krishnagiri, S., & Bilics, A. (2015). The issue is—Energizing occupation as the center of teaching and learning. *American Journal of Occupational Therapy, 69*(Suppl. 2), 6912360010. doi:10.5014/ajot.2015.018242

Krishnagiri, S., Hooper, B., Price, P., Taff, S. D., & Bilics, A. (2017). Explicit or hidden? Exploring how occupation is taught in occupational therapy curricula in the United States. *American Journal of Occupational Therapy, 71*(2), 7102230020p1-7102230020p9.

Kristensen, H. K., & Petersen, K. S. (2016). Occupational science: An important contributor to occupational therapists' clinical reasoning. *Scandinavian Journal of Occupational Therapy, 23*(3), 240-243.

Law, M., Cooper, B., Strong, S., Stewart, D., Rigby, P., & Letts, L. (1996). The person-environment-occupation model: A transactive approach to occupational performance. *Canadian Journal of Occupational Therapy, 63*(1), 9-23.

Mitcham, M. D. (2014). Education as engine (Eleanor Clarke Slagle Lecture). *American Journal of Occupational Therapy, 68*, 636-648. doi:10.5014/ajot.2014.686001

Molineux, M. (2004). *Occupation for occupational therapists.* Malden, MA: Blackwell Publishing, Inc.

Molineux, M. (2010). Occupational science and occupational therapy: Occupation at center stage. In C. Christiansen & E. Townsend (Eds.), *Introduction to occupation: The art and science of living* (pp. 359-384). Upper Saddle River, NJ: Pearson.

Paul, R. W. (1995). *Critical thinking: What every person needs to survive in a rapidly changing world.* Rohnert Park, CA: Foundation for Critical Thinking.

Pierce, D. (1999). Putting occupation to work in occupational therapy curricula. *Education Special Interest Section Quarterly, 9*(3), 1-4.

Pierce, D. E. (Ed.). (2014). *Occupational science for occupational therapy.* Thorofare, NJ: SLACK Incorporated.

Price, P., Hooper, B., Krishnagiri, S., Taff, S., & Bilics, A. (2017). A way of seeing: How occupation is portrayed to students when taught as a concept beyond its use in therapy. *American Journal of Occupational Therapy, 71*(4), 7104230010p1-7104230010p9. doi:10.5014/ajot.2017.024182

Price, P., Hooper, B., Krishnagiri, S., Wood, W., Taff, S. D, & Bilics, A. (In press). Toward robust assessments of student knowledge of occupation. *American Journal of Occupational Therapy.*

Rodger, S., & Turpin, M. (2011). Using threshold concepts to transform entry level curricula. 34th HERDSA Annual International Conference, Gold Coast, QLD, Australia, 4-7 July 2011. Milperra, NSW, Australia: Higher Education Research and Development Society of Australasia

Schaber, P. (2014). Conference proceedings—Keynote address: Searching for and identifying signature pedagogies in occupational therapy education. *American Journal of Occupational Therapy, 68*, S40-S44. doi:10.5014/ ajot.2014.685S08

Schell, J. (2018). Teaching for reasoning in higher education. In B. Schell & J. Schell (Eds.), *Clinical and professional reasoning in occupational therapy* (2nd ed., pp. 417-438). Philadelphia, PA: Wolters Kluwer.

Taff, S. D., Price, P., Krishnagiri, S., Bilics, A., & Hooper, B. (2018). Traversing hills and valleys: Exploring doing, being, becoming and belonging experiences in teaching and studying occupation. *Journal of Occupational Science, 25*(3), 417-430.

Weimer, M. (2011). Defining active learning. Faculty Focus, Teaching Professor Blog. Magna Publications.

Wenger, E. (2009). A social theory of learning. In K. Illeris (Ed.), *Contemporary theories of learning: learning theorists—in their own words* (pp. 209-218). New York, NY: Routledge.

Whiteford, G. E., & Hocking, C. (Eds.). (2011). *Occupational science: Society, inclusion, participation.* Hoboken, NJ: John Wiley & Sons.

Whiteford, G. E., & Wilcock, A. A. (2001). Centralizing occupation in occupational therapy curricula: Imperative of the new millennium. *Occupational Therapy International, 8*(2), 81-85.

Wiggins, G. (1998). *Educative assessment: Designing assessments to inform and improve student performance.* San Francisco, CA: Jossey-Bass.

Wiggins, G. P., & McTighe, J. (2011). *The understanding by design guide to creating high-quality units.* Alexandria, VA: ASCD.

Wood, W., Nielson, C., Humphry, R., Coppola, S., Baranek, G., & Rourk, J. (2000). A curricular renaissance: Graduate education centered on occupation. *American Journal of Occupational Therapy, 54*(6), 586-597.

Yerxa, E. J. (1998). Occupation: The keystone of a curriculum for a self-defined profession. *American Journal of Occupational Therapy, 52*(5), 365-372.

Young, M. F. (1993). Instructional design for situated learning. *Educational Technology Research and Development, 41*(1), 43-58.

Section III

Future

11

Internationalizing
Occupational Therapy Education
Designing Opportunities for
Critical Engagement Across Cultures

Rebecca M. Aldrich, PhD, OTR/L

Chapter Objectives

By the end of this chapter, the reader will be able to:

1. Define internationalization and identify examples of internationalization of the curriculum and internationalization at home in occupational therapy education.
2. Explain how ideas about cultural responsiveness can guide learning goals for internationalized occupational therapy education.
3. Describe format, structure, and evaluation considerations for designing internationalized education activities.

INTRODUCTION

Internationalized occupational therapy education can take a variety of forms (Horton, 2009; Shimmel et al., 2016), including service learning (Cipriani, 2017), immersion experiences (Elliot, 2015), fieldwork placements (Humbert, Burket, Deveney, & Kennedy, 2012; Kinsella, Bossers, & Ferreira, 2008; Sim & Mackenzie, 2016), and virtual interactions (Aldrich & Grajo, 2017; Aldrich & Johansson, 2015; Aldrich & Peters, 2019; Asher, Estes, & Hill, 2014; Cabatan & Grajo, 2017; Grajo & Aldrich, 2016; Sood et al., 2014). International educational experiences can "promote nuanced and complex understandings of culture, worldviews, and occupational therapy" (Aldrich & Peters, 2019, p. 7303205100p7) by fostering engagement with diverse ways of doing, being, becoming, and belonging. By thoughtfully adding international components to educational experiences, educators can help make students aware of unexamined assumptions and interpersonal uncertainties (Swartz, 2007); they can also inspire questioning of the status quo and "the structural constraints that patients and [health care providers] operate within" (Metzl & Hansen, 2014, p. 128). This chapter reviews relevant definitions and uses brief examples from the author's experiences to build readers' capacities for internationalizing occupational therapy education.

Taff, S. D., Grajo, L. C., & Hooper, B. R. (Eds.). *Perspectives on Occupational Therapy Education: Past, Present, and Future* (pp. 131-141).

What Is Internationalization?

Internationalization is a process of "understanding and exploring multiple national identities and contexts" given the belief that "societies and nations are unique … and [we can] learn from each other irrespective of the level of development that has occurred" (Nagarajan & McAllister, 2015, p. 89). This definition underscores the parity of knowledge from different parts of the world—a recognition that has emerged slowly in occupational therapy scholarship and curricula (Hammell, 2011, 2015; Kantartzis & Molineux, 2011). Diverse perspectives are essential to occupational therapy education because the profession operates across international contexts and serves people with varying needs, circumstances, and worldviews (Dsouza, Galvaan, & Ramugondo, 2017; Hammell, 2013; Iwama, 2007). By providing opportunities to engage with diverse perspectives, internationalization can help students think broadly and inclusively as they learn to design and deliver services.

Educational internationalization can involve increasing international student enrollment, facilitating teaching and learning in other countries, or incorporating global perspectives into courses or curricula (Nagarajan & McAllister, 2015). These activities can be categorized as internationalization of curriculum (IoC), which entails "integrating an international, intercultural, or global dimension into the purpose, functions or delivery of postsecondary education" (Nagarajan & McAllister, 2015, p. 89), or internationalization at home (IaH), which includes "any internationally related activity with the exception of outbound student mobility" (Nagarajan & McAllister, 2015, p. 91). Cabatan and Grajo (2017) identified fieldwork, immersion, and global service learning experiences in occupational therapy education as IoC and virtual interactions and local service learning as IaH.

Selecting Internationalization Activities

Internationalization begins with the identification of learning goals. Relevant goals can range from exposure to other perspectives, to developing increased self-awareness and reflexivity, to demonstrating more nuanced habits of thinking and acting. The suitability of particular goals for an internationalized experience depends on both students' and instructors' positioning, and the activities that constitute an internationalized experience must link to feasible goals for both learners and educators.

For example, when designing previous internationalized educational experiences (see Aldrich, 2015; Aldrich & Grajo, 2017; Aldrich & Johansson, 2015; and Aldrich & Peters, 2019, for descriptions), I determined that 50% to 60% of my students had studied abroad, most students had at least one experience with people of backgrounds different from their own, and students were being educated in a department and university that emphasized global connections. Yet, I also knew that few students had critically reflected on their personal biases, the occupational therapy curriculum was largely structured around Northern/Anglophone ideas, and adding international travel to the degree program was not feasible. In light of this knowledge, my collaborators and I designed IaH learning experiences to facilitate critical reflexivity about core occupational therapy ideas ideas, with a secondary focus on exposure to global perspectives. We developed activities, such as guided video-conferencing discussions (Aldrich & Johansson, 2015) and student-led cross-cultural presentations (Aldrich & Peters, 2019), to work toward those identified learning goals. As an educator who lived, trained, and worked only in the United States, I needed to reflect on whether or not my epistemological and pedagogical assumptions made sense in the context of the internationalized learning experience. I sought help from my international collaborators as well as an instructional designer to help me consider whether or not identified learning goals were feasible given the time frame for the internationalized experience and the positioning of students and faculty members involved in the collaboration.

Using this brief example as a guide, educators can consider the following questions when designing their internationalized educational experiences:

- What level of exposure to global perspectives do students and faculty members have, both in general and relative to the profession?
- To what degree have students already interrogated or critiqued their own perspectives?
- How are faculty members prepared to arrange and facilitate internationalized experiences?
- How important are global perspectives in explicit and implicit program curricula?
- How feasible are IoC vs IaH activities within the program and university?

THE EVOLVING DISCOURSE ON
CULTURALLY RELEVANT PRACTICE

During the conceptualization phase, educators must carefully consider what terminology defines their internationalized learning goals. In occupational therapy education, such goals usually relate to practice competencies; for example, accreditation standards in the United States require entry-level practitioners to develop culturally relevant interventions (Brown, Muñoz, & Powell, 2011; Wells, Black, & Gupta, 2016) and draw on pertinent international evidence (Accreditation Council for Occupational Therapy Education, 2017). For many years, competency-related internationalization learning goals used the term *cultural competence*, which Awaad (2003) defined as the process of "seek[ing] a comprehensive understanding both of the cultural norms and variances of the societal group(s) with which [a therapist] is working ... and of the personal philosophical and theoretical background that [the therapist] brings to the service" (p. 357). However, as Black (2016) noted, a range of terms have since supplanted *competence* to describe the ongoing learning, skill development, and critical reflection necessary for culturally relevant practice (Table 11-1 provides terms and definitions). These terms "differ in identification of the problem or issue; relationship to existing power structures ... ; the degree to which they have encompassed multiple forms of diversity, beyond ethnicity; and how well established they are in occupational therapy" (Beagan, 2016, p. 278).

Far from being purely semantic, this discourse about terminology is important for defining the format and scope of internationalized education. When focused primarily on "acquiring knowledge about 'other' cultures," internationalized education "runs the risk of objectifying individuals ... different from the majority into overly simplistic categorical descriptions of character and behavior" (Kumagai & Lypson, 2009, p. 783). Therefore, although cultural sensitivity can be developed through repeated real-time (or synchronous) engagement with people who have different perspectives, mere exposure to those perspectives without associated reflexive activities may lead to problematic generalizations. At the other end of the spectrum, "international educational experiences can serve as an excellent vehicle ... [for] critiquing processes of oppression and power relations and enacting moral agency" (Kirkham, van Hofwegen, & Pankratz, 2009, p. 11). However, developing critical consciousness (Kumagai & Lypson, 2009) or structural competency (Metzl & Hansen, 2014) requires a baseline knowledge, openness, and depth and duration of engagement that may not be realistic within every IaH or IoC experience. Developing appropriate learning goals and activities for internationalized education requires defining the goals using appropriate terminology and considering what is logistically feasible; what kinds of knowledge, skills, and dispositions particular activities can engender in particular students; and what programmatic and educational priorities an internationalized experience aims to satisfy.

Drawing on another example, in my first attempt at internationalization, I used the language of cultural competence (Aldrich, 2015) to frame learning goals for 4 weeks of synchronous video discussions between occupational therapy students from the United States and Sweden (Aldrich & Johansson, 2015; Grajo & Aldrich, 2016). I asked students to provide examples of their own and

Table 11-1

TERMS RELATED TO CULTURALLY RELEVANT HEALTH CARE PRACTICES

TERM	DEFINITION	EXAMPLE TEACHING/ LEARNING ACTIVITIES
Cultural sensitivity	"Employing one's knowledge, consideration, understanding, respect, and tailoring after realizing awareness of self and others and encountering a diverse group or individual" (Foronda, 2008, p. 210).	• Discussions with people of different backgrounds • Reflective journal assignment examining own/others' assumptions and worldviews
Cultural competence	"The development of awareness, knowledge, and skills" where "awareness includes developing insight into one's own cultural values, attitudes, and biases as well as developing awareness of and sensitivity to the potentially distinct values, beliefs, and attitudes of clients unlike oneself. Knowledge entails learning about other cultures" and skills "include effective communication, rapport building across differences, respect, active listening, advocacy … use of culturally appropriate occupations, and thinking outside the box to adapt practices, assessments, and interventions" (Beagan, 2016, p. 274).	• Research assignment about own/others' cultures • Case studies about how a situation might be understood from a variety of cultural orientations
Cultural effectiveness	"The ability to interact with people from different cultures so as to optimize the probability of mutually successful outcomes" (Stone, 2006, p. 338 as cited in Black, 2016, p. 58).	• Practical exams focused on intercultural communication and interaction skills
Cultural humility	"A process of openness, self-awareness, being egoless, and incorporating self-reflection and critique after willingly interacting with diverse individuals" (Foronda, Baptiste, Reinholdt, & Ousman, 2016, p. 213).	• Reflective journal assignment critiquing implicit knowledge hierarchies on a given topic • Demonstration of increased openness and desire for multicultural experiences via standardized assessments

Table 11-1 (continued)

TERMS RELATED TO CULTURALLY RELEVANT HEALTH CARE PRACTICES

TERM	DEFINITION	EXAMPLE TEACHING/ LEARNING ACTIVITIES
Cultural safety	"Giving voice to members of society who are typically silenced and marginalized" (Black, 2016, p. 51) by recognizing that "social relations of power in society and healthcare specifically influences what counts as knowledge and evidence" and "that health beliefs and practices that differ from the dominant society are viewed as equally valid and relevant" (Gerlach, 2016, p. E98).	• Coconstructed narrative assignment that amplifies marginalized ways of knowing • Presentations of nondominant perspectives on key evidence in a field • Practical examinations focused on validating a variety of beliefs and practices
Critical consciousness	"A reflective awareness of the differences in power and privilege and the inequities that are embedded in social relationships" (Kumagai & Lypson, 2009, p. 783).	• Discussions about inequitable power relations in clinical case examples • Reflective journal assignment identifying and critiquing power relations in fieldwork experiences
Structural competency	"The trained ability to discern how a host of issues defined clinically as symptoms, attitudes, or diseases … also represent the downstream implications of a number of upstream decisions" (Metzl & Hansen, 2014, p. 128).	• Rewriting a clinical case description to foreground discourses and policy decisions • Discussions of infrastructure and economic issues that impact a clinical case

others' perspectives on a topic to demonstrate their progress toward cultural competence through the internationalized discussions. However, this approach did not facilitate deep or critical learning for students. A new partnership with a South African colleague prompted a restructuring of the internationalized experience around 7 weeks of student-led presentations. Changes to the duration, format, and content of this second internationalized experience created an opportunity for different learning goals related to critical consciousness (Aldrich & Peters, 2019). For that second experience, my students demonstrated their learning through applying concepts and analyzing real-life examples of concepts from different contexts. Through in-class presentations, the students verbally described how their worldviews shaped their interpretation and application of concepts.

Based on these examples, when designing learning activities for internationalized experiences, educators can consider the following questions:

- What internationalization activity and format will best meet teaching and learning goals?
- What kind and degree of change can realistically be accomplished given the duration of an experience and students' baseline knowledge, skills, and attitudes?
- In what ways will students be expected to apply knowledge and skills or demonstrate habits of thinking and acting following an internationalized educational experience?

REFLECTING ON AND EVALUATING INTERNATIONALIZED EDUCATION

As Bender and Walker (2013) argued, internationalized experiences can foster "an often uncomfortable and troubling re-examination of deeply rooted beliefs" (p. e1029) within students. Yet, as Swartz (2007) noted, "there may well be great benefits for allowing some space in which it is possible for [students] to acknowledge a visceral but probably somewhat shameful experience" of feeling incompetent when engaging with diverse perspectives (p. 36). Therefore, it is important to create opportunities for students to debrief during and after internationalized learning experiences and for reflection to be part of evaluation processes.

Opportunities to reflect on learning (Aldrich, 2015) and process interpersonal interactions (Aldrich & Peters, 2019) have been core features of the internationalized learning experiences I have codesigned. My collaborators and I have asked students to reflect verbally through in-class discussions and process their understandings and questions through an anonymous written survey. Through these mechanisms, students have reflected on and shared what and how they learned, where they struggled, and what we ought to adjust in future internationalized experiences. Aside from qualitative reflections and evaluations, I have also used standardized questionnaires as pre- and postinteraction assessments to understand how internationalized learning may relate to students' development (Aldrich & Grajo, 2017).

Because internationalized education can have a number of aims, it can be evaluated in a number of ways. Evaluation can focus on student learning objectives, or it may measure the achievement of programmatic, departmental, or institutional goals (Green, 2012); in many internationalization efforts, it may make sense to evaluate both. The following questions can help educators identify which evaluation approaches might be most relevant for an international experience:

- Does the evaluation aim to assess students' content learning, knowledge application, or reflective habit development?
- Does the evaluation aim to assess the design or structure of the learning experience or compare it with other kinds of learning experience?

Table 11-2 illustrates sample approaches for evaluating students' learning and reflective development through internationalized educational experiences.

Table 11-2

APPROACHES FOR EVALUATING INTERNATIONALIZED EDUCATIONAL EXPERIENCES

PRIMARY OUTCOME	TOOLS/METHODS TO ASSESS OUTCOMES	EXAMPLES OF USE IN THE LITERATURE
Students' cultural sensitivity	• Cultural Sensitivity and Awareness Questionnaire (CASQ) (Cheung, Shah, & Muncer, 2002) • Intercultural Sensitivity Scale (ISS) (Chen & Starosta, 2000)	• Murden et al., 2008 (CASQ): study aimed to explore development of cultural awareness through classroom instruction • Wimpenny et al., 2016 (ISS): study aimed to understand shifts in cultural sensitivity following an internationalized online discussion module
Students' cultural competence	• Inventory for Assessing the Process of Cultural Competence Among Health Care Professionals—Student Version (IAPCC-SV; Campinha-Bacote, 2007) • Open-ended interviews • Quantitative surveys	• Sood et al., 2014 (IAPCC-SV): study aimed to explore the impact of an internationalized learning experience on students' cultural competence • Hyett et al., 2018 (interviews and quantitative surveys): study aimed to understand how an IaH intercultural learning activity facilitated cultural competency

continued

Table 11-2 (continued)

APPROACHES FOR EVALUATING INTERNATIONALIZED EDUCATIONAL EXPERIENCES

PRIMARY OUTCOME	TOOLS/METHODS TO ASSESS OUTCOMES	EXAMPLES OF USE IN THE LITERATURE
Students' multicultural desires	• Multicultural Experiences Questionnaire (MEQ; Narvaez, Endicott, & Hill, 2009)	• Aldrich & Grajo, 2017 (MEQ): study aimed to understand how the number of IaH experiences in a curriculum might influence students' multicultural desires
Students' content learning	• Qualitative surveys • Content analysis of audio/video class recordings • Content analysis of educational artifacts	• Aldrich & Peters, 2019 (qualitative survey): study aimed to understand what and how students learned through an IaH experience in relation to occupational justice • Cabatan & Grajo, 2017 (qualitative survey, educational artifacts): study aimed to understand how a pilot IaH experience facilitated learning about occupation and what teaching and learning strategies were most/least useful within the IaH experience • Aldrich & Johansson, 2015 (qualitative survey, audio analysis): study aimed to understand what and how students learned through an IaH experience

CONCLUSION

As the chapters in Section III illustrate, educators around the world are thinking innovatively about how to develop future occupational therapists. The occupational therapy students of today and tomorrow will practice, research, and teach in contexts where global perspectives are ever more relevant. Internationalization requires more than an interest in creating global connections; it necessitates embracing a range of educational norms and approaches, honoring a variety of cultural perspectives, and developing collaborations that benefit all parties involved. Although internationalization may not be appropriate for every learning outcome in educational programs, it can help develop students' dispositions, appraisal abilities, and practice approaches in ways that build bridges, celebrate diversity, and reinforce the need for criticality and equity within occupational therapy.

Implications for Occupational Therapy Education

- Internationalizing occupational therapy education can take many forms, all of which requires dedication, time, intention, and openness from faculty and students. Educators planning on integrating internationalization activities must be explicit about learning objectives and expected outcomes of the activity.
- International educational partnerships must incorporate opportunities for meaningful student and faculty reflection and evaluation.
- Students' and faculty members' baseline understandings, as well as programmatic and professional competency expectations, must inform the development of international educational experiences.

Key Reflection Questions

1. After reading this chapter, what element(s) of your course(s) or curriculum might be appropriate for internationalization?
2. Given existing infrastructure, what kind of internationalization (IoC or IaH) is most realistic in your educational setting?
3. What partnerships can you build or leverage to internationalize your course or curriculum?

What led you to become an occupational therapy educator?

I have known for most of my life that I wanted to be an educator, thanks to several inspiring teachers who encouraged and stimulated my love of learning and thirst for knowledge. When I discovered occupational science and occupational therapy, I knew I had found my intellectual and professional home, and I felt compelled to accompany others as they discovered their passions within the discipline and profession. As an educator, I want to help students develop dispositions toward lifelong learning, critical questioning, and engagement with the complexity of the world. In short, I hope to help students answer a question that the late Dr. Dallas Willard once asked me and my classmates, "What makes you rub your mental tummy and say, 'Ahh'?"

Rebecca M. Aldrich, PhD, OTR/L

REFERENCES

Accreditation Council for Occupational Therapy Education. (2017). 2011 ACOTE standards and interpretive guide: 2017 interpretive guide version. Retrieved from https://www.aota.org/~/media/Corporate/Files/EducationCareers/Accredit/Standards/2011-Standards-and-Interpretive-Guide.pdf

Aldrich, R. (2015). Course redesign to promote local and global experiential learning about human occupation: Description and evaluation of a pilot effort. *South African Journal of Occupational Therapy, 45*(1), 56-62.

Aldrich, R., & Johansson, K. (2015). U.S. and Swedish student learning via online synchronous international interactions. *American Journal of Occupational Therapy, 69*(Suppl. 2), 1-5. doi: 10.5014/ajot.2015.018424

Aldrich, R., & Peters, L. (2019). Using occupational justice as a "linchpin" of international educational collaborations. *American Journal of Occupational Therapy, 73*(3), 7303205100p1-7303205100p10. doi: 10.5014/ajot.2019.029744

Aldrich, R. M., & Grajo, L. C. (2017). International educational interactions and students' critical consciousness: A pilot study. *American Journal of Occupational Therapy, 71*, 7105230020p1-7105230020p10. doi:10.5014/ajot.2017.026724

Asher, A., Estes, J., & Hill, V. (2014). International outreach from the comfort of your classroom! *Educational Special Interest Section Quarterly, 24*(4), 1-4.

Awaad, T. (2003). Culture, cultural competency, and occupational therapy: A review of the literature. *British Journal of Occupational Therapy, 66*, 356-362. doi:10.1177/030802260306600804

Beagan, B. L. (2016). Approaches to culture and diversity: A critical synthesis of occupational therapy literature. *Canadian Journal of Occupational Therapy, 82*(5), 272-282. doi:10.1177/0008417414567530

Bender, A., & Walker, P. (2013). The obligation of debriefing in global health education. *Medical Teacher, 35*, e1027-e1034. doi:10.8019/0142159X.2012.733449

Black, R. M. (2016). The changing language of cross-cultural practice. In S. A. Wells, R. M. Black, & J. Gupta (Eds.), *Culture and occupation: Effectiveness for occupational therapy practice, education, and research* (3rd ed., pp. 51-61). Bethesda, MD: AOTA Press.

Brown, E. V. D., Muñoz, J. P., & Powell, J. M. (2011). Multicultural training in the United States: A survey of occupational therapy programs. *Occupational Therapy in Health Care, 24*(2-3), 178-193. doi:10.3109/07380577.2011.560240

Cabatan, M. C. C., & Grajo, L. C. (2017). Internationalization in an occupational therapy curriculum: A Philippine-American pilot collaboration. *American Journal of Occupational Therapy, 71*, 1-9. doi:10.5014/ajot.2017.024653

Campinha-Bacote, J. (2007). *Inventory for assessing the process of cultural competence among healthcare professionals–student version (IAPCC-SV)*. Cincinnati, OH: Transcultural C.A.R.E Associates.

Chen, G. M., & Starosta, W. J. (2000). The development and validation of the intercultural sensitivity scale. *Human Communication, 3*, 1-15.

Cheung, Y., Shah, S., & Muncer, S. (2002). An exploratory investigation of undergraduate students' perception of cultural awareness. *British Journal of Occupational Therapy, 65*(12), 543-550. doi:10.1177/030802260206501203

Cipriani, J. (2017). Integration of international service learning in developing countries with occupational therapy education: Process and implications. *Occupational Therapy in Health Care, 31*(1), 61-71. doi:10.1080/07380577.2016.1244734

Dsouza, S., Galvaan, R., & Ramugondo, E. (2017). *Concepts in occupational therapy: Understanding Southern perspectives*. Karnataka, India: Manipal University Press.

Elliot, M. L. (2015). Critical ethnographic analysis of "doing good" on short-term international immersion experiences. *Occupational Therapy International, 22*(3), 121-130.

Foronda, C. L. (2008). A concept analysis of cultural sensitivity. *Journal of Transcultural Nursing, 19*(3), 207-212. doi:10.1177/1043659508317093

Foronda, C. L., Baptiste, D.-L., Reinholdt, M. M., & Ousman, K. (2016). Cultural humility: A concept analysis. *Journal of Transcultural Nursing, 27*(3), 210-217. doi:10.1177/1043659615592677

Gerlach, A. J. (2016). Shifting our gaze: Thinking critically about 'culture'. *Israeli Journal of Occupation Therapy, 25*(4), E92-E107.

Grajo, L. C., & Aldrich, R. M. (2016, January 18). Cross-cultural learning experiences: Using international collaborations as an educational tool. *OT Practice, 21*(1), 13-16.

Green, M. F. (2012). Measuring and assessing internationalization. *NAFSA: Association of International Educators*. Retrieved from http://www.usask.ca/secretariat/governing-bodies/council/committee/international/reports-archive/NAFSAMeasuringInternationalization.pdf

Hammell, K. W. (2011). Resisting theoretical imperialism in the disciplines of occupational science and occupational therapy. *British Journal of Occupational Therapy, 74*(1), 27-33. doi:10/4276/030802211X12947686093602

Hammell, K. W. (2013). Occupation, well-being, and culture: Theory and cultural humility. *Canadian Journal of Occupational Therapy, 80*(4), 224-234. doi:10.1177/0008417413500465

Hammell, K. W. (2015). Respecting global wisdom: Enhancing the cultural relevance of occupational therapy's theoretical base. *British Journal of Occupational Therapy, 78*(11), 718-721. doi:10.1177/0308022614564170

Horton, A. (2009). Internationalising occupational therapy education. *British Journal of Occupational Therapy, 72*(5), 227-230.

Humbert, T. K., Burket, A., Deveney, R., & Kennedy, K. (2012). Occupational therapy students' perspectives regarding international cross-cultural experiences. *Australian Occupational Therapy Journal, 59*, 225-234. doi:10.1111/j.1440-1630.2011.00987.x

Hyett, N., Lee, K. M., Knevel, R., Fortune, T., Yau, M. K., & Borkovic, S. (2018). Trialing virtual intercultural learning with Australian and Hong Kong allied health students to improve cultural competency. *Journal of Studies in International Education, 23*(3), 389-406. doi:10.1177/1028315318786442

Iwama, M. (2007). Culture and occupational therapy: Meeting the challenge of relevance in a global world. *Occupational Therapy International, 14*(4), 183-187.

Kantartzis, S., & Molineux, M. (2011). The influence of Western society's construction of a healthy daily life on the conceptualization of occupation. *Journal of Occupational Science, 18*(1), 62-80. doi:10.1080/14427591.2011.566917

Kinsella, E. A., Bossers, A., & Ferreira, D. (2008). Enablers and challenges to international practice education: A case study. *Learning in Health and Social Care, 7*(2), 79-82. doi:10.1111/j.1473-6861.2008.00178.x

Kirkham, S. R., van Hofwegen, L., & Pankratz, D. (2009). Keeping the vision: Sustaining social consciousness with nursing students following international learning experiences. *International Journal of Nursing Education Scholarship, 6*(1), 1-16. doi:10.2202/1548-923X.1635

Kumagai, A. K., & Lypson, M. (2009). Beyond cultural competence: Critical consciousness, social justice, and multicultural education. *Academic Medicine, 84*(6), 782-787. doi:10.1097/ACM.0b013e3181a42398

Metzl, J. M., & Hansen, H. (2014). Structural competency: Theorizing a new medical engagement with stigma and inequality. *Social Science & Medicine, 103*, 126-133. doi:10.1016/j.socscimed.2013.06.032

Murden, R., Norman, A., Ross, J., Sturdivant, E., Kedia, M., & Shah, S. (2008). Occupational therapy students' perceptions of their cultural awareness and competency. *Occupational Therapy International, 15*(3), 191-203. doi:10.1002/oti.253

Nagarajan, S., & McAllister, L. (2015). Internationalisation of curriculum at home: Imperatives, opportunities and challenges for allied health education. *Journal of Teaching and Learning for Graduate Employability, 6*(1), 88-99.

Narvaez, D., Endicott, L., & Hill, P. (2009). *Guide for using the Multicultural Experiences Questionnaire (MEQ): For college students and adults.* Notre Dame, IN: Moral Psychology Laboratory, University of Notre Dame.

Shimmel, L., Al-Helo, H., Demille, K., Kandel-Lieberman, D., Kremenovic, M., Roorda, K., ... Baptiste, S. (2016). Targeting the globe: Internationalisation in occupational therapy education. *World Federation of Occupational Therapists Bulletin, 71*(1), 16-23. doi:10.1080/14473828.2016.1149980

Sim, I., & Mackenzie, L. (2016). Graduate perspectives of fieldwork placements in developing countries: Contributions to occupational therapy practice. *Australian Occupational Therapy Journal, 63*, 244-256. doi:10.1111/1440-1630.12282

Sood, D., Cepa, D., Dsouza, S., Saha, S., Aikat, R., & Tuuk, A. (2014). Impact of international collaborative project on cultural competence among occupational therapy students. *The Open Journal of Occupational Therapy, 2*(3), 1-18. doi:10.15453/2168-6408.1111

Swartz, L. (2007). The virtues of feeling culturally incompetent. *Monash Bioethics Review, 26*(4), 36-46.

Wells, S. A., Black, R. M., & Gupta, J. (2016). *Culture and occupation: Effectiveness for occupational therapy practice, education, and research* (3rd ed.). Bethesda, MD: AOTA Press.

Wimpenny, K., Lewis, L., Roe, S., Désiron, H., Gordon, I., & Waters, S. (2016). Preparation for an uncertain world: international curriculum development for mental health occupational therapy. *World Federation of Occupational Therapists Bulletin, 72*(1), 5-15. doi:10.1080/14473828.2016.1161960

12

Perspectives on Occupational Therapy Education in Southeast Asia

*Maria Concepcion Cabatan, MHPEd, OTRP, OTR, FPAOT
and R. Lyle Duque, MSc, OTRP, FPAOT*

Chapter Objectives

By the end of this chapter, the reader will be able to:

1. Critically examine the impact of the beginnings of occupational therapy in Southeast Asia on its present and future.
2. Present a comprehensive and in-depth picture of occupational therapy education in Southeast Asia through the integration of information regarding the evolving historical, political, economic, and educational landscapes within which it exists.
3. Create visions of possible futures for occupational therapy in Southeast Asia as influenced by social, political, and economic, and educational trends in the region.

SHARED BEGINNINGS FROM THE WEST

The development of occupational therapy education in Southeast Asia (SEA) shares a common heritage—that of being spurred largely by the needs of survivors of World War II and being imported from the West. In most SEA countries, occupational therapy education programs were established by returning occupational therapists educated in the West or foreign occupational therapists who were part of a program by a government or nongovernment agency (e.g., the U.K. Colombo Plan and Peace Corps). Because of differences in educational and regulatory laws in each country, exit award levels (i.e., diploma vs bachelor's) differed (Table 12-1). The "Western origin" of occupational therapy and differences in award levels would have far-reaching implications on the development of occupational therapy education as well as the harmonization and mutual recognition of credentials in the region (discussed later in the chapter).

The Philippines exemplifies this developmental trajectory. The University of the Philippines Manila—College of Allied Medical Professions (formerly known as the School of Allied Medical Professions) opened in 1962, offering a bachelor of science in occupational therapy (BSOT) degree

Taff, S. D., Grajo, L. C., & Hooper, B. R. (Eds.). *Perspectives on Occupational Therapy Education: Past, Present, and Future* (pp. 143-151).

Table 12-1				
DEVELOPMENT OF OCCUPATIONAL THERAPY EDUCATION IN SOUTHEAST ASIA				
1960s	1970s	1980s	1990s	2000 (ONWARD)
First occupational therapy education program opened in the Philippines (bachelor's program)	Setting up occupational therapy practice in hospitals and establishment of the Occupational Therapy Association of the Philippines	Occupational therapy programs opened in Malaysia (diploma) and Thailand (bachelor's)	Occupational therapy programs opened in Malaysia and Thailand (both diploma programs)	Program in Singapore transitioned into a bachelor's degree (2016); second program in Thailand opens (2007) and gets WFOT approval; postprofessional master programs opens in the Philippines (2014); first bachelor's degree in Malaysia opens (2004)

(Bondoc, 2005). Two U.S. educated practitioners, Charlotte Floro and Conchita Abad, developed the curriculum and got it approved by the World Federation of Occupational Therapists (WFOT) in 1968 (Bondoc, 2005).

AN EVOLVING PAST

Current occupational therapy education in SEA can be viewed as part of an evolving past—a narrative that revolves around upgrading of education programs and faculty qualifications, managing the challenges of migration, and the Association of Southeast Asian Nations (ASEAN) context of collaborations.

Upgrading of Education Programs

It can be argued that the revolution in occupational therapy education leading to the upgrading of programs was instigated mainly by two factors: the profession's "refocusing" on occupation and the move to higher entry-level qualifications.

The 2002 version of the Minimum Standards for the Education of Occupational Therapists (WFOT, 2002) underscored the need for occupation therapy education programs to have occupation as the central focus and be relevant to local health needs (Carswell, 2009). It provided the impetus for educational programs to revisit and redesign their curricula to be more occupation based. This increased emphasis on occupation internationally led to a profound examination of what "occupation" meant for the different people in SEA, resulting in an "occupational revolution" (Duque, 2005). Ensuing changes included curricular revisions and innovations (Coronel & Cabatan, 2007), the melding of occupational therapy concepts with local practices and concepts (Satiansukpong, Pongsaksri, & Sasat, 2016), collaborations between occupational therapists in SEA and those from other world regions (Coppola, 2009; Hocking, Wright-St. Clair, & Bunrayong, 2002), and an examination of the validity of assessment approaches from the West in the Asian context (Chan, Ng, & Chan,

2014). The 2016 version of the Minimum Standards for the Education of Occupational Therapists (WFOT, 2016) continues to drive further changes in both policies and curricula (Commission on Higher Education, 2017).

The transition to higher entry-level qualifications was a response to both an evolving educational landscape and a changing employment market requirement, particularly in the United States and Canada—two major destinations for migrating occupational therapists from SEA. There was growing recognition of the importance for occupational therapists to be ready for postgraduate education and have entry-level qualifications that were on par with similar health professions (WFOT, 2018). Postprofessional programs have likewise been developed (e.g., the Philippines) to produce a cadre of practitioners ready to engage in research, assume leadership positions, and develop more specialized practice (Table 12-2).

Evolving student demographics impact the development of occupational therapy education as well. In general, students in SEA enter college immediately after secondary school. The relatively young age (typically 16 or 17 years) and technology-savvy culture (e.g., social media) of SEA students may prove pivotal in shifting pedagogical practices. Face-to-face lectures are still common, but with current technology, the use of blended learning and flipped classrooms are emerging. There is increased engagement of occupational therapy students in professional activities such as attendance in national and international conferences and participation in global initiatives (e.g., World Occupational Therapy Day and Global Day of Service), indicating early exposure to research, service, and scholarship. Virtual interactions using social media platforms between students from different cultures to promote cultural competence and broaden worldviews are becoming popular (Cabatan & Grajo, 2017).

Practice placements, although mostly still in traditional settings such as hospitals, clinics, and schools, are expanding to include emerging and innovative areas of practice, such as exposure to work in professional associations (e.g., the Philippine Academy of Occupational Therapists internship program) and international exchange of students (e.g., 6-week placement at University of Alberta in Indonesia). Innovative models of student supervision are likewise being explored to address the issue of limited faculty.

Upgrading faculty qualifications continue to be a challenge for many education programs. Because of the lack of qualified faculty, as well as legal and regulatory constraints, among other factors, it has taken decades for Malaysia and Singapore to develop their bachelor's programs. A number of occupational therapy educators in these countries pursued higher degrees in occupational therapy or other disciplines locally or abroad (e.g., Australia and Hong Kong; Yang, Shek, Tsunaka, & Lim, 2006). After earning their advanced degrees, they came back and led the transformation of the transformation of education and practice in their respective countries. In certain instances, such as in the Philippines, it has been observed by the authors that a majority of those who left chose to stay abroad, whereas those who came back often did not pursue a career in the academe. An interesting recent development in the Philippines is that practitioners and academicians who have retired or are close to retirement abroad have expressed willingness to assist in the development of new programs or the strengthening of existing ones.

Challenges Due to Migration

International labor markets influenced and continue to influence the development of occupational therapy practice and education in SEA. For example, in the late 1980s to the 1990s, the huge demand for therapists in other regions of the world, particularly in the United States, the United Kingdom, and Australia, resulted in a marked increase in student enrollment in the Philippines. During this time, there were as many as 30 programs in the country. In the same period, the acute migration of Filipino occupational therapists to other countries resulted in a high turnover of practitioners and educators. Those who opted to stay were often stretched thin because they had to take on multiple roles, including teaching and leadership roles in their institutions, the national professional association, and regulatory body. This slowed the development of occupational therapy practice and education in the Philippines, resulting in a lack of advanced occupational therapy programs and

Table 12-2

PROFILE OF OCCUPATIONAL THERAPY EDUCATION IN SOUTHEAST ASIAN COUNTRIES

COUNTRY	YEAR FIRST OCCUPATIONAL THERAPY EDUCATION PROGRAM OPENED	WHO INTRODUCED OCCUPATIONAL THERAPY EDUCATION?	CURRENT NUMBER OF EDUCATION PROGRAMS	CURRENT NUMBER OF WORLD FEDERATION OF OCCUPATIONAL THERAPISTS APPROVED PROGRAMS	OCCUPATIONAL THERAPY DEGREES CONFERRED
Indonesia	1994	Australian- and New Zealand-trained Indonesian occupational therapists	2	1	Diploma and bachelor's
Malaysia	1984	British-trained Malaysian occupational therapist	6	4	Diploma and bachelor's
Philippines	1962	U.S.-trained Filipino occupational therapists	21	6	Bachelor's, postprofessional master's
Singapore	1992	British and Australian occupational therapists	1	1	Bachelor's (beginning 2016; prior diploma)
Thailand	1981	U.S. trained occupational therapists	2	2	Bachelor's

ASEAN member countries without occupational therapy education programs: Brunei Darussalam, Cambodia, Laos, Myanmar, and Vietnam.
Adapted from Santoso, T. B. (2016). The development of occupational therapy in Indonesia. *World Federation of Occupational Therapists Bulletin, 43*(1), 42-43. doi:1
0.1080/20566077.2001.1180026; Malaysian Occupational Therapy Educational Institution Training History. (n.d.). Retrieved from http://www.ot-malaysia.my/history/;
Philippine Commission on Higher Education Data Manager (personal communication, October 30, 2017); Singapore Association of Occupational Therapists. (n.d.).
Occupational therapy education in Singapore. Retrieved from https://www.saot.org.sg/ot-education; and World Federation of Occupational Therapists. (2017). *WFOT
list of recognized entry level OT educational programs, 2017*. Retrieved from https://www.wfot.org/programmes/education/wfot-approved-education-programmes

inequitable distribution of therapists in the country (Duque & De Leon, 2006). Today, migration continues, albeit at a slower pace. Although demand for occupational therapists in many Western countries (e.g., the United States) is still high, higher entry-level requirements in these countries have somewhat stemmed the exodus of occupational therapists from SEA. However, other regions such as the Middle East have opened up employment opportunities (Lorenzo, Dela Rosa, Ronquillo, Mercado, & Villegas, 2012).

The Association of Southeast Asian Nations Context of Regional Integration and Collaborations

An important development in the region is the ASEAN regional integration, which includes the harmonization of higher education institutions (HEIs) to encourage student mobility, address human resource needs for socioeconomic development, and promote academic, research, and cultural collaborations (Sirat, 2017). One effort toward harmonization is the ASEAN Qualifications Reference Framework (AQRF; Association of Southeast Asian Nations Secretariat, 2014). The AQRF enables the comparison of qualifications across national frameworks. It provides a mechanism for facilitating the mobility of skilled persons in the region, in the process addressing human resource gaps and enriching the professions through the exchange of ideas and resources.

The ASEAN regional integration can be viewed as a platform for education programs to forge partnerships to address higher education challenges, such as shortage of qualified faculty, need to improve instructional quality, and financial constraints for lower- and middle-income countries (Asian Development Bank, 2011). The ASEAN University Network is an initiative aimed at promoting cooperation and collaboration, currently largely through faculty and student visits (Rezasyah, Konety, Rifawan, & Wardhana, 2017). Of the 30 member universities of the ASEAN University Network, five (Chang-Mai University and Mahidol University [Thailand], National University of Malaysia [Malaysia], and De La Salle University and University of the Philippines [Philippines]) offer an occupational therapy education program.

Based on an examination of patterns of academic/research collaborations of 16 ASEAN universities, Sirat (2017) found that collaborations between HEIs within SEA were confined to select countries such as Malaysia, Indonesia, Thailand, and Singapore. There was also a predilection toward academic/research collaborations with HEIs in East Asian countries (e.g., Japan, China, and South Korea), North America, and Europe (Sirat, 2017). Although Sirat's study did not identify specific disciplines, it can be inferred that collaborations, specifically in teaching and research, among occupational therapy education programs in ASEAN have not yet been realized and optimized.

Several challenges to the implementation of the AQRF in particular (Table 12-1) and regional integration in general remain. So far, mutual recognition agreements have been established for only eight professions (e.g., architecture, engineering, and nursing), and there have been no observed large-scale movements of these professionals (Fukunaga, 2015).

THE FUTURE FOR SOUTHEAST ASIA: OCCUPATION, INNOVATION, LEADERSHIP, AND INTEGRATION

The challenge for occupational therapy education in SEA is two-fold: (1) ensuring the continuing relevance and influence of programs on occupational therapy practice, scholarship, policy development, social welfare, and health care delivery, and (2) producing a critical mass of practitioners to meet the diverse and evolving needs of both the profession and society. It can be argued that meeting this challenge largely rests with compelling educator leaders. Educator leaders are key persons who are not just intellectually sophisticated but also are politically savvy and serve as an inspiration and model to their students and peers. With competition for recognition and limited resources within

Table 12-1

Constraints on Implementation of the ASEAN Qualification Reference Framework

- Uneven degrees of development of education programs across Southeast Asian countries
- Lack of comprehensive understanding of the nature and processes of the framework by occupational therapy leaders
- Lack of stature of the profession at the national policy level
- Legal and regulatory limitations/constraints

and outside the academe becoming more intense, and issues impacting education and practice becoming more varied and complex, educator leaders are key to the survival of occupational therapy education programs.

There is a global recognition of the scarcity of health professionals (Global Health Workers Alliance, 2008; WFOT, 2018; World Health Organization, 2017). This requires occupational therapy education to respond both quantitatively and qualitatively, producing a critical number of not only clinicians but also educators, researchers, entrepreneurs, and leader advocates.

Furthermore, it is not enough for education programs to be simply responsive to changing educational, political, regulatory, practice, and socioeconomic landscapes; they need to demonstrate leadership. Occupational therapy academic departments need to demonstrate leadership and excellence, not just in teaching, research, and extension/community services but also in policy and program development. In order to fulfill all these functions, education programs need sufficient resources. However, resources within the academe are becoming more rationalized. To tap into more resources that may be outside the university and the profession, curricula must align not just with the priorities of the profession but also with the thrusts of relevant government institutions and other stakeholders (e.g., World Health Organization and funding agencies). Competencies aligned with national and international priorities—such as those related to disaster risk reduction and response, occupational therapy for persons displaced by war and other geopolitical tensions, utilization of research to inform clinical practice, cultural competence, interprofessional education and practice, and establishing practice in areas where the profession does not currently exist, such as health and wellness programs—need to be increasingly represented in curricula.

Furthermore, collaboration with other disciplines can facilitate access to more resources. Educator leaders should position occupational therapy to influence the direction of educational policies at all levels and relevant areas (e.g., education, health, social welfare, and justice system). Advanced degrees are needed to develop educator leaders who will advance scholarship and compelling leadership to move occupational therapy forward as an academic discipline in the region.

Practice placement in emerging areas of practice (e.g., community centers for the elderly, local health units, and organizational and leadership positions) need to be developed and strengthened to prepare students to work in diverse settings and broaden their worldviews on health care and social welfare systems. Practice placement should serve as an impetus for graduates to develop competencies that will enable them to become pioneers in areas/settings/countries where occupational therapy is just starting or does not yet exist (e.g., in rural areas or countries like Vietnam). This will be a way of addressing the problem of inequitable access to occupational therapy services.

Harnessing the potentials of technology to facilitate learning and make graduate education more accessible is an important consideration. This positions programs to connect better with the changing student demographics and culture, while at the same time expanding teaching-learning strategies and addressing each country's health human resource needs.

Finally, in order to contribute to the ASEAN regional integration and harness its potentials, occupational therapy education programs need to work collaboratively. As Duque (2016) asserted, "working together is crucial, if not imperative, in contexts where resources are scarce, and the stakes high; and where the socio-cultural, economic, educational and political landscapes continually evolve" (p. 13). Several areas of collaboration and resource sharing between programs exist, such as curriculum and instruction, faculty and student exchange, practice placement education, and research and technology.

CONCLUSION

This chapter has shown that, as in the past, the development of occupational therapy education (and consequently practice) in SEA rests on strong leadership and collaborative effort. To move the profession forward, educator leaders need to focus on both the quantity and quality of their graduates. The opportunity and challenge offered by ASEAN regional integration needs to be recognized, addressed, and harnessed. It is by learning from the developmental trajectory of occupational therapy education in SEA that we can assure the continuing relevance, influence, and advancement of occupational therapy scholarship.

Implications for Occupational Therapy Education

Occupational therapy education in SEA needs to:

- Be led by educator leaders who will strategically position the profession within and beyond their educational institutions to influence policies.
- Ensure continuing evolution of curricula to keep it relevant vis-à-vis the needs of society and national and regional health and social welfare goals and priorities.
- Produce a critical mass of practitioners who are ready to take on and develop diverse roles to address society's occupational needs.
- Increase and expand collaborations among education programs to enrich curricula and upgrade faculty credentials.

Key Reflection Questions

1. How do you think lessons learned from the establishment of occupational therapy programs in SEA can inform or influence the development of programs in other countries or regions of the world? Alternatively, given these insights, what factors would you consider crucial if you were to assist with developing an education program in this region of the world?

2. Aside from those identified in this chapter, what other challenges to occupational therapy education do you see in SEA or in other regions where occupational therapy is in its infancy?

3. How can programs from SEA and your part of the world collaborate? What are the most feasible areas of collaboration?

What led you to become an occupational therapy educator?

I was lured to the academe for its relative freedom, flexibility, and collegial environment. It is also a privilege and joy to engage with young people and to have intellectual discussions with peers.

Maria Concepcion Cabatan, MHPEd, OTRP, OTR, FPAOT

I suppose it was serendipity. I never imagined that I would become passionate about teaching until I was invited to be a member of the faculty by a former professor.

R. Lyle Duque, MSc, OTRP, FPAOT

REFERENCES

Asian Development Bank. (2011). *Higher education across Asia: An overview of issues and strategies.* Mandaluyong City, Philippines: Author.

Association of Southeast Asian Nations Secretariat. (2014). *ASEAN qualifications reference framework.* Jakarta, Indonesia: Author.

Bondoc, S. (2005). Occupational therapy in the Philippines: From founding years to the present. *Philippine Journal of Occupational Therapy, 1*(1), 9-22.

Cabatan, M. C., & Grajo, L. C. (2017). Centennial topics—Internationalization in an occupational therapy curriculum: A Philippine–American pilot collaboration. *American Journal of Occupational Therapy, 71,* 7106100010. doi:10.5014/ajot.2017.024653

Carswell, A. (2009). Minimum standards for the education of occupational therapists: Building occupational therapy communities in WFOT member countries. *Asian Journal of Occupational Therapy, 7,* 23-26.

Chan, P., Ng, S., & Chan, D. (2014). Psychometric properties of the Chinese version of the Kid-KINDLR Questionnaire for the measuring of the health-related quality of life of school-aged children. *Hong Kong Journal of Occupational Therapy, 24*(1), 28-34. doi:10.1016/j.hkjot.2014.05.001

Commission on Higher Education. (2017). *Policies, standards, and guidelines for the Bachelor of Science in Occupational Therapy Education (BSOT) program* (CMO No. 52, Series of 2017). Retrieved from https://ched.gov.ph/wp-content/uploads/2018/04/CMO-No.-52-Series-of-2017-Policies-Standards-and-Guidelines-for-the-Bachelor-of-Science-in-Occupational-Therapy-Education-BSOT-Program.pdf

Coppola, S. (2009). Thailand University collaborations. Retrieved from https://docplayer.net/4642445-Thailand-university-collaborations-s-coppola-2009.html

Coronel, C. M., & Cabatan, M.C. (2007). Curriculum redesign—The UP Manila experience. *Philippine Journal of Occupational Therapy, 3,* 20-31.

Duque, R. L. (2005). *A grounded theory of occupation from a Filipino perspective* (Unpublished master's thesis). University of Plymouth, Plymouth, UK.

Duque, R. L. (2016). Tsuyoshi Sato Lecture Award: Bayanihan: Doing together, achieving together. *New Zealand Journal of Occupational Therapy, 63,* 15-19.

Duque, R. L., & De Leon, C. (2006). Occupational therapy in the Philippines: Where have we been and where are we headed? *Philippine Journal of Occupational Therapy, 1*(2), 57-67.

Fukunaga, Y. (2015). Assessing the progress of ASEAN MRAS on professional services. *ERIA Discussion Paper, 21,* 1-43. Retrieved from http://www.eria.org/ERIA-DP-2015-21.pdf

Global Health Workers Alliance. (2008). Health workers for all and all for health workers: An agenda for global action. Retrieved from http://www.who.int/workforcealliance/forum/1_agenda4GAction_final.pdf

Hocking, C., Wright-St. Clair, V., & Bunrayong, W. (2002). The meaning of cooking and recipe work for older Thai women and New Zealand Women. *Journal of Occupational Science, 9,* 117-127.

Lorenzo, F., Dela Rosa, J., Ronquillo, K., Mercado, R., & Villegas, S. (2012). *Philippines Mobility of Health Professionals.* Manila, Philippines: Institute of Health Policy and Development Studies, National Institutes of Health, University of the Philippines Manila.

Malaysian Occupational Therapy Educational Institution Training History. (n.d.). Retrieved from http://www.ot-malaysia.my/history/

Rezasyah, T., Konety, N., Rifawan, A., & Wardhana, W. (2017). Higher education integration in the ASEAN: ASEAN University Network Case. *Journal of ASEAN Studies, 5*(1), 51-59. doi:10.21512/jas.v5i1.962

Satiansukpong, N., Pongsaksri, M., & Sasat, D. (2016). Thai elephant-assisted therapy programme in children with Down syndrome. *Occupational Therapy International, 2,* 121-131.

Singapore Association of Occupational Therapists. (n.d.). *Occupational therapy education in Singapore.* Retrieved from https://www.saot.org.sg/ot-education

Santoso, T. B. (2016). The development of occupational therapy in Indonesia. *World Federation of Occupational Therapists Bulletin, 43*(1), 42-43. doi:10.1080/20566077.2001.11800266

Sirat, M. (2017). ASEAN's flagship universities and regional integration initiatives. *Higher Education Evaluation and Development, 11*(2), 68-80. doi:10.1108/HEED-07-2017-0004

World Federation of Occupational Therapists. (2002). *Revised Minimum Standards for the Education of Occupational Therapists 2002.* Perth, Western Australia: Author.

World Federation of Occupational Therapists. (2016). *Minimum standards for the education of occupational therapists.* Australia: Author.

World Federation of Occupational Therapists. (2017). WFOT list of recognized entry level OT educational programs, 2017. Retrieved from https://www.wfot.org/programmes/education/wfot-approved-education-programmes

World Federation of Occupational Therapists. (2018). Human resources project. Retrieved from www.wfot.org/ResourceCenter

World Health Organization. (2017). Rehabilitation 2030: A call for action. Retrieved from http://www.who.int/disabilities/care/Rehab2030MeetingReport_plain_text_version.pdf

Yang, S., Shek, M. P., Tsunaka, M., & Lim, H. B. (2006). Cultural influences on occupational therapy practice in Singapore: a pilot study. *Occupational Therapy International, 13*(3), 176-192. doi:10.1002/oti.217

13

Perspectives on Occupational Therapy Education in South America
Case of Brazil

Daniel Marinho Cezar da Cruz, PhD, OT;
Mirela de Oliveira Figueiredo, OT, PhD;
and Maria Luísa Guillaumon Emmel, OT, PhD

Chapter Objectives

By the end of this chapter, the reader will be able to:
1. Describe a brief history of occupational therapy in Brazil from 1956 to the present.
2. Describe how occupational therapy education and practice have changed in Brazil over the years.
3. Identify the challenges in occupational therapy training in Brazil.

South America encompasses the southern portion of the Americas with an area of 8,515,759,090 km², comprising 12% of the Earth's surface and 6% of the world's population (Instituto Brasileiro de Geografia e Estatistica, 2018). Brazil is the most influential country in South America with its growing economic power and a highly diverse population, including indigenous Americans, descendants of African slaves, and European settlers (British Broadcasting Corporation [BBC], 2017). It has deep social inequalities, including a wide gap between the rich and poor, despite improvements in recent decades with the objective of reducing poverty (BBC, 2017; Paim, Travassos, Almeida, Bahia, & Macinko, 2011). Advances in the health field include investments in human resources, science and technology, and primary health care (Paim et al., 2011).

Brazil currently represents half the population and gross domestic product of South America (Schenoni, 2015), with the city of São Paulo having almost 21 million inhabitants and being the most populous of all metropolitan regions in South America. Its demographic profile between 1950 and 2050 with estimated values by age indicates a growth in the population over 65 years as well as reduced fertility, increased life expectancy at birth, and decreased mortality below 5 years of age (United Nations, 2017).

These demographics pose certain challenges for health and education. Poverty associated with aging has important implications for the health of the population, including access to health services

Taff, S. D., Grajo, L. C., & Hooper, B. R. (Eds.). *Perspectives on Occupational Therapy Education: Past, Present, and Future* (pp 153-158).
© 2020 Taylor & Francis Group.

and diminished participation in important activities such as work, study, leisure, and taking care of themselves and others. Therefore, public health constitutes a vast and challenging field of interventions for occupational therapy. This chapter describes the history of occupational therapy education in Brazil and discusses current issues, and future perspectives, opportunities, and challenges.

THE OCCUPATIONAL THERAPY UNDERGRADUATE PROGRAM IN BRAZIL

Occupational therapy in Brazil did not result from the need for rehabilitation, unlike in North America and Europe, where it occurred as a result of the two World Wars. Rather, occupational therapy was one of the professions recommended by the United Nations Organization; the International Labor Organization; and the United Nations Educational, Scientific and Cultural Organization to be deployed in Latin America following the international movement of rehabilitation (Drummond & Cruz, 2018; Emmel, Cruz, & Figueiredo, 2015; Soares, 1991).

Technical training in occupational therapy (i.e., training focused on the application of methods and techniques) responded most directly to the societal needs at that time, such as the poliomyelitis epidemic and the rehabilitation of workers who suffered accidents at work, but these approaches were distinct from public policies and social and economic issues of the clients assisted by the occupational therapists (Emmel & Lancman, 1998, 2003; Soares, 1991).

Until 1968, occupational therapy was not recognized by the Ministry of Education of the Brazilian government as a higher education program because it was a 2-year technical course centered on training in some methods and techniques for interventions in physical rehabilitation and mental health. In this modality, the professional was dependent on the physician, who was the one directing and controlling the work that the occupational therapists should perform.

The first set of occupational therapists in Brazil were required to adapt the profession to their needs and demands and the inequalities present in the Brazilian context, such as poverty, unemployment, and low levels of education (Barros & Oliver, 2003; Drummond & Cruz, 2018; Emmel & Lancman, 1998, 2003). Thus, changes ensued in the Brazilian curriculum of occupational therapy education. By 1969, occupational therapy began to be recognized as a higher educational degree. The first occupational therapy program was offered at the University of São Paulo, with a course duration of 2160 hours to be completed in 3 academic years (Emmel & Lancman, 1998, 2003). From 1969 until the end of the 1970s, training was focused only on professional practice in physical rehabilitation, with limited possibilities for any other area of practice or research generation. This training proved to be insufficient to meet the demands of the labor market, which led professionals to seek improvement and specialization courses through certification, such as the Bobath method, sensory integration, hand therapy, and upper extremity rehabilitation (Lopes, 1991; Soares, 1991).

Between the 1970s and 1980s, the concept of health was broadened; the understanding of health evolved from the absence of disease to the pursuit of quality of life—a more humanitarian and preventative approach. Consequently, occupational therapy expanded to other work areas and fields of practice as well, such as psychosocial occupational therapy, gerontology, and intervention for people without disabilities through the knowledge of the potential of human occupation by understanding people's doing from a developmental perspective. At the same time, occupational therapists began to join multidisciplinary teams by working in therapeutic communities in mental health care, forensic settings in the social field, and kindergartens in the area of education (Emmel & Lancman, 2003). As a result of this, Brazilian occupational therapists also began critically analyzing their practices in workplaces involving "social exclusion" (e.g., asylums, rehabilitation centers, nursing homes, special education schools, and institutions of permanent hospitalization for people with physical, mental, social, and educational issues; Emmel & Lancman, 1998, 2003; Moreira, 2008).

The changes, promoted by the expansion of fields of practice, the introduction of lecturing, and research in occupational therapy, reinforced the need for modifications in the profile of professional occupational therapy education. At that time, professional occupational therapy education still lacked the theoretical and practical knowledge required in the new and expanding fields of practice. This indicated the importance of developing and providing knowledge in undergraduate education with a focus on aspects of practice beyond the medical model (Lopes, 1991, 1996; Rocha, Nicolau, & De Souza, 2013).

From 1982 to 1984, there was a reformulation of the minimum undergraduate curriculum in occupational therapy for all 13 existing programs in Brazil. This new curriculum involved an increased course duration from 3 to 4 years. The new curriculum reduced the emphasis on medical disciplines (e.g., anatomy, physiology, and kinesiology) and introduced disciplines of humanities (e.g., anthropology, philosophy, psychology, and sociology) as well as more specific knowledge disciplines (e.g., human occupation, occupational thearpy applied to different fields of practice, therapeutic resources). These changes made the integration of biological, psychological, and social contents more homogeneous and enhanced the importance of occupational therapy contents in the course, giving a distinct framework to this training. Thus, the contents of the foundations of occupational therapy were increased, and the professional contents of the different practices were included (Emmel & Lancman, 1998, 2003). As a result, between 1977 and 1984, at least five more undergraduate programs were created (Emmel & Lancman, 1998, 2003). The urgency for lecturers for these new programs encouraged many occupational therapists to explore an academic career that included research generation.

The increase in the number of occupational therapy programs was undoubtedly a milestone in the history of occupational therapy in Brazil. According to the survey conducted by Emmel et al. (2015), there were eight occupational therapy programs in 1978, 15 in 1986, 24 in 1999, and 35 in 2003. The most recent survey reported that there are now 40 undergraduate programs in the country, 20 in public universities and 20 in private universities (Drummond & Cruz, 2018). This new reality required more lecturers and researchers, in addition to the generation of a national knowledge base given that the research performed in universities was strictly based on international literature and published in the English language.

In 2004, the Ministry of Education approved the curricular guidelines in occupational therapy education with revisions to the undergraduate minimum curriculum. The undergraduate program began to have a minimum course load of 3600 hours to be completed in 4 or 5 academic years. Consequently, in recent years, the profession went through a process of rapid expansion in terms of emerging areas of practice, specialty areas, and availability of advanced degrees.

THE GRADUATE PROGRAM IN OCCUPATIONAL THERAPY IN BRAZIL (MSC AND PHD)

The creation of a master's and doctorate program in occupational therapy is recent and was intended to address the need for knowledge in the Brazilian context. The first and only master's program (the graduate program in occupational therapy) in Brazil was founded in 2009 at the Federal University of São Carlos, São Paulo, Brazil (Malfitano, Matsukura, Martinez, Emmel, & Lopes, 2013). In 2010, the first Master of Science (MSc) class in occupational therapy began, and in 2015, the first doctoral program was offered; this was the only Doctor of Philosophy (PhD) program in South America (Emmel, 2017). As of 2018, 85 MSc students have graduated, and 23 MSc and 31 PhD research projects are in progress. The program is organized to include research about processes of intervention in occupational therapy and aims to describe an epistemological perspective of the field and intrinsic aspects of the practices developed by occupational therapists. The program has two lines of research entitled Promotion of Human Development in Contexts of Daily Living and Social Networks and Vulnerability. These two lines of research are focused on studies related to (a) typical and atypical development of humans, (b) analysis and adaptation of daily activities for people with special needs with temporary or permanent disability, (c) development of new technologies for occupational therapy interventions that minimize dependence and facilitate autonomy in various contexts of daily life (at home, school, and work and in social life), (d) inclusion of populations in cases of rupture of the social support networks, (e) study of public policies directed at the target population of occupational therapy, and (f) research on the production and application of new knowledge and technologies for intervention in occupational therapy to address social problems (Matsukura et al., 2010).

Conclusion

This chapter outlined a brief history of occupational therapy education in Brazil, where occupational therapy has been influenced by many political and cultural factors. Occupational therapy education follows the current trends of an expanded view of health and is integrated with the establishment of fundamental rights (e.g., health, leisure, education, freedom of expression, social interaction); diversity of fields, experienced therapeutic processes, and multiplicity of workplaces occupied; and theoretical and practical applications in line with the objective and subjective needs of the treated population.

In the past decades, occupational therapy undergraduate programs have focused on the acquisition and mastery of techniques for practice and the fundamental knowledge for research, including theoretical and methodological procedures. Because the development of occupational therapy practitioners is connected with the complex demands in different contexts, the teaching-learning process has been carried out in a reflexive and proactive way based on an expanded view of the concept of health and integration with fundamental rights (Della Barba et al., 2017).

Concerning specific occupational therapist publications in Brazil from the three existing journals in the country, the *Brazilian Journal of Occupational Therapy* is the first journal in South America to be indexed in Scopus and Web of Science databases (Emerging Sources Citation Index). These two accomplishments indicate the effort of a group of scholars in public universities to enhance the quality of Brazilian occupational therapy publications. The *Brazilian Journal of Occupational Therapy* is a quarterly publication with open access and publishes articles with no publication fees in the languages of Brazilian Portuguese, English, and Spanish (Lopes, Cruz, & Malfitano, 2017, 2018).

Finally, because of the changes that occurred and were reported here, the potential for consolidation of the professional and research fields of Brazilian occupational therapy has been observed. Nevertheless, certain challenges must be addressed, and there is a considerable scope for development in the future.

Implications for Occupational Therapy Education

- The constant revision of minimum curricula upsurge demands is needed for occupational therapy educators because it is associated with an increase in the number of courses in the country.
- The bachelor's degree in occupational therapy with a general focus challenges occupational therapy educators to constantly update curriculum, and at the same time, develop a current critical and political practice in Brazilian occupational therapy.
- The investment in education and training of researchers in graduate programs specific to occupational therapy may contribute to the increase in specific knowledge in occupational therapy.

Key Reflection Questions

1. Some occupational therapists still do not base their professional practice on evidence. How can scientific reasoning/thought be adopted among occupational therapists, and what approaches could be adopted in the process of education and training?

2. Brazilian occupational therapy is still in the process of legitimization of its scientific status. How can Brazilian occupational therapy researchers enhance international recognition of their nationally conducted research?

3. How can education in ocupational therapy train professionals to promote social change from a reflexive teaching-learning process?

What led you to become an occupational therapy educator?

I worked for 4 years as an occupational therapist in hospitals and always had an interest in supervising students. After completing my master's degree, I was interested in being an educator given the possibility of researching and training professionals engaged in the advocacy and development of the profession in my country.

Daniel Marinho Cezar da Cruz, PhD, OT

I worked 10 years in the area of physical, sensory, and cognitive dysfunctions in childhood. After my doctorate, I became an educator with the purpose of developing teaching and research focused on interventions in occupational therapy, history, and fundamentals of the profession.

Mirela de Oliveira Figueiredo, OT, PhD

I came from a family of teachers, and they were examples who influenced me. Thus, after undergraduate training, I sought training for the teaching of occupational therapy, which did not exist in the 1970s. The master's degree was for me the path to doing occupational therapy research and also to start lecturing. In the southeast, I also created the first occupational therapy program in a public federal university.

Maria Luísa Guillaumon Emmel, OT, PhD

REFERENCES

Barba, P. C. S. D., Silva, R. F., Joaquim, R. H. V. T., & Brito, C. M. D. (2012). Formação inovadora em Terapia Ocupacional. *Interface—Comunicação, Saúde, Educação, 16*(42), 829-842. https://dx.doi.org/10.1590/S1414-32832012000300019

Barros, D. D., & Oliver, F. C. (2003). Contributing for the discussion of the Qualis classification in occupational therapy in Brazil. *Revista de Terapia Ocupacional da Universidade São Paulo, 14*(2), 52-63.

British Broadcasting Corporation. (2017). Brazil: country profile. Retrieved from http://www.bbc.co.uk/news/world-latin-america-18909529

Drummond, A. F., & Cruz, D. M. C. (2018). History of occupational therapy in Brazil: Inequalities, advances, and challenges. *Annals of International Occupational Therapy, 1*(2), 103-112.

Emmel, M. L. G. (2017). Tracked ways and contributions for the development of occupational therapy in Brazil. *Cadernos de Terapia Ocupacional da UFSCar, 25*(1), 235-242.

Emmel, M. L. G., Cruz, D. M. C., & Figueiredo, M. O. (2015). An historical overview of the development of occupational therapy educational institutions in Brazil. *South African Journal of Occupational Therapy, 45*(2), 63-67.

Emmel, M. L. G., & Lancman, S. (1998). Quem são nossos mestres e doutores? O avanço da capacitação docente em Terapia Ocupacional no Brasil. *Cadernos de Terapia Ocupacional da UFSCar, 7*(1), 29-38.

Emmel, M. L. G., & Lancman, S. (2003). La recherche en ergothérapie: Développement de la formation des enseignants au brésil. *Canadian Journal of Occupational Therapy, 70*(2), 97-102.

Instituto Brasileiro de Geografia e Estatistica. Áreas dos Municípios. (2018). Retrieved from https://www.ibge.gov.br/geo-ciencias-novoportal/organizacao-do-territorio/estrutura-territorial/15761-areas-dos-municipios.html?=&t=o-que-e

Lopes, R. E. (1991). *A formação do terapeuta ocupacional. O currículo: Histórico e propostas alternativas* (Unpublished master's thesis). Universidade Federal de São Carlos, São Carlos, Brazil.

Lopes, R. E. (1996). A direção que construímos: Algumas reflexões sobre a formação do Terapeuta Ocupacional. *Revista de Terapia Ocupacional Universidade de São Paulo, 4*(7), 27-35.

Lopes, R. E., Cruz, D. M. C., & Malfitano, A. P. S. (2017). Estamos no nosso melhor momento. *Brazilian Journal of Occupational Therapy, 25*(3), 447-448.

Lopes, R. E., Cruz, D. M. C., & Malfitano, A. P. S. (2018). Em tempos difíceis, compartilhando boas notícias em meio a muito trabalho. *Brazilian Journal of Occupational Therapy, 26*(3), 519-510.

Malfitano, A. P. S., Matsukura, T. S., Martinez, C. M. S., Emmel, M. L. G., & Lopes, R. E. (2013). Stricto sensu postgraduate program in occupational therapy: Strengthening and expanding production of knowledge in the field. *Revista Brasileira de Atividade física e Saúde, 18*(1), 105-111.

Matsukura, T. S., Malfitano, A. P., Martinez, C. M. S., Emmel, M. L. G., & Lopes, R. E. (2010). Programa de Pós-Graduação Stricto Sensu em Terapia Ocupacional no Brasil: Avanços e Desafios no Fortalecimento e na Expansão da Produção de Conhecimento na Área. In: XII Encontro Nacional de Docentes de Terapia Ocupacional, 2010, Curitiba. Terapia Ocupacional e Docência: Articulação e Gestão nos Desafios e Conquistas. São Carlos: Cadernos de Terapia Ocupacional da UFSCar, 2010. p. 432-439.

Moreira, A. B. (2008). Terapia Ocupacional: História crítica e abordagens territoriais comunitárias. *Vita et Sanitas, 2*(2), 79-81.

Paim, J., Travassos, C., Almeida, C., Bahia, L., & Macinko, J. (2011). The Brazilian health system: History, advances, and challenges. *Lancet, 377*(9779), 1778-1797.

Rocha, E. F., Nicolau, S. M., & De Souza, C. S. B. (2013). As pessoas com deficiência e a produção de conhecimento no campo da Terapia Ocupacional no Brasil. Anais do I Simpósio Internacional de Estudos sobre a Deficiência. SEDPcD/Diversitas/USP Legal. São Paulo. Retrieved from http://www.memorialdainclusao.org.br/ebook/Textos/Eucenir_Fredini_Rocha.pdf

Schenoni, L. L. (2015). *The Brazilian rise and the elusive South American balance.* Rochester, NY: Social Science Research Network.

Soares, L. B. T. (1991). *Occupational Therapy: logic of capital or work?* São Paulo, Brazil: Hucitec.

United Nations. (2017). World population prospects: The 2017 population division. Retrieved from https://esa.un.org/unpd/wup/

14

Perspectives on Occupational Therapy Education in Canada

Sue Baptiste, OTDip, MHSc, FCAOT

Chapter Objectives

By the end of this chapter, the reader will be able to:

1. Describe the evolution of occupational therapy education in Canada, highlighting major points of innovation.
2. Identify occupational therapy educational enrichment from a cross-country perspective.
3. Articulate potential next steps in the educational evolution of occupational therapy as a profession in Canada.

INTRODUCTION

When exploring the literature for this chapter, I was reminded strongly of the close ties between American and Canadian colleagues through the years of the emergence of occupational therapy as a powerful societal presence. This closeness existed through many cross-border exchanges in the waning years of the 19th century and the beginning of the 20th century, in which key foundational figures had an impact on both sides of the border (Friedland, 2003). Given that the genesis of occupational therapy as a profession stemmed from a common seed in the United Kingdom (England), United States, and Canada, little time here will be spent detailing with the theoretical foundations of the profession overall because space does not permit. However, I recognize and accept passionately and gratefully the immense importance of the values and ethics clearly exemplified during that time and welcome their return in more recent years to provide guidance to practitioners, educators, and researchers in occupational therapy. Current Canadian society is developing along a pathway of consonance between the past, present, and future; congruence between and among educational offerings, societal needs, and globalization is becoming ever more in concert. This kind of environment comes as a gift to occupational therapists in so many ways. The values and initiatives from which our original professional philosophy emerged have been revisited and seen as worthy. This rich historical

Taff, S. D., Grajo, L. C., & Hooper, B. R. (Eds.). *Perspectives on Occupational Therapy Education: Past, Present, and Future* (pp. 159-168). © 2020 Taylor & Francis Group.

foundation is detailed in all Canadian occupational therapy educational programs at the time of the writing of this chapter (Canadian Association of Occupational Therapists, 2012).

Chapter Framework

As vice president of the World Federation of Occupational Therapists (WFOT), I have been involved for 6 years in building relationships between many countries as they move forward in establishing occupational therapy as a fully fledged profession within their own cultures and societies. WFOT works directly with potential members to develop a constitution to guide the development of an emerging professional association and then to assist with ensuring that occupational therapy education programs are developed according to the Minimum Standards for the Education of Occupational Therapists and gain WFOT approval.

The emergence of a profession graphic (Figure 14-1) represents a timeline for the journey undertaken by a professional group as they strive to move from skilled technician status to that of contributor to global health leadership (WFOT, 2015). This evolutionary path is bracketed between environmental press from the profession on one side and society on the other. Stages of development are defined as skilled technician, preprofessional, professional, advanced professional, and global health leader. Education is an essential element of the growth of a profession and can be the instigator of and vehicle for change and growth or the response to opportunities for change as they arise. By distilling this graphic, one can see the relationships between the stages of professional development and the evolving needs of society that require ever-increasing educational knowledge and skills.

Skilled Technician

This first stage is exemplified through the role models of early pioneers who shaped the foundations of what would become occupational therapy. Their work was based on established theories with clear and powerful examples of application. Leaders in the development of the occupational therapy profession in the United States, such as Jessie Luther and Thomas Kidner (Rompkey, 2001; Friedland & Davids-Brumer, 2007), were emigrants from the United States and England, settling for periods of time in Canada while making their more permanent homes in America. They, and others, imprinted their mark clearly and firmly on emerging Canadian society, awakening a clear awareness of the power of "hand and mind to health." Thus, by the start of World War I, several ideas about the use of crafts in occupational therapy were already in place, as shown through a 1989 survey undertaken by Roland of a highly successful occupational therapy department in North Battleford, Saskatchewan (Friedland, 2003). These occupational goals were to preserve immigrants' identities and self-image, to learn skills for work, to enhance children's learning, to invoke the art spirit for promoting health, to relieve stress and restore the soul, and to reduce the need for physical restraints (Friedland, 2003, p. 209).

When World War I began, assistance was needed in the theater of conflict and the front lines in establishing equilibrium for the wounded and injured. Medical leaders determined the value of having young women to work with the soldiers in order to bring a sense of normalcy and purpose; thus, the role of ward aide was established. In 1918, the University of Toronto launched a short course for ward aides (6 weeks to 6 months), with the curriculum focused on working with the injured soldiers of World War I. These ward aides were employed by the Military Hospitals Commission of Canada to provide the soldiers with occupations, generally in the form of crafts, to "rehabilitate" their spirit during long periods of convalescence (Friedland, 2006). By the end of World War I, there were 350 graduates, most of whom were deployed postconflict across Canada to provide services within tuberculosis sanitaria and rehabilitation hospitals (Friedland, 2003). This was a time of important changes for women: they had just been given the right to vote, there were only small numbers in universities, and they were being received in less than a welcoming manner into the workforce. Therefore, the pioneering occupational therapists chose to forge strong relationships with medical leaders who

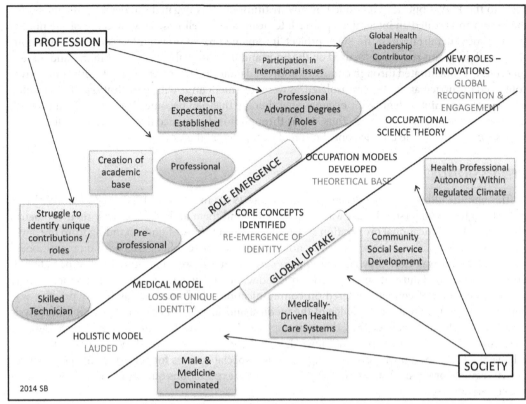

Figure 14-1. Emergence of a profession. (Reprinted with permission from World Federation of Occupational Therapists Chronicle: 2002-2012 [2015]. *Emergence of a profession.* Retrieved from https://www.wfot.org/resources/chronicle-of-the-world-federation-of-occupational-therapists-part-iv-2002-2012.)

formed the first advisory council of the Ontario Occupational Therapy Society. These men provided advice and influenced the formation of the Canadian Association of Occupational Therapy. In 1926, the first formal 2-year diploma program was established at the University of Toronto. This heralded the beginning of occupational therapy as a viable health profession viewed as a skilled technical field.

This first phase of occupational therapy professional evolution was happening during a time of male and medical dominance in society; the early therapists built alliances with male and medical leadership well into the 20th century. This was wise and assisted in establishing credibility to the contributions of this embryonic profession. This facilitated the development of skilled technical curricula followed by programs from undergraduate to postgraduate studies and qualifications, as exemplified within the early 21st century.

Preprofessional

The medical model dominated society despite a particularly innovative occupational therapy initiative early in World War II, thus enabling preprofessional status. Canadian occupational therapists came together to send ideas, patterns, materials, and guidance to the many thousands of prisoners of war (POWs) held in German internment camps (Cockburn, 2005). Parcels were split up across all prison camps so everyone had the chance of receiving something, with embroidering regimental crests being by far the most popular (Cockburn, 2005, p. 186). This volunteer effort spearheaded by the Ontario Society and the Canadian Association of Occupational Therapists became institutionalized through the Federal Department of War Services, which arranged to send ample supplies to POWs for the duration of the war (Cockburn, 2005, p. 183). This effort was recognized as being of value to the POWs but not sanctioned by any institutions. This negated the need for diagnoses for the POWs and created an integrated approach to healing and wellness. Sadly, because of the nonacceptance or generalization of the POW project, it remained based on volunteerism. The existing institutional programs remained focused on the body and the observable features of injury and disease that could be ameliorated through cure, care, and/or adaptation. Whatever mental health content was contained in curricular models was isolated, as were treatment units within institutions. This resulted in a loss of the unique identity for occupational therapy that had become clear and valued through the work of the original founders. Thus, it was through this dissonance that the seeds of discontent were sown relative to the unique contribution of occupational therapy.

Professional

Through the following three decades, from the late 1940s to the early 1980s, occupational therapists struggled to understand what was happening around them and where exactly their ecological niche was. Their educational preparation still gave them a wide base of understanding from the physical to the social sciences, but their role was not easy to describe to others. Demands on practitioners were such that it was clear they needed to gain comfort at a more conceptual level of narrative in order to explain and illustrate their practice role. Educational curricula expanded to an increasingly sophisticated level of content centered on communication. The "meat" of day-to-day practice was demanding a much greater knowledge of the medical and social sciences coupled with basic physical and psychological sciences; thus, the steps to professional status became clearer. Firm credentials were established to illustrate proven knowledge, skills, and abilities earned by academic effort and achievement. This began with creating diplomas and special courses for skilled technicians that reflected regional or national standards. These courses and expectations quickly became diplomas and undergraduate degrees.

University programs shored up their credibility through the inclusion of courses on evidence, which settings were most valuable for therapists to work in and make a difference, and the establishment of a sophisticated understanding related to social systems, power, and change. The original identity of occupational therapy encompassing medical, psychological, and social knowledge and skills was reemerging with the creation of a clearly recognizable academic base. This base determined that all programs should be striving for a bachelor's level and for this to be delivered within a university environment. This was a key juncture at which educational and academic clarity for occupational therapy became definitive. The tide for the profession turned in Canada by the end of the 1970s and the start of the 1980s. Research expectations were made very clear through statements in program accreditation standards; faculty members were advised a master's degree would be needed to teach, and then a PhD was essential for academic leadership. Practice remained the hub of what we did, recognizing practice needed facts, knowledge, and skills to address the needs of patients/clients and their families. Concepts and models of health care arose that spoke to clients being partners in their own health care decision making; client-centered practice became the core construct for service delivery as well as for health professional education. Interprofessional health care practice, education, and research came alive, thus encouraging occupational therapists to exhibit confidence in their unique contributions to health care. Occupational therapists partnered with researchers and social scientists to create tools addressing the evaluation of occupational therapy services. Some of these tools became known to other health disciplines, the results of which were valued increasingly by treatment teams.

Professional Advanced Degrees/Roles

Regulatory colleges were initiated across Canada, beginning in Ontario. From the middle of the 1980s to the present, each province has worked to gain synchrony to enable ease of transition for registrants across provincial boundaries. This was a cultural shift for the profession that has reached relative equilibrium between regulators and registrants across the country. Resources to assist in understanding the Canadian regulatory experience can be obtained through the website of the Association of Canadian Occupational Therapy Regulatory Organizations (https://www.acotro-acore.org/).

Within the academic environment, advanced roles emerged for occupational therapists to pursue thesis master's degrees and consider undertaking a PhD. Concurrently, "occupational science" was offered as a different approach to understanding and exploring concepts inherent within the human connection to occupation. This cutting-edge idea arose out of California posited by Yerxa (1990). Further, Yerxa defined occupational science as "the science of everyday living.... As an academic discipline, it focuses on the benefits of productive, social and physical activity (called 'occupations') in people's everyday lives" (USC Chan Division of Occupational Science and Occupational Therapy, n.d.).

One of the massive gains achieved through the occupational science partnership is the development of vibrant relationships across multiple disciplines, thus expanding occupational therapists' worldviews. This innovative worldview provided new opportunities for educational experiences that now can culminate in equally innovative degree studies and collaborations.

Areas for special skill development burgeoned, expanding the scope for occupational therapy practice. From the 1990s to the 2010s, professional ownership became a priority through provincial regulatory colleges protecting the public and ensuring quality and ethical practice. Through the inclusion of entrepreneurship with traditional and familiar practice models, professional thinking was reframed, seeing the profession's contribution within a competency framework. The growth of private practices provided choice for obtaining professional services through personal payment or insurance coverage. Occupational therapists populated all work environments and were based in institutions, community agencies, business, industry, government and policy, prisons, technology, manufacturing, and marketing. Roles and settings for practice continue to expand.

Global Health Leadership Contributor

Globalization was making a critical impact on Canadian society, with increased demands for refugee and immigrant claims and applications. International relationships were essential in academic work and also within health care programs to ensure currency in approaches to assessment and intervention. Academics belonged to international research teams as a matter of course, and occupational therapists were invited to participate in research trials that often crossed continents.

The Canadian population saw an expanded role for themselves in understanding health care delivery in general and personal health in particular. Health care consumers became vocal in their claims of wanting more information and to be partners in the enterprise of seeking support, cure, or care. Understanding research became an everyday expectation. Commitment to the central concept of "occupation" spoke to occupational therapy's uniqueness in the health care team and was heard everywhere. Notions of activities of daily living and holism being occupational therapy's special skills were questioned. Some advocate that reductionism is still the central approach in being an occupational therapist; however, when considering the overall global picture of what occupational therapists do, there is no doubt that the trigger for input is meaningful engagement and occupation. Occupational therapy educational preparation has enabled expanded roles for occupational therapists, assistants, and aides.

CONCLUSION

The journey from 1880 to the present has been astonishing. The seed of a good idea for the benefit of society has grown into a forest of uncountable trees, representative of a multitude of species that reside harmoniously together under the umbrella of "tree." This is how I see the occupational therapy profession looking down its evolutionary timeline in Canada. The professional education pathway follows closely with social changes, new insights into health, and concepts uncovered in the interest of "from hand and heart to health." Despite our fears, it appears that our growth has been synchronous with and responsive to societal growth and that the graduates of the current programs are indeed prepared to move forward and face new challenges such as technology, cultural differences, political priorities, and social and environmental disasters (Table 14-1).

Implications for Occupational Therapy Education

- Reinforce mutual regard and support for the evolution of a profession that, at the start, had yet to be recognized and valued.
- Realize the critical difference between collaboration vs copying, sharing of effort vs the protection of intellectual property, and combined curriculum creation vs loss of individual accomplishment.

Key Reflection Questions

1. When thinking about what you have just read, what are the areas of new knowledge that you feel were helpful to you in some way?
2. What do you believe were the milestones for the development of occupational therapy in Canada based on this chapter?
3. Do the ideas expressed here seem familiar to you in any way? If so, what and how?
4. Are there places within this narrative that you are tempted to explore more?

What led you to become an occupational therapy educator?

After immigrating to Canada from England in response to a long-standing wish to walk on tundra and after gaining several years of rich professional experience in practice and management, I leapt at the chance to move and assume a combined role of occupational therapy practitioner, manager, and teacher at McMaster University Medical Centre. I found my niche in an environment that welcomed those who tended to leave the mainstream and take risks in order to experiment, explore, and innovate. And so began 5 decades of amazing experiences, four of which were spent educating student occupational therapists, completing graduate work, and learning about facilitating learning. Now, as a professor emerita, I choose how and where I am involved, knowing full well that the privileges of teaching and learning are not relinquished easily. So, how did I get here? Being open to innovation perhaps and being supported so well by my father and my husband—"Do you want to do it? Then, of course, you should go for it." Bless them for that.

Sue Baptiste, OTDip, MHSc, FCAOT

Table 14-1

CANADIAN EDUCATION PROGRAMS FOR OCCUPATIONAL THERAPY PROFESSIONAL PREPARATION

UNIVERSITY	INAUGURAL YEAR	ACADEMIC AWARD	COMMENTS
British Colombia	1961: occupational therapy/physical therapy 1969/1970 1983: occupational therapy 2007: occupational science and occupational therapy	Certificate BSc(BSR) BScOT MSc(OT)	Several steps along the way for easing in academic change
Alberta	1960: occupational therapy/physical therapy 1976: occupational therapy 1986: occupational therapy	BSc BSc(OT) MSc(OT)	Physical therapy began several years before occupational therapy First in Canada
Manitoba	1960: occupational therapy/physical therapy 1964: occupational therapy/physical therapy 1966: occupational therapy 1976: occupational therapy 2003: master of occupational therapy	2.5-year certificate 3-year certificate BOT with optional 4th year BOT degree only	
Ottawa	1986: occupational therapy 2004: occupational therapy 2005: occupational therapy	BScOT MScOT	Only bilingual program Entry-level degree Indigenous program began
Queen's	1967: occupational therapy 1968: occupational therapy 2000: occupational therapy 2004: occupational therapy	Diploma 3 years BSc(OT) 4 years PhD in rehabilitation science MScOT	During the development process, a short course was offered to prepare occupational therapy practitioners to meet societal demand

continued

Table 14-1 (continued)

CANADIAN EDUCATION PROGRAMS FOR OCCUPATIONAL THERAPY PROFESSIONAL PREPARATION

UNIVERSITY	INAUGURAL YEAR	ACADEMIC AWARD	COMMENTS
Toronto	1918: occupational therapy 1926: occupational therapy 1946: occupational therapy 1950: occupational therapy/physical therapy 1974: occupational therapy 2000: occupational therapy	Short course for ward aides Diploma 2 years Diploma 3 years BSc(OT) MScOT	Began as 6 weeks and then became 6 months "POTS" in faculty of medicine Separated occupational therapy from physical therapy entry-level master's
McMaster	1978: occupational therapy 1980: occupational therapy 1989: occupational therapy occupational therapy 2000: occupational therapy	Diploma 3 years BHSc(OT) BHSc(OT) 3 years MSc(OT)	Combined program between McMaster University and Mohawk College One more semester at McMaster University Moved fully to McMaster University 2 years after honors undergrad
Western Ontario	1971: occupational therapy 1972: occupational therapy 1999: occupational therapy 2003: occupational therapy 2011: occupational therapy	BScMR(OT) BSc(OT) MClSc MSc(OT) MSc(OT)/PhD	MR stands for medical rehabilitation
Montreal	1954: occupational therapy/physical therapy 1962: occupational therapy	Diploma 3 years Individual programs 2 years following general year	Francophone
McGill	1919: occupational therapy 1950: occupational therapy/physical therapy 1954: occupational therapy 2007: occupational therapy	Short courses for ward aides Diploma 3 years combined BSc in occupational therapy and physical therapy MSc Applied (occupational therapy)	First in Canada Nonpracticing undergrad, then 2 years

continued

Table 14-1 (continued)

CANADIAN EDUCATION PROGRAMS FOR OCCUPATIONAL THERAPY PROFESSIONAL PREPARATION

UNIVERSITY	INAUGURAL YEAR	ACADEMIC AWARD	COMMENTS
Sherbrooke	1987: occupational therapy 2007: occupational therapy	Faculty of medicine MSc(OT)	Problem-based curriculum
Quebec at Trois Rivieres	Data pending		
Laval	Data pending		
Dalhousie	1982: occupational therapy 1998: occupational therapy 2006: occupational therapy	BScOT 3 years MSc(OT) MSc(OT)	Distance education/thesis Entry level

REFERENCES

Canadian Association of Occupational Therapists. (2012). *Occupational therapy profile*. Ottawa, Canada: Author.

Cockburn, L. (2005). Canadian occupational therapists' contributions to prisoners of war in World War II. *Canadian Journal of Occupational Therapy, 72*(3), 183-188.

Friedland, J. (2003). Muriel Driver memorial lecture. Why crafts? Influences on the development of occupational therapy in Canada between 1890 and 1930. *Canadian Journal of Occupational Therapy, 70*(4), 204-212.

Friedland, J. (2006). *Canadian occupational therapy education begins at U of T.* Retrieved from http://ot.utoronto.ca/about/program-history/

Friedland, J., & Davids-Brumer, N. (2007). From education to occupation: The story of Thomas Bessell Kidner. *Canadian Journal of Occupational Therapy, 74*(1), 27-37.

Rompkey, R. (Ed.). (2001). *Jessie Luther at the Grenfell Mission*. Montreal, Canada: McGill-Queen's University Press.

USC Chan Division of Occupational Science and Occupational Therapy. (n.d.). *What is occupational science?* Retrieved from http://chan.usc.edu/about-us/os-and-ot/what-is-os

World Federation of Occupational Therapists Chronicle: 2002-2012 (2015). *Emergence of a profession*. Retrieved from https://www.wfot.org/resources/chronicle-of-the-world-federation-of-occupational-therapists-part-iv-2002-2012

Yerxa, E. (1990). An introduction to occupational science: a foundation for occupational therapy in the twenty-first century. *Occupational Therapy in Health Care, 6*(4), 1-17.

15

Perspectives on Occupational Therapy Education in Europe

*Lyn Westcott, MSc, BSc, DipCOT, MRCOT, HCPC Registered
and Hanneke van Bruggen, BSc OT, Hon. Dscie, FWFOT*

Chapter Objectives

By the end of this chapter, the reader will be able to:
1. Describe the origins of occupational therapy education in Europe.
2. Discuss how occupational therapy education is shaped by the complex historical, political, and economic landscape of European nations, including the European Union.
3. Examine current and possible future trends for occupational therapy education in Europe.

INTRODUCTION: SETTING A CONTEXT

The historical, ongoing, and future development of occupational therapy education in Europe is tied to the complexity of the region. Although a geographically small continent, it claims a rich, diverse cultural and political heritage across 50 nations. Many Western European countries enjoy robust economies, whereas some Eastern European states are still developing their potential. Nations vary in size from Russia (6.6 million square miles) to Vatican City, with less than 500 inhabitants. At the time of writing, the European Union (EU) has grown to 28 nations, and 24 of these are part of the Schengen Area (with free movement of citizens and no passport controls). Alongside this, 19 EU nations share a single currency, the euro. Non-EU nations are independently governed, although some are transposing their legislation to prepare for membership, like Serbia, whereas at the time of writing, the United Kingdom has been working towards exit from the EU to gain greater legislative autonomy. The EU officially recognizes 23 languages, and many Europeans are multilingual, although English is often used for international discussion, professional dialogue, and publication within academia (EU, 2017).

Furthermore, there is a wide variety of health and social care systems across Europe, reflecting the range of economic and political structures. Some services are insurance based and others

Taff, S. D., Grajo, L. C., & Hooper, B. R. (Eds.). *Perspectives on Occupational Therapy Education: Past, Present, and Future* (pp. 169-176).
© 2020 Taylor & Francis Group.

government funded, meaning some Europeans pay for their health and social care while others have state provision (free of charge).

Although complex and ever changing, an appreciation of these political and cultural factors is important for people working throughout and liaising with Europe as curricula come to reflect these multiple realities. Not surprisingly, educational systems hosting occupational therapy programs have evolved in different ways. Some nations have programs that offer students full scholarships, whereas substantive tutorial fees are required elsewhere. Occupational therapy curricula are still not offered in all European countries and have emerged over a period of time, some very recently. This can impact the demographics of learners; for example, there can be more mature students in some nations than others because of funding. Importantly, the EU supports initiatives for sharing good practice throughout its nations and supports the occupational therapy education community throughout Europe to work together.

Political change in Europe has influenced many systems and the way emerging professions like occupational therapy develop their philosophy, practice, and education. This includes how they have grown and regulated their professional organizations, educational standards, and affiliations, as well as how they continue to develop. This is illustrated in this chapter.

OCCUPATIONAL THERAPY EDUCATION:
EARLY DEVELOPMENTS AND INFLUENCES

The development of occupational therapy in Europe was informed and inspired by events on its own shores. The pioneering 18th-century move to moral treatment of mentally ill people by William Tuke at the Retreat in York, England, and Phillippe Pinel at Hospice de Bicêtre in Paris, France, during the French Revolution are well-known and inspiring influences on occupational therapy. They introduced kinder regimens than those common at the time, like creating homey environments and involving inmates in occupations such as horticulture and domestic work, noting how the environment and occupation improved mental health (Wilcock, 2001). Following the emergence of the Arts and Crafts movement in England at the turn of the 20th century, the value of artistic and creative endeavours further influenced the treatment of the mentally ill. For example, Van de Scheer in Santpoort, the Netherlands, developed the nonrestraint approach of Conolly, a 19th century English psychiatrist who removed physical fetters from the insane, helping to change the attitudes of the times.

In the treatment of physical conditions, occupation was also being used to a curative effect. Clement Tissot had already published a book in 1780 with detailed regulations for the use of craft and recreational activities for the treatment of muscle and joint disorders (Luitse, 1970). In 1822, a small book titled *Enchiridion: A Hand for the One-Handed* was published by Captain George Webb de Renzy. It described assistive devices for the replacement of the right hand informed by de Renzy's own experience. In 1910, Philip introduced a farm colony to treat patients recovering from tuberculosis (Wilcock, 2001). Medicine over Europe was starting to see the value of using occupation as therapy, and "active therapy" was advocated through the first half of the 20th century (Aan de Stegge, 2014).

Within Europe, occupational therapy grew in the wake of the human devastation from both World Wars. Massive numbers of men returned home needing rehabilitation for both physical and psychological issues. These wars were a significant trigger to enable large numbers of women to enter the professional workforce, including in hospitals. For those fighting in World War I, occupation emerged as an effective treatment for both body and mind, with craftwork used for treating shell shock as well as physically injured soldiers in services like orthopedics (Wilcock, 2002). These largely biomedical settings required staff cognizant of medical treatments and terminologies to work under the direction of doctors. Occupational therapy became one of the professions to fill this gap. It is of note that the legacy of the Nazi occupation of World War II and the Russian occupation of Eastern European countries has influenced how the profession has grown with different names in Europe. *Ergotherapie* or *arbeitstherapie* is used rather than *occupational therapy* in the majority of nations, including France and Germany (Kinébanian, Nierstrasz, & van de Velde, 2017). Occupational therapy education developed in Europe after Henderson, a Scottish psychiatrist, introduced the first occupational therapy instructor at Glasgow's Gartnavel Royal Hospital, influenced by the work of Dr. Adolf Meyer in Chicago, IL (Paterson, 2014). Although psychiatric nursing had begun training schemes in Europe at the start of the 20th century, the first European school of occupational therapy, Dorset House, was developed by Dr. Elizabeth Casson in 1930 alongside her private psychiatric clinic for women in Bristol, United Kingdom (Wilcock, 2002). In Denmark, the first formal occupational therapy education started soon after in 1935 in Copenhagen, whereas in most other European countries, including France, Germany, the Netherlands, Norway, Spain, and Sweden, formal education started in the 1950s and 1960s. In the early days, especially before World War II, training was for psychiatric or physical health settings or both (Wilcock, 2002). Awards given were at the diploma level, with some national professional bodies guiding standards for these (e.g., the United Kingdom Association [not Scotland] set an examination syllabus back in 1938). The World Federation of Occupational Therapists (WFOT) standards influenced all curricula when their education standards were first formally published in 1958. These early curricula were rich in placement time, practical skills, and craftwork rather than theory or evidence driven as we know today. Without any real research element, such programs limited the development of an independent evidence base for the profession, impeding the evolution of innovative theory and tying the profession to the apron strings of medicine (Turner, 2011).

MOVING TOWARD CONTEMPORARY TIMES

During the 1980s to mid-1990s, occupational therapy education in the United Kingdom, Sweden, Ireland, Finland, Denmark, the Netherlands, and Belgium moved to a bachelor of science (BSc) entry level. This happened under the influence of the Sorbonne Joint Declaration (1998), which was the first step to harmonize the architecture of the European higher education system. By this time, "training" had turned the tide from technical education toward professional values, encouraging understanding and reflection on emerging theories and the need to generate and use evidence for practice. In the 1990s, some new postgraduate programs also evolved in the United Kingdom for people to become occupational therapists, initially a postgraduate diploma and then a master of science (MSc). These programs often used problem-based learning, a pedagogy first introduced to the diploma program at the West London Institute of Higher Education in 1984 by Sadlo (1994). This key educational approach drew attention in Europe when used by the medical school in Maastricht, the Netherlands, for encouraging deep levels of reasoning and problem solving (Matheson & Haas, 2010). Importantly for occupational therapy education, problem-based learning enabled a professional identity that owned the concept of occupation informed by occupational science and occupational therapy theory. Through facilitated exploration and discussion, problem-based learning encouraged students to develop greater ownership of their unique professional identity and a means to articulate this. This pedagogy has now become even more widespread, especially in the United Kingdom, the Netherlands, Sweden, and Denmark, although not universally within occupational therapy education in Europe.

Education elsewhere in Europe has largely followed this pattern of development, with diplomas of at least 3 years being widely offered initially, followed by BSc awards that are now the baseline standard set by the latest WFOT (2016) curriculum guidelines. It may be that this pattern of transition has helped retain the important place of practical skills within many European programs. It will be interesting to reflect on future developments and see how the ever-increasing literature base for occupational science and occupational therapy will impact on this trend for learning through doing.

THE CONSEQUENCES OF THE EUROPEAN UNION OPEN LABOR MARKET AND THE BOLOGNA PROCESS FOR OCCUPATIONAL THERAPY EDUCATION

Freedom of movement for workers is one of the founding principles of the EU. It is laid down in Article 45 of the Lisbon Treaty (2007) on the functioning of the EU and is a fundamental right of working people, including occupational therapists. It entails the abolition of any discrimination based on nationality between workers of member states. Besides freedom of movement, there was a need to recognize occupational therapy diplomas and degrees throughout Europe and align regulations for professional practice, resulting in the founding of the Council of Occupational Therapists for the European Countries (COTEC). This began with nine occupational therapy associations in 1986 and has grown to 30 national associations, representing more than 130,000 European occupational therapists (van Bruggen, 2012). COTEC supports national professional associations in working together on innovations to develop, harmonize, and improve standards of professional practice and advance the theory of occupational therapy throughout Europe to best address the social and health issues affecting European citizens. Another influential body, the European Network of Occupational Therapy in Higher Education (ENOTHE), was founded in 1995. Like COTEC, membership stretches to European nations beyond the EU. ENOTHE arose from continued discussions among occupational therapy educators on EU directives about the recognition of professional qualifications. It was known that there were obstacles for occupational therapy migrants within Europe and also marked differences in approaches to occupational therapy education. Some small, private vocational schools with occupational therapy intakes of 20 students coexisted alongside programs in larger universities with annual intakes of 100 or more. The majority of occupational therapy education in Europe was not embedded in the higher education system at that time, and it was seriously thought that EU ministers may decide that the profession in the whole of Europe would be at the lower vocational level (van Bruggen, 2016). There was a need to work together to embrace the opportunities of standardizing higher education for occupational therapists, advancing the research agenda, and optimizing the potential of the unified European labor market. It is of note that at that time in most countries (except Sweden, Finland, and the United Kingdom), occupational therapists had little opportunity to enter formal continuing education at the doctoral or master's level.

With increasing mobility of students that highlighted national differences, more and more problems for recognition of education and degrees among occupational therapy and other professions arose because of the little unity in the education systems. In 1999, the ministers of 29 European countries agreed on the Bologna Declaration, which outlined the main goals for higher education known as the Bologna Process. These included the following:

- Adoption of a system of easily readable and comparable degrees
- Establishing two main study cycles (undergraduate and graduate), although a third doctoral cycle was added later
- Beginning a "credits" system (i.e., the European Credit Transfer System [ECTS]) that represents student workload (60 ECTS per full study year), assessing defined learning outcomes of what the individual knows, understands, and is able to do
- Promoting mobility by overcoming obstacles to the free movement of students, educators, researchers, and administrative staff
- Advocating European cooperation in quality assurance
- Supporting the necessary European dimensions in higher education

These six objectives formed the essence of the Bologna Process and have since been developed further in the creation of the European Higher Education Area of 47 countries. The European Higher Education Area insists that higher education should link directly to society and its needs. Connected to the Bologna Process, the European Tuning Project is a university-driven initiative within Europe. It offers a concrete approach to implementing the Bologna Process. *Tuning* is a methodology to redesign, develop, implement, and evaluate degree programs for each of the Bologna cycles while allowing for diversity and flexibility in a lifelong learning context (Conzález & Wagenaar, 2006).

Diversity is a vital characteristic of European society and influences the need for and practice of occupational therapy. As a continent that enjoys a rich range of culture and historical influences, the current mobility of European citizens means that a wealth of skills, talents, and perspectives are available for the benefit of all. At a political and organizational level, acknowledging and managing that diversity to use the enormous benefits that it can bring the workplace are essential for all organizations and professions.

Since its foundation, ENOTHE set objectives and began work closely related to the Bologna Process. Several publications emerged reflecting collaborative work linked to the implementation of ECTS and competence-based learning outcomes (Howard & Lancée, 2000).

In 2003, ENOTHE collaborated with COTEC to start the Occupational Therapy Tuning Project (2008), which resulted in establishing occupational therapy education at an academic level, with shared graduate competencies and credits for the three levels of occupational therapy education in Europe. These competencies clearly indicate the skills, knowledge, and attitudes that graduate occupational therapists offer society, especially highlighting cultural knowledge, communication skills, and social reform, such as improving rights, inclusion, and participation. These competencies were translated in 24 languages, which facilitated the process of consultation during their development.

The European Network is aware of the importance of using culturally appropriate language in occupational therapy. With that in mind, ENOTHE created a multinational, multilingual terminology group, which developed the European dynamic framework of core concepts. "The framework does not attempt to simplify the complexity of human doing by using words that lock activities and occupations into static categories. Rather it captures the dynamism and unpredictability of occupation in all its manifestation" (Creek, 2010, pg. 12). The book is written in English, French, and Spanish, each using their own terminology from both a participant's and observer's perspective on occupation. The discourse of occupational therapy is still open to debate, and at its heart the title of the profession in Europe is not united, emerging either as occupational therapy or ergo therapy because of a legacy of territorial occupation in the last century.

The EU has been influential in promoting an increasing mobile workforce and joint educational courses in occupational therapy. A notable example is the European master of science in occupational therapy offered from 1999 as a joint master's degree by four (later five) partner higher education institutions in the Netherlands, United Kingdom, Sweden, Denmark, and Switzerland. This European master of science in occupational therapy is primarily aimed at qualified occupational therapists who wish to continue their academic and professional development at a higher degree level. Students rotate to attend modules in each country.

The enlargement of the EU has also influenced the development of occupational therapy practice and education. As Eastern European countries joined the EU, they underwent social and educational reform, leading to initiatives to develop new disciplines, including occupational therapy. Before 1989 (the fall of the Berlin Wall), the new accession states formed part of the communist former Soviet Union, which provided cradle-to-grave protection to the whole population. A major aspect of the changes was the enlargement of human choices in all areas of life and a transition to a market economy (van Bruggen, 2011). The European Commission's commitment to human rights, equal opportunities, and democracy was an opportunity for occupational therapy education and practice in these new accession countries and to reflect these values in their work. Programs have developed in many of these nations, supported by occupational therapy educators from elsewhere in Europe who are experts in the European context of provision. Some countries have also received input from elsewhere in the world, although this is not always so mindful of the European context.

One year after its founding in 1996, ENOTHE made the enlargement of Europe and the collaboration with the so-called new accession countries a specific objective in its policy plans for the following reasons:

- The EU was fundamentally committed to ensuring the welfare of all its members and minimizing disparities.
- EuroHealthNet (2007) published a strategy to tackle health inequalities in Europe titled "Closing the Gap: Strategies for Action to Tackle Health Inequalities in Europe. A European Project From 2004 to 2007."
- The Bologna Process called for a single European higher education area with compatible degrees and effective sharing of knowledge, research, and expertise.

Within the framework of these policies, ENOTHE received European grants to undertake several projects aimed to facilitate the participation of disadvantaged groups in Eastern and Central European countries and to contribute to social and educational reform. This needed to be achieved by developing occupational therapy education and practice. For ENOTHE, it was important to uphold two general principles. First was the need to ensure occupational therapy curricula were at least developed by a participatory action approach that included future local occupational therapists working in partnership with a wide range of stakeholders. It also included working to relevant national and international standards from WFOT and ENOTHE. The second principle required education of student occupational therapists to focus on the facilitation of occupational participation of marginalized populations, people with disabilities, and their caregivers and families in both their physical and social environments and within a framework of occupational justice and human rights (van Bruggen, 2011). As a result, to develop education modules in occupational therapy, ENOTHE members collaborated with local staff, students, client groups, caregivers, and families, leading to the implementation of small projects.

Developing occupational therapy education for social reform is not just implementing a good curriculum, training lecturers, or allocating skills, but it needs organizational engagement, strategic thinking, creativity, and willingness to change (van Bruggen, 2011). This system's change or reform can be seen in terms of social reform, and following the 2020 strategy of the European Commission, it should lead to inclusive growth. This reform means empowering people through investing in education, employment, fighting poverty, and exclusion to build a cohesive society. Therefore, the priority competencies required of occupational therapy students in these countries focus on many areas. They need to know how to instigate occupation-based community development, work with occupational justice, promote their profession, and be leaders, taking active part in planning, implementing new systems, and redesigning the old ones in health and social care. One of the outcomes of these ENOTHE projects has been the establishment of at least 10 occupational therapy schools, each with their own identity and functioning under the jurisdiction of different universities and faculties (placed in facilities of medicine, social sciences, and education).

CONCLUSION

Although there have been positive developments of the profession and occupational therapy education in Europe, considerable variation still exists. Although helpful, underlying core principles are evident because of a wide range of factors that include variations in the way higher education has developed and been governed in each nation, local traditions of health and social care services, and differences regarding the founding and development of the profession in each country. Social changes in Europe are influencing the need for occupational therapy, as elsewhere in the world. The demographics of an aging population, cultural diversity, family changes, caregiver burden, information accessibility, increased education levels, economic changes, poverty, and social and health inequality all impact European nations and are shaping the world in which occupational therapy seeks to reach out and improve the health and well-being of individuals, groups, and the wider population.

Typically, characteristics of the European occupational therapy practice and education focus on diversity, the use of practical activities including crafts in modern practice and academic settings (Dehnerdt et al., 2004), and the focus on inclusion and participation in community or occupation-based community development.

Implications for Occupational Therapy Education

- Despite the cultural and political diversity of Europe, occupational therapy education needs to be relevant to its context while relating to the same terminology and principles of occupational therapy and occupational science.
- Occupational therapy program will continue to grow as Europe develops, new countries engage in the EU, and the aspirations of greater equalities throughout Europe are realized.
- As the undergraduate portfolio of occupational therapy education becomes more established in Europe as the entry level for the profession, the opportunities for postgraduate degrees at the master's and doctoral levels is anticipated to grow generally as part of the development of already qualified practitioners.

Key Reflection Questions

1. There are large differences across the EU in how long people live and how many years they enjoy good health. How can occupational therapists contribute to occupational justice?
2. Experiences from Eastern European countries show how occupational therapy education was focused on working with communities on capability development through engagement in occupation and occupational justice; is such a role also important in other countries?
3. Respecting the health, social, and education context of a country, what does that mean for developing occupational therapy education?

What led you to become an occupational therapy educator?

I studied at Dorset House School of Occupational Therapy, Oxford, United Kingdom, qualifying as an occupational therapist in 1984. After working in various mental health settings for the U.K. National Health Service, I was inspired to enter education because I had enjoyed taking student occupational therapists on placement within my practice. Working with undergraduate and postgraduate learners, I have always been inspired by the wealth of enthusiasm and creativity of students for their chosen career. As Chair of the Learning and Development Board for the Royal College of Occupational Therapists in the United Kingdom, I am able to link my educational practice with a more strategic role in supporting the work of my national professional body.

Lyn Westcott, MSc, BSc, DipCOT, MRCOT, HCPC Registered

I studied at Institute Leffelaar, School for Occupational Therapy Amsterdam, the Netherlands, qualifying as an occupational therapist in 1969. After working in general hospitals in the Netherlands and several years in Kenya for the International Labour Organisation and Ministry of Social Affairs, I felt attracted to share my experience with student occupational therapists and to develop occupational therapy education from diploma to bachelor's level. The strategical development of the occupational education in Europe has always fascinated me. First as Chair of COTEC and later as Director of ENOTHE, I have intensively worked on tuning the occupational therapy education in Europe and the development of 10 new occupational therapy schools in Eastern and Central European countries.

Hanneke van Bruggen, BSc OT, Hon. Dscie, FWFOT

REFERENCES

Aan de Stegge, C. (2014). Changing attitudes towards 'non-restraint' in Dutch psychiatric nursing 1897-1994. In M. Gijswijt-Hofstra, M. H. Harry Oosterhuis, & J. Vijselaar (Eds.), *Psychiatric cultures compared: Psychiatry and mental health care in the twentieth century*. Amsterdam, Netherlands: Amsterdam University Press

Conzález, J., & Wagenaar, R. (2006). *Tuning educational structures in Europe, universities' contribution to the Bologna process*. Bibao, Spain: Publicaciones de la Universidad de Deusto.

Creek, J. (2010). *The core concepts of occupational therapy: A dynamic framework for practice*. London, UK: Jessica Kingsley Publishers.

Dehnerdt, S., Ferreire, M., Gilbert, M., le Granse, M., Himschoot, P., Isachsen, S. G., ... Dudakova, Z. (2004). *Occupational therapy education in Europe: Approaches to teaching and learning 'practical' occupational skills*. Amsterdam, Netherlands: The European Network of Occupational Therapy in Higher Education.

EuroHealthNet. (2007). *Closing the gap: Strategies for action to tackle health inequalities in Europe, A European project from 2004 to 2007* (Final report 1/06/2004-31/05/2007). Retrieved from https://neaygeia.gr/wp/wp-content/uploads/2017/06/2003_3_15_frep_en.pdf

European Union. (2017). *About the EU: Countries*. Retrieved from https://europa.eu/european-union/about-eu/countries_en#countries_using_the_euro

Howard, R., & Lancée, J. (2000). *Occupational therapy education in Europe: Curriculum guidelines*. Amsterdam, Netherlands: The European Network of Occupational Therapy in Higher Education.

Kinébanian, A., Nierstrasz, H., & van de Velde, D. (2017). De beroepsvorming van de ergotherapie. In M. le Granse, M. van Hartingsveldt, & A. Kinébanian (Eds.), *Grondslagen van de ergotherapie*. Houten, Netherlands: Bohn Stafleu van Loghum.

Lisbon Treaty. (2007). Retrieved from https://eur-lex.europa.eu/legal-content/EN/TXT/?uri=celex%3A12012E%2FTXT

Luitse, W. J. (1970). Theorie arbeidstherapie. In A. Kinébanian, H. Nierstrasz, & D. van de Velde (Eds.), *De beroepsvorming van de ergotherapie*. Houten, Netherlands: Bohn Stafleu van Loghum.

Matheson, R., & Haas, B. (2010). Exploring the foundations for problem base learning. In T. J. Clouston, L. Westcott, S. W. Whitcombe, J. Riley, & R. Matheson (Eds.), *Problem based learning in health and social care*. Chichester, UK: Wiley-Blackwell.

Paterson, C. (2014). A short history of occupational therapy in mental health. In W. Bryant, J. Fieldhouse, & K. Bannigan (Eds). *Creek's occupational therapy and mental health*. Edinburgh, Scotland: Churchill Livingstone Elsevier.

Publicaciones de la Universidad de Deusto (2008). Tuning educational structures in Europe: Reference points for the design and delivery of degree programmes in occupational therapy. Retrieved from http://tuningacademy.org/wp-content/uploads/2014/02/RefOccupationalTherapy_EU_EN.pdf

Sadlo, G. (1994). Problem-based learning in the development of an occupational therapy curriculum. Part 2: The BSc at the London School of Occupational Therapy. *British Journal of Occupational Therapy, 57*(3), 79-84.

Sorbonne Joint Declaration. (1998). *Joint declaration on harmonisation of the architecture of the European higher education system*. Retrieved from http://www.ehea.info/cid100203/sorbonne-declaration-1998.html

Turner, A. (2011). The Elizabeth Casson Memorial Lecture 2011: Occupational therapy—A profession in adolescence. *British Journal of Occupational Therapy, 74*(7), 314-322.

van Bruggen, H. (2011). Eastern European transition countries: Capacity development for social reform. In F. Kronenberg, N. Pollard, & D. Sakellariou (Eds.), *Occupational therapy without borders* (Vol. 2), 295-303. London, UK: Churchill Livingstone/ Elsevier.

van Bruggen, H. (2012). The European employment strategy and opportunities for occupational therapy. *Work, 41*(4), 425-431.

van Bruggen, H. (2016). Strategic thinking and reasoning in occupational therapy. In M. B. Cole & J. Creek (Eds.), *Global perspectives in professional reasoning*. Thorofare, NJ: SLACK Incorporated.

Wilcock, A. (2001). *Occupation for health volume 1: A journey from self help to prescription*. London, UK: British Association and College of Occupational Therapists.

Wilcock, A. (2002). *Occupation for health volume 2: A journey prescription to self help*. London, UK: British Association and College of Occupational Therapists.

World Federation of Occupational Therapists. (2016). *Minimum standards for the education of occupational therapists*. London, UK: Author.

16

Perspectives on Occupational Therapy Education in Australia

Melanie Roberts, BAppSc (OccThy), MClinRehab;
Matthew Molineux, BOccThy, MSc, PhD, MBA;
and Barbara R. Hooper, PhD, OTR/L, FAOTA

Chapter Objectives

By the end of this chapter, the reader will be able to:

1. Identify the themes present across the Australian education literature.
2. Identify opportunities and challenges for education suggested by the themes.
3. Draw implications from the themes for future education research in Australia and beyond.

INTRODUCTION

Occupational therapy began in Australia in response to growing rehabilitation needs after World War II, and now there are over 20,000 registered occupational therapists (Occupational Therapy Board of Australia, 2018). The first educational programs began in the 1940s (Cusick, 2017), and today there are two entry degrees—the 4-year bachelor's degree and the 2-year graduate-entry master's degree. The number of education programs in Australia has increased from 14 in 2010 to 42 individual degrees in 2018 (Occupational Therapy Council, 2019); this growth is significant given there are 43 universities in Australia (Australian Trade and Investment Commission, 2017).

The increased number of programs creates challenges for the profession, including the need for more academic staff who are appropriately qualified, more placements for students, and more employment for graduates (Cusick, 2017). However, the growth in programs also provides opportunities. More practicing occupational therapists may increase awareness of the profession. More programs and academics increase the opportunities to deepen and broaden the evidence base of the profession and better understand the educational process of becoming an occupational therapist. Indeed, the scholarship of occupational therapy education has been growing. However, the increasing body of

Taff, S. D., Grajo, L. C., & Hooper, B. R. (Eds.). *Perspectives on Occupational Therapy Education: Past, Present, and Future* (pp. 177-182).
© 2020 Taylor & Francis Group.

literature on education has not been mapped to determine emphases, research methods, outcomes targeted, and key themes.

Therefore, a systematic mapping review of Australian education literature published between 2000 and 2017 was undertaken. This chapter presents a small portion of that review, the education-related themes that cut across many articles in the review.

APPROACH TO IDENTIFYING AND PRESENTING EDUCATION THEMES

Systematic mapping reviews describe and categorize a body of scholarship to identify gaps and guide future enquiry (Grant & Booth, 2009). The term *scholarship* refers to descriptive, conceptual, and research publications that address teaching and learning. The protocol for this study was largely based on the approach taken by Hooper, King, Wood, Bilics, and Gupta (2013). For the wider review, we asked the following question: What is the state of scholarship on entry-level occupational therapy education in Australia? One subquestion, which is the focus of this chapter, was the following: What themes are evident across the education literature?

We identified 123 articles published between 2000 and 2017. Sixty-one focused primarily on practice education and were excluded. Practice education is a particular concern in Australia warranting a separate review. Data were extracted from the remaining 62 articles using a tool that provided a detailed analysis of each article. One element of the data extraction tool identified the broad themes. We identified areas of emphasis in the education scholarship using the teaching framework and acronym MAKER developed by Fenstermacher and Solits (2004), which captures the following transactive elements of teaching and learning:

M—Methods, skills, techniques

A—Awareness of students' characteristics, histories, and former knowledge

K—Knowledge of the content (the educator's knowledge)

E—Ends or the goals and motivations for educating students

R—Relationships educators have with students

THEMES IN AUSTRALIAN EDUCATION SCHOLARSHIP

The common themes across the articles included the content that is and should be taught, the characteristics of occupational therapy students, making scholarship relevant to practice education, examining education through student perceptions, and faculty development.

The Content That Is and Should Be Taught

Several articles addressed the issue of what content is and should be taught. This theme relates to the K in the MAKER acronym (i.e., the knowledge to be imparted). Although this element in the framework refers specifically to educators, the articles coded under this theme addressed knowledge or content apart from the educators who teach it, students who learn it, and evidence-based teaching processes that convey it. In other words, content was addressed from an objectivist, deductive perspective, not a transactive perspective in which content is shaped within the interactions between faculty, students, context, and the content itself. The articles made recommendations for particular standalone content for curricula, including (a) person-related factors like neurology (McCluskey, 2000) and mental health (Scanlan et al., 2015), (b) environmental factors such as technology (Hills et al., 2016) and cultural awareness (Rasmussen, Lloyd, & Wielandt, 2005), and

(c) occupation-related content such as conceptual practice models (Ashby & Chandler, 2010) and threshold concepts (Nicola-Richmond, Pépin, & Larkin, 2016). Some articles went beyond addressing specific content to considering how challenging it is to decide what curricular content to include and exclude (Farnworth, Rodger, Curtin, Brown, & Hunt, 2010).

The Characteristics of Occupational Therapy Students

Scholarship assigned to this theme sought to understand student characteristics, histories, prior knowledge, and experience, which is the A in the MAKER acronym (i.e., awareness of students' characteristics, histories, and former knowledge). Articles emphasized student characteristics and prior experience. For example, in a study comparing students' values of inclusive education based on their country of origin, Mu et al. (2010) discussed how prior experience with inclusion likely shaped how much students valued it. Articles studied the characteristics of students, such as approaches to learning (Brown et al., 2017), levels of altruism (Byrne, 2008), and Generation Y students (Hills, Boshoff, Gilbert-Hunt, Ryan, & Smith, 2015). Some articles also compared students across programs, disciplines, or countries (Brown et al., 2017). The rationale given for this research was that understanding student characteristics will help tailor student-centered teaching and learning. However, how to apply the findings from these studies to teaching remained largely implicit and general.

Making Scholarship Relevant to Practice Education

Although articles that primarily focused on practice education were excluded, many remaining articles included some consideration of it. This theme related to the E, or the end result in the MAKER acronym (i.e., helping students succeed in or actually change their practice was sometimes presented as the end goal of practice education). Other articles represented practice education as a method, the M in MAKER (i.e., methods, skills, and techniques used in teaching), a strategy to teach students about different topics. For example, placement was considered a method to teach and convey professional identity (Ashby, Adler, & Herbert, 2016). Ashby and Chandler (2010) identified occupation-focused practice models taught in curricula and suggested practice education as an additional strategy to teach and disseminate these models to students.

Examining Education Through Student Perceptions

Articles documented students' perspectives on aspects of education, including awareness of their own characteristics and their experience of specific educational methods. This theme crosses the method, awareness, ends, and relationship elements of the MAKER acronym. Articles about perspectives of learning techniques fall within M (teaching methods). Articles seeking student perspectives on learning outcomes fall within E (ends of teaching). It could also be said that believing in the value of students' perspectives of their education constitutes a particular kind of relationship between educators and students, the R in MAKER. Articles in this theme explored student perspectives on preparation for practice (Doherty, Stagnitti, & Schoo, 2009), the ability to describe the profession (Turpin, Rodger, & Hall, 2012), receiving feedback on assessment tasks (Strong et al., 2012), and interprofessional learning (Larkin, Hitch, Watchorn, Ang, & Stagnitti, 2013). This group of articles contributed valuable knowledge about the student experience in a range of areas. However, student responses to understanding the core philosophy of the profession and teaching methods and approaches that impart this philosophy have not been investigated in Australia.

Faculty Development

This theme includes both K and M in the MAKER acronym, educator knowledge and methods. Some articles addressed knowledge of subject matter specifically, such as educators' knowledge of and confidence with teaching indigenous content (Melchert, Gray, & Miller, 2016) and threshold concepts (Rodger, Turpin, & O'Brien, 2015). Other articles addressed educators' knowledge and experience beyond the content they teach, e.g., the development of scholarship (Fortune et al., 2016), benchmarking of research output (Broome & Gray, 2017), and transition from clinician to academic (Murray, Stanley, & Wright, 2014). This group of articles was largely focused on capturing the range of roles academics are required to complete and how they develop those roles. However, for the majority of academics, teaching and learning are significant parts of their responsibilities. No articles explored profession-specific teaching methods and approaches to assist academics in performing this aspect of their job.

DISCUSSION

Reflecting on the themes using the MAKER acronym, the Australian occupational therapy education scholarship has rarely studied the R, the relationships educators have with students. Similarly, the M was not a predominant focus, with few articles addressing what educators do (i.e., the skills, processes, and techniques they use). It is often argued that due to occupational therapists' education of clients, they are well positioned to be educators. However, it cannot be assumed that occupational therapists know how to effectively educate university students without additional knowledge and skills or what has been called "pedagogical content knowledge" (Shulman, 2013). Just as students must integrate theory and skills into practice, occupational therapists must integrate education theory and skills to become effective educators. Furthermore, academics must integrate educational theory, methods, and evidence with the profession's core philosophy (Hooper & Rodger, 2016).

Overall, with little attention given to methods in general, profession-specific teaching methods, theory, and processes appear to be taken for granted or overlooked in Australian education scholarship. This oversight was apparent given the themes that were more prominent across the articles (i.e., content, characteristics of students, practice education, student perceptions, and faculty development). For example, the content theme included studies of "related knowledge" (Kielhofner, 2009) but did not discuss such knowledge in terms of how it relates to occupation. Very few articles in the content theme addressed teaching the concept of occupation beyond teaching conceptual practice models and threshold concepts. Thus, profession-specific teaching has not been adequately addressed in Australian education scholarship.

Similarly, articles in the student perceptions theme provided information about how students perceive learning but have not explored how students perceive profession-specific teaching methods and processes. Articles in the *faculty development* theme have elucidated aspects of becoming educators. However, little work has addressed how to support educators in delivering evidence-based education that is centered on the core philosophy of the profession. Articles in the *practice education* theme sought to use practice education as a means for learning certain content and to change practice. Few articles examined profession-specific teaching and learning in the practice context.

Therefore, there is a need to conduct inquiry in profession-specific teaching methods and approaches as they relate to the following themes identified: content, student characteristics, practice education, student perceptions, and faculty development. Future inquiry can support evidence-based, occupation-centered education and how programs develop curricula that are congruent with the profession's organizing concept of occupation.

Implications for Occupational Therapy Education

- There is a need for occupational therapy academics to inquire into discipline-specific teaching and learning methods and approaches across multiple aspects of education.

Key Reflection Questions

1. How can occupational therapy academics broaden research to study, develop, and share profession-specific teaching practices nationally and internationally?

2. How should occupational therapy academics integrate educational literature so that it is contextualized within the profession?

3. What might occupational therapy scholars investigate about profession-specific teaching and learning to support current and future academics?

4. How do occupational therapy educators design learning congruent with the profession's organizing concept of occupation?

What led you to become an occupational therapy educator?

I grew up surrounded by family members who worked in education, so it is no surprise that I ended up educating my first student 6 months postgraduation. After this, I continued to educate students on placement, and then I had the opportunity to work as an educator in a health service and then in new occupational therapy programs. Through these experiences, I have gained a great deal of professional satisfaction and growth from working with students, which is ultimately what drew me to teaching in the first place and still does!

Melanie Roberts, BAppSc(OccThy), MClinRehab

When deciding what to do after high school, occupational therapy was my first choice, but teaching was on my short list, so it has always been an interest. As a clinician, I worked with students on placements and fairly early on became a clinical lecturer when I was working in London, U.K. This role enabled me to work with students both on placement and also in university-based courses, which I designed and taught. It was not long after that when an opportunity came to move into education full time, and I have pretty much stayed there ever since—without regrets.

Matthew Molineux, BOccThy, MSc, PhD, MBA

REFERENCES

Ashby, S., & Chandler, B. (2010). An exploratory study of the occupation-focused models included in occupational therapy professional education programmes. *British Journal of Occupational Therapy, 73*(12), 616-624. doi:10.4276/0308 02210X12918167234325

Ashby, S. E., Adler, J., & Herbert, L. (2016). An exploratory international study into occupational therapy students' perceptions of professional identity. *Australian Occupational Therapy Journal, 63*(4), 233-243. doi:10.1111/1440-1630.12271

Australian Trade and Investment Commission (Austrade). (2017). Universities and higher education. Retrieved from https://www.studyinaustralia.gov.au/english/australian-education/universities-and-higher-education

Broome, K., & Gray, M. (2017). Benchmarking the research track record and level of appointment of Australian occupational therapy academics. *Australian Occupational Therapy Journal, 64*(5), 400-407. doi:10.1111/1440-1630.12387

Brown, T., Fong, K. N. K., Bonsaksen, T., Lan, T. H., Murdolo, Y., Gonzalez, P. C., & Beng, L. H. (2017). Approaches to learning among occupational therapy undergraduate students: A cross-cultural study. *Scandinavian Journal of Occupational Therapy, 24*(4), 299-310. doi:10.1080/11038128.2016.1229811

Byrne, N. (2008). Differences in types and levels of altruism based on gender and program. *Journal of Allied Health, 37*(1), 22-29.

Cusick, A. (2017). Editorial: How many courses for how many jobs? Enduring questions in need of research-based answers. *Australian Occupational Therapy Journal, 64*(1), 1-2. doi:10.1111/1440-1630.12361

Doherty, G., Stagnitti, K., & Schoo, A. M. M. (2009). From student to therapist: follow up of a first cohort of bachelor of occupational therapy students. *Australian Occupational Therapy Journal, 56*(5), 341-349. doi:10.1111/j.1440-1630.2008.00751.x

Farnworth, L., Rodger, S., Curtin, M., Brown, T., & Hunt, S. G. (2010). Occupational therapy entry-level education in Australia: Which path(s) to take? *Australian Occupational Therapy Journal, 57*(4), 233-238. doi:10.1111/j.1440-1630.2010.00862.x

Fenstermacher, G. D., & Solits, J. F. (2004). *Approaches to teaching* (4th ed.). New York, NY: Teachers College Press.

Fortune, T., Ennals, P., Bhopti, A., Neilson, C., Darzins, S., & Bruce, C. (2016). Bridging identity "chasms": Occupational therapy academics' reflections on the journey towards scholarship. *Teaching in Higher Education, 21*(3), 313-325. doi:10.1080/13562517.2016.1141289

Grant, M., & Booth, A. (2009). A typology of reviews: An analysis of 14 review types and associated methodologies. *Health Information and Libraries Journal, 26,* 91-108. doi:10.1111/j.1471-1842.2009.00848.x

Hills, C., Boshoff, K., Gilbert-Hunt, S., Ryan, S., & Smith, D. R. (2015). The future in their hands: The perceptions of practice educators on the strengths and challenges of "Generation Y" occupational therapy students. *Open Journal of Occupational Therapy, 3*(4), 1-16. doi:10.15453/2168-6408.1135

Hills, C., Ryan, S., Smith, D. R., Warren-Forward, H., Levett-Jones, T., & Lapkin, S. (2016). Occupational therapy students' technological skills: Are 'generation Y' ready for 21st century practice? *Australian Occupational Therapy Journal, 63*(6), 391-398. doi:10.1111/1440-1630.12308

Hooper, B., King, R., Wood, W., Bilics, A., & Gupta, J. (2013). An international systematic mapping review of educational approaches and teaching methods in occupational therapy. *British Journal of Occupational Therapy, 76*(1), 9-22. doi:10.4276/030802213X13576469254612

Hooper, B., & Rodger, S. (2016). She said, she said: A conversation about growing education research in occupational therapy. *Open Journal of Occupational Therapy, 4*(3). doi:10.15453/2168-6408.1307

Kielhofner, G. (2009). *Conceptual foundations of occupational therapy practice* (4th ed.). Philadelphia, PA: F.A. Davis.

Larkin, H., Hitch, D., Watchorn, V., Ang, S., & Stagnitti, K. (2013). Readiness for interprofessional learning: a cross-faculty comparison between architecture and occupational therapy students. *Journal of Interprofessional Care, 27*(5), 413-419. doi:10.3109/13561820.2013.779233

McCluskey, A. (2000). Collaborative curriculum development: Clinicians' views on the neurology content of a new occupational therapy course. *Australian Occupational Therapy Journal, 47*(1), 1-10. doi:10.1046/j.1440-1630.2000.00200.x

Melchert, B., Gray, M., & Miller, A. (2016). Educator perspectives on indigenous cultural content in an occupational therapy curriculum. *Australian Journal of Indigenous Education, 45*(1), 100-109. doi:10.1017/jie.2016.3

Mu, K., Brown, T., Peyton, C. G., Rodger, S., Huang, Y., Wu, C., … Hong, C. S. (2010). Occupational therapy students' attitudes towards inclusion education in Australia, United Kingdom, United States and Taiwan. *Occupational Therapy International, 17*(1), 40-52. doi:10.1002/oti.285

Murray, C., Stanley, M., & Wright, S. (2014). Weighing up the commitment: A grounded theory of the transition from occupational therapy clinician to academic. *Australian Occupational Therapy Journal, 61*(6), 437-445. doi:10.1111/1440-1630.12146

Nicola-Richmond, K. M., Pépin, G., & Larkin, H. (2016). Transformation from student to occupational therapist: Using the Delphi technique to identify the threshold concepts of occupational therapy. *Australian Occupational Therapy Journal, 63*(2), 95-104. doi:10.1111/1440-1630.12252

Occupational Therapy Board of Australia. (2018). Occupational Therapy Board of Australia registrant data. 1st April 2018–30th June 2018. Retrieved from http://www.occupationaltherapyboard.gov.au/About/Statistics.aspx

Occupational Therapy Council. (2019). Accreditation status of Australian Occupational Therapy Programs. Retrieved from http://otcouncil.com.au/accreditation/

Rasmussen, T. M., Lloyd, C., & Wielandt, T. (2005). Cultural awareness among Queensland undergraduate occupational therapy students. *Australian Occupational Therapy Journal, 52*(4), 302-310. doi:10.1111/j.1440-1630.2005.00508.x

Rodger, S., Turpin, M., & O'Brien, M. (2015). Experiences of academic staff in using threshold concepts within a reformed curriculum. *Studies in Higher Education, 40*(4), 545-560. doi:10.1080/03075079.2013.830832

Scanlan, J. N., Pépin, G., Haracz, K., Ennals, P., Webster, J. S., Meredith, P. J., … Bruce, R. (2015). Identifying educational priorities for occupational therapy students to prepare for mental health practice in Australia and New Zealand: Opinions of practising occupational therapists. *Australian Occupational Therapy Journal, 62*(5), 286-298. doi:10.1111/1440-1630.12194

Shulman, L. S. (2013). Those who understand: Knowledge growth in teaching. *Journal of Education, 193*(3), 1-11. doi.org/10.1177/002205741319300302

Strong, J., Hughes, C., Wilson, W., Arnott, W., Isles, R., & Bennison, A. (2012). Perceptions of feedback among undergraduate and postgraduate students of four health science disciplines. *Internet Journal of Allied Health Sciences and Practice, 10*(4), 11.

Turpin, M. J., Rodger, S., & Hall, A. R. (2012). Occupational therapy students' perceptions of occupational therapy. *Australian Occupational Therapy Journal, 59*(5), 367-374. doi:10.1111/j.1440-1630.2011.00988.x

17

Perspectives on Occupational Therapy Education in Africa

Liesl Peters, BSc (OccTher), MSc (OccTher)
and Roshan Galvaan, PhD, MSc (OccTher), BSc (OccTher)

Chapter Objectives

By the end of this chapter, the reader will be able to:

1. Describe the evolution and structure of occupational therapy education within the South African and, more broadly, the African context.
2. Discuss the challenges associated with the development of occupational therapy education in Africa and the opportunity that exists in the decolonization of curricula.
3. Discuss the critical contribution of Southern perspectives for the ongoing development of occupational therapy education in Africa.

INTRODUCTION

Recognizing that the African continent consists of 54 countries, with complex histories, cultures, beliefs, people, and systems influencing the character of occupational therapy education in each one, this chapter begins with key information about occupational therapy education on the African continent and then draws on a more detailed perspective from one country, namely, South Africa.

Most countries in Africa require a bachelor's degree for entry-level practice as an occupational therapist. Seven of the countries whose programs are accredited by WFOT were started between 2000 and 2018 (with one program per country). The remaining four countries started between 1948 and 1999. Notably, the four countries with the longest history of occupational therapy have 11 programs collectively. South Africa has the highest concentration of bachelor's degree occupational therapy programs ($N = 8$) on the African continent.

Taff, S. D., Grajo, L. C., & Hooper, B. R. (Eds.). *Perspectives on Occupational Therapy Education: Past, Present, and Future* (pp. 183-190).

There is also an increase in candidates pursuing master's- and doctoral-level programs, with all of the eight South African universities that offer undergraduate degree programs also offering master's and doctoral programs in occupational therapy. In most African countries, postgraduate qualifications are not formally recognized by the regulatory body for health professions; however, academic staff members are commonly required to have or acquire these postgraduate qualifications to fulfill their roles as educators. Many clinicians also pursue postgraduate studies.

Despite the similarities in degrees offered and pursued, occupational therapy education is diverse across the continent. It is asserted that representing perspectives of occupational therapy education across Africa would require a substantially larger, more collaborative endeavor, well beyond the scope of a single chapter. Therefore, this chapter draws on available literature and our experiences in occupational therapy education to highlight emergent trends in occupational therapy programs from the vantage point of South Africa.

Developing Occupational Therapy
Education in Africa: A Critique

Occupational therapy education in South Africa, similar to elsewhere in Africa, has been shaped by the way that the profession developed in the Global North. For example, the influence of patriarchy on the profession (Frank, 1992), together with biomedical, individualized epistemologies in occupational therapy, has continued to shape practice and education (Dsouza, Galvaan, & Kaushik, 2017). Although the need for a profession such as occupational therapy develops in response to a need for services, it appears that, at the introduction of education programs, less attention is given to the way that contexts may shape such programs. In this way social, political, and economic factors that influence education curricula and occupational therapy practice are given insufficient attention (Dsouza et al., 2017).

The development of educational programs in African countries has been largely through forging international partnerships with universities or organizations in the Global North. Occupational therapy education in South Africa was initiated by British occupational therapists in 1944 (Crouch, 2016), and a review of the OTARG newsletters between 2005 and 2017 reveals numerous other examples of educational program development through the support of international partners. For instance, the educational program in Rwanda has continued to develop with the support of Belgian partners (Engelen, 2014), and there are plans to begin a program in Malawi with the support of international partners in 2019 (Loveday, 2014). Similarly, Morocco began a program in 2017 with the sponsorship of Handicap International (Nafai, 2017), an organization situated in the Global North, and Madagascar has been supported by the Christian Blind Mission International. Although the support of international partners may be necessary and helpful, it can result in the imposition of ideologies that do not serve contextually relevant curricula development given the global centralization of Euro-American ways of understanding and knowing the world within occupational therapy (Hammell, 2011).

Findings from a qualitative research project exploring African occupational therapists' views on the support of international partnerships in the development of the profession (Hansen, Ndaa, Piora, Weigand, & Munoz, 2018) highlighted the many mistakes that international partners make when they assume that they already know what curricula and practice foci are important within various African countries. These assumptions fail to acknowledge that their ways of knowing have developed through practice in the Global North. Engaging the views of Kenyan, Ghanaian, Ugandan, South African, and Zimbabwean occupational therapists and educators, this study powerfully indicated the importance of avoiding a form of "paradigmatic arrogance" that forces the views of the international partners onto situations and contexts about which they know little (Hansen et al., 2018).

In South Africa, importing occupational therapy knowledge and methods from the Global North continue to shape what occupational therapists are taught and use in their practice. For instance,

Table 17-1

PERSONAL REFLECTIVE JOURNAL

On this specific session that I had with my block partner (who happened to be a White female), the theme was finding balance in your life, and we gave the group members a pie chart for them to "guesstimate" how much time they spend in each area of their lives. The pie chart had different life areas, and the participants had to color in how much time they figure they spend in each area of life.

I also feel the need to mention that in the group seated next to me were about four to five Black Xhosa women. The instruction was then given, and so the group participants were given a chance to reflect on their pie chart. One of the areas in the pie chart was "Miscellaneous Use"; one of the ladies seated next to me asked what this miscellaneous use of time meant, and my block partner spoke up and said, not in direct words, but something along the lines of it's free time we have to do things we want, like going out with your friend to go get coffee. My first thoughts were, Black women don't call their friends to go buy coffee, but that was a random thought and I brushed it off quickly.

After they got the reply from my block partner, I saw some of the women shaking their heads, and they had unimpressed looks on their faces; I myself was very unimpressed with what my block partner said, and I quickly cleared it from them and thought what does my mother/aunt/the aunt who helps around the house do in her free time and gave them those examples, and that's when they said they understood. My thinking at the time was that it's so unfortunate that there are no Black occupational therapists here that will actually understand a Black woman's life, in this case a Black Xhosa woman's life, and clear up things like this. The ladies then started having a little conversation among them; their conversation was them saying that sitting in a circle every day and hearing people talk to them about what they need to do with their lives will not help them. I quote "zizinto zabelungu ezi," which translates to "this is White people stuff."

Reprinted with permission from Awonke Mpokela.

therapists working in mental health settings commonly make use of the Model of Human Occupation, the KAWA model, or the Vona du Toit Model of Creative Ability (Owen, Adams, & Franszen, 2014). These models are taught as part of occupational therapy curricula across South African universities. Although the Model of Creative Ability was developed by a South African occupational therapist, it does not aim to engage African ways of knowing and being, and in this way it is similar to other models. As a way of illustrating the implications and challenges emerging as a result of the importation of theories, we share Awonke Mpokela's reflections in Table 17-1. Ms. Mpokela, a recent BSc graduate from the Division of Occupational Therapy at the University of Cape Town, shared her experience as a Black student while at a practice learning placement at a psychiatric unit during her third year of study. She recounts the difficulties associated with having to engage the Eurocentricity of theories, approaches, and ideas within occupational therapy and questions the value of services that do not consider or resonate with the lived experiences of those whom they serve. Her reflection on the discomfort of the interchange highlights the importance of developing contextually relevant occupational therapy curricula that prompt a practice that resonates with the lived realities within a particular place.

As exemplified in Table 17-1, our view is that the development of curricula for both emerging and current occupational therapy programs in Africa requires critical thinking about the philosophical orientation, fit, and selection of epistemologies and pedagogies in order for practice and education to respond to and resonate with local needs. In order to avoid a situation in which inappropriate knowledge is imposed, partnerships that intend to support program development should prioritize African ways of understanding, teaching, and researching occupational therapy and allow African occupational therapists and educators to lead the development of these programs.

Decolonizing Occupational Therapy Curricula in South Africa: An Opportunity

The historical development of occupational therapy curricula within African institutions has resulted in the reproduction of the dominant global voice in the profession. The profile of the majority of occupational therapists is female, White, and middle class (Frank, 1992), and until very recently the demographic profile of most occupational therapy students also reflected this race, class, and gender profile. As Ms. Mpokela's experience illustrates (Table 17-1), occupational therapy students holding identities beyond these often struggle to find themselves within curricula and can experience epistemic violence. Janse van Rensburg and Kapp (2014) conducted a longitudinal case study of a Black, first-generation occupational therapy student from a rural background at a university in South Africa and found that successful navigation of the occupational therapy curriculum required a reworking of this student's identity over time and a reframing of their subject position in order to survive this experience. This requires students to distance themselves from their own identities and ways of knowing. Epistemic violence occurs when the curriculum is structured in ways that do not challenge the inherent dominance of ways of knowing and being that excludes people based on their marginalized identities. In this way, knowledge is imposed on students and the beneficiaries of services, and their identities and ways of being are othered. The epistemological commitment to change such educational practices should be prioritized. The calls for decolonizing the curriculum in higher education in South Africa provides an opportunity for this to occur within occupational therapy education.

Student protests in South Africa between 2015 and 2017 have consistently highlighted the injustices faced by Black students from working class backgrounds within higher education and have called for a decolonized, free education. A decolonized education is based on an ideology that actively rejects curricula that perpetuate the ongoing subjugation of marginalized identities as well as norms and practices that are based on and related to colonial ideologies (UCT Curriculum Change Working Group, 2018). Instead, such an education centralizes issues of social justice as critical in the transformation of the academy. Since 2015, students and academics have fervently highlighted the racially skewed staff profile at South African higher education institutions and have called for more Black staff who are representative of the population and who interrogate the ideological positions that have traditionally been taught and reinforced through the academy. South African universities are engaging with this call in different ways. There is no doubt that the shifting higher education landscape has magnified the need for occupational therapy departments across South Africa to critically evaluate their stance, values, and ways of teaching and learning occupational therapy, which is long overdue. Although there has previously been reorientation of the curricula of different occupational therapy programs at universities in South Africa, the curriculum change processes, where they have occurred, have not adopted a decolonial agenda.

We support the argument that decoloniality should not be avoided, and occupational therapy programs will have to engage with this process in the immediate future if they are to remain relevant

(Ramugondo, 2017). One way of doing this would be to initiate a process of contesting the usual ways occupational therapy is taught in which a biomedical focus is prioritized and issues of equity and justice are placed on the periphery (Galvaan, 2018). Doing so would open up spaces for critical dialogue that allows for the repositioning of an occupational therapy education that serves students and the beneficiaries of the profession in more relevant ways (UCT Curriculum Change Working Group, 2018). Examples of how this may occur is demonstrated in instances of occupational therapy education where a social justice orientation to engaged scholarship has been applied. The chapter authors have been involved for many years (19 years for Galvaan and 14 years for Peters at time of publication of this text) in developing an occupational therapy practice demonstration site in Lavender Hill, Cape Town (Galvaan & Peters, 2013), where issues of equity and justice are engaged with actively through practices framed within occupation-based community development (Galvaan & Peters, 2017). This scholarship has resulted in the evolution of an occupational therapy practice that moves away from a biomedical approach toward a humanizing approach that allows people to build on their agency. The development of this approach has continued through work in occupational therapy education that is focused on community development and an approach to teaching such practice has been developed (Richards, Galvaan, & Peters, 2018).

THE IMPORTANCE OF SOUTHERN PERSPECTIVES FOR THE ONGOING GROWTH OF OCCUPATIONAL THERAPY EDUCATION IN AFRICA

Despite the fact that concepts and theories of and in occupational therapy theory have extensively originated in the Global North, there is acknowledgment that the early history of occupational therapy includes links to Egypt (Gordon, 2009), which illustrates ancient understandings of the relationship between health and occupation as originating in Africa. However, the acknowledgment of how such views and understanding have contributed to the global knowledge base of the profession have been absent. Knowledge and ideas that originate in the Global South have an important contribution to make toward an occupational therapy education that prioritizes contextually relevant practice and engages actively with issues of equity and justice. These kinds of knowledges are referred to as Southern occupational therapies (Guajardo, Kronenberg, and Ramugondo, 2015) and are influencing the education of both undergraduate and postgraduate students on the continent. Table 17-2 captures some examples of contributions of occupational therapy texts that draw on and include authors who offer Southern perspectives. These texts have influenced or are influencing occupational therapy education in Africa and include a number of authors from Africa. More importantly, they prioritize diverse voices from the Global South.

Using organically generated knowledge from the Global South allows occupational therapy programs on the continent to enact the WFOT minimum standards ideal of recognizing that occupational therapy education has to be "constantly updated to address the changing conditions and expectations in the society it serves and that regional and national differences are acknowledged within local programmes while meeting a defined standard" (WFOT, 2016, p. 11).

Table 17-2

EXAMPLES OF OCCUPATIONAL THERAPY BOOKS INFLUENCING OCCUPATIONAL THERAPY EDUCATION IN AFRICA

EDITORS	YEAR PUBLISHED	BOOK TITLE	PUBLISHER
Dsouza, S.E.; Galvaan, R.; Ramugondo, E.L.	2017	*Concepts in Occupational Therapy: Understanding Southern Perspectives*	Manipal University Press
Sakellariou, D.; Pollard, N.	2016	*Occupational Therapies Without Borders: Integrating Justice With Practice (2nd ed.)*	Elsevier
Pollard, N.; Sakellariou, D.; Kronenberg, F.	2011	*Occupational Therapies Without Borders: Volume 2. Towards an Ecology of Occupation-Based Practices*	Churchill Livingstone; Elsevier
Pollard, N.; Sakellariou, D.; Kronenberg, F.	2009	*A Political Practice of Occupational Therapy*	Churchill Livingstone; Elsevier
Lorenzo, T.; Duncan, M.; Buchanan, H.; Alsop, A.	2006	*Practice and Service Learning in Occupational Therapy: Enhancing Potential in Context*	John Wiley and Sons
Watson, R.; Swartz, L.	2004	*Transformation Through Occupation*	Whurr
Note: Examples listed are not exhaustive.			

Implications for Occupational Therapy Education

This chapter has described the challenges associated with the development of occupational therapy education in Africa. The importance of engaging African ways of understanding the world in our curricula has been illustrated as being of importance, taking into consideration the complex African identities of our students and the imposition of prevailing ideologies from the Global North. In order to continue to develop occupational therapy education on the continent, we propose the following:

- The call for a decolonial occupational therapy education is engaged with critically and authentically. Occupational therapy programs on the continent should consider how to use Global Southern knowledge and scholarship as we decolonize occupational therapy curricula by centralizing equity and justice.
- The strong focus on sociopolitical aspects of occupational engagement in African occupational therapy practice (Occupational Therapy Africa Regional Group Conference Publication Sub-commitee, 2017) is used as an important foundation for further engagement with such issues.
- International partnerships support the development of curricula that respond to local issues and give priority to African ways of knowing, positioning these as important for the development of the occupational therapy knowledge base in the Global South.

Key Reflection Questions

1. Where does the knowledge that supports occupational therapy education in your region come from?

2. What do you see as the potential for Global Southern perspectives to influence your own curricula given the people whom occupational therapy practice is intended to serve in your region?

3. What opportunities exist for applying a decolonial lens to occupational therapy education in your region?

What led you to become an occupational therapy educator?

My journey with occupational therapy education began concurrently with my journey with practice within community development in 2006. I hold the view that it is both an honor and a privilege to work with young and developing occupational therapy practitioners, particularly through the field of community development practice where we challenge and interrogate our usual ways of thinking about and viewing the world. I am inspired by the opportunities this offers to shape the profession of occupational therapy, given the urgent need for transformation that I have witnessed in the profession. I wish, through my work with students, to build occupational therapy contributions that respond to the issues of social justice in society.

Liesl Peters, BSc (OccTher), MSc (OccTher)

My interest in promoting social justice through education and scholarship has shaped my role and contributions as an occupational therapy educator. Being in this role is a privileged position because it allows me to teach and learn from students, recognizing the innovation and leadership that they bring to the profession and academy. Together through our research and teaching, we are able to work toward critical occupational therapy practices.

Roshan Galvaan, PhD, MSc (OccTher), BSc (OccTher)

REFERENCES

Crouch, R. (2016). *OTASA—A remarkable story*. Cape Town: Shorten Publishers.

Dsouza, S., Galvaan, R., & Kaushik, A. (2017). History of occupational therapy in India and South Africa. In S. Dsouza, R. Galvaan, & E. Ramugondo (Eds.), *Concepts in occupational therapy: Understanding Southern perspectives*. Manipal, India: Manipal University Press.

Engelen, A. (2014) Progress of OT education in Rwanda. OTARG Newsletter. http://www.otarg.org.za/Newsletters/ Newsletter%202014.pdf

Frank, G. (1992). Opening feminist histories of occupational therapy. *American Journal of Occupational Therapy, 46*(11), 989-999.

Galvaan, R. (2018). *Perspective on positioning for public good: Occupational therapy practice learning in South Africa*. Paper presented at the World Federation of Occupational Therapists Congress, 2018, Cape Town, South Africa.

Galvaan, R., & Peters, L. (2013). Open education resource: A strategy for occupation-based community development. Retrieved from http://hdl.handle.net/11427/6651

Galvaan, R., & Peters, L. (2017). Occupation-based community development: A critical approach to occupational therapy. In S. Dsouza, R. Galvaan, & E. Ramugondo (Eds.), *Concepts in occupational therapy: Understanding Southern perspectives*. Manipal, India: Manipal University Press.

Gordon, D. M. (2009). The history of occupational therapy. In E. B. Crepeau, E. S. Cohn, & B. A. B. Schell (Eds.), *Willard & Spackman's occupational therapy* (11th ed., pp. 202-215). Philadelphia, PA: Lippincott Williams & Wilkins.

Guajardo, A., Kronenberg, F., & Ramugondo, E. (2015). Southern occupational therapies: Emerging identities, epistemologies and practices. *South African Journal of Occupational Therapy, 45*(1), 3-10.

Hammell, K. W. (2011). Resisting theoretical imperialism in the disciplines of occupational science and occupational therapy. *British Journal of Occupational Therapy, 74*(1), 27-33.

Hansen, A. M. W., Ndaa, P., Piora, A., Weigand, S., & Munoz, J. (2018). *A qualitative study of how African occupational therapists perceive, describe and experience effective and sustainable global partnerships.* Paper presented at the World Federation of Occupational Therapists Congress, 2018 Cape Town, South Africa.

Janse van Rensburg, V., & Kapp, R. (2014). "So I have to be positive, no matter how difficult it is": A longitudinal case study of a first-generation occupational therapy student. *South African Journal of Occupational Therapy, 44*(3), 29-33.

Lorenzo, T., Duncan, M., Buchanan, H., & Alsop, A. (2006). *Practice and service learning in occupational therapy: Enhancing potential in context.* Chichester, England, New York: John Wiley & Sons.

Loveday, K. (2014). Occupational therapy education in Malawi. *OTARG Newsletter.* http://www.otarg.org.za/Newsletters/Newsletter%202014.pdf

Nafai, S. (2017). OT in Morocco. *OTARG Newsletter.* https://www.wfot.org/assets/resources/OTARG-NEWSLETTER.-MARCH-2017.pdf

OTARG Conference Publication Sub-Commitee. (2017). OTARG 2017, Accra-Ghana: come, learn and enjoy the gold coast. *OTARG Newsletter.* https://www.wfot.org/assets/resources/OTARG-NEWSLETTER.-MARCH-2017.pdf

Owen, A., Adams, F., & Franszen, D. (2014). Factors influencing model use in occupational therapy. *South African Journal of Occupational Therapy, 44*(1), 41-47.

Pollard, N., Sakellariou, D., & Kronenberg, F. (2009). *A political practice of occupational therapy.* Edinburgh; New York: Churchill Livingstone/Elsevier.

Pollard, N., Sakellariou, D., & Kronenberg, F. (2011). *Occupational therapies without borders. Vol. 2: towards an ecology of occupation-based practices.* Edinburgh; New York: Churchhill Livingstone/Elsevier.

Ramugondo, E. (2017). OT@100 years: A piece on decoloniality for OTARG. In: Maphosa, T (Ed). OTARG Newsletter, March 2017. https://www.wfot.org/assets/resources/OTARG-NEWSLETTER.-MARCH-2017.pdf

Richards, L., Galvaan, R., & Peters, L. (2018). *Occupational therapy curriculum: Promoting the development of socially-transformative practice.* Paper presented at the World Federation of Occupational Therapists Congress, 2018 Cape Town, South Africa.

Sakellariou, D., & Pollard, N. (Eds). (2017). *Occupational therapies without borders: Integrating justice with practice* (2nd ed.). Edinburgh, England: Elsevier.

UCT Curriculum Change Working Group. (2018). UCT curriculum change framework. Retrieved from https://www.news.uct.ac.za/images/userfiles/downloads/media/UCT-Curriculum-Change-Framework.pdf

Watson, R., & Swartz, L. (2004). *Transformation through occupation.* London, England: Whurr.

World Federation of Occupational Therapists. (2016). Minimum Standards for the Education of Occupational Therapists. Revised 2016. https://www.wfot.org/assets/resources/COPYRIGHTED-World-Federation-of-Occupational-Therapists-Minimum-Standards-for-the-Education-of-Occupational-Therapists-2016a.pdf

18

Educational Technologies
Enhancing Learning, Engagement, and Global Connectedness

Amanda K. Giles, OTD, OTR/L
and William E. Janes, OTD, MSCI, OTR/L

Chapter Objectives

By the end of this chapter, the reader will be able to:

1. Define educational technology from a holistic approach by considering the intentional combination of tool, method, and theory.
2. Examine current research on the use of educational technology within occupational therapy education.
3. Identify barriers that should be considered when implementing educational technology.
4. Implement best practices when using educational technology within an occupational therapy curriculum.
5. Conduct research on the application of educational technology within occupational therapy education.

WHAT IS EDUCATIONAL TECHNOLOGY?

Technology as a Building Block of Students' Occupations

"Technology has a role in occupation so fundamental, it must be considered an essential building block of occupation" (Smith, 2017, p. 7). For today's student, technology is an integral part of everyday life. From checking e-mail to watching recorded lectures, students move easily from one technology to another. Beyond the classroom, students use technology for social interaction, leisure pursuits, health needs, and even sleep/wake routines. Educators must acknowledge that technology is a large component of students' daily occupations and, therefore, consider how to integrate technology into the learning environment as a means of engaging meaningful participation.

Taff, S. D., Grajo, L. C., & Hooper, B. R. (Eds.). *Perspectives on Occupational Therapy Education: Past, Present, and Future* (pp. 191-200).

Educational Technology as the Intentional Combination of Tool, Method, and Theory

In this chapter, *educational technology* refers specifically to electronic methods of enhancing student engagement and understanding. A wide variety of electronic tools are now available to assist in the acquisition, application, integration, and innovation of knowledge (Table 18-1). However, the success of educational technology is determined by the intentional, theory-driven interaction between the tool and the method. For example, a cutting-edge computerized medical simulator (a tool) may positively affect learning in an anchored instruction approach but could lose its effect if students are not encouraged to reflect on the experience afterward (method). In the same way, low-quality preclassroom videos (tool) may negatively impact a well-thought-out flipped classroom design (method). Educational technology must be understood as more than an accumulation of tools, but as the practice of using those tools within a sound pedagogical approach (see Chapter 4 on Signature Pedagogies and Learning Designs in Occupational Therapy Education for specific learning outcomes).

USES OF EDUCATIONAL TECHNOLOGY WITHIN OCCUPATIONAL THERAPY EDUCATION

The rise in technology over the past few decades has dramatically influenced the occupational therapy classroom (Gee, Porter, Clark, & Peterson, 2017). Instructors use educational technology to teach clinical skills, deliver educational content, simulate clinical environments, engage students in interprofessional virtual reality, and facilitate international collaboration among students. The following are just some examples of educational technology used within occupational therapy curricula as reported in the literature.

Audience Response Systems

An audience response system (ARS), or student response system, allows students to individually and simultaneously answer questions using a wireless remote control, such as a clicker, mobile device, or laptop. An ARS promotes active and equal student participation, provides immediate feedback, and fosters a sense of classroom community, all of which can be particularly useful with large class sizes. In a study by Taylor, Benson, and Szucs (2017), occupational therapy students perceived an ARS as easy to use and demonstrated improved test scores. Mernar (2015) found that occupational therapy students prepared differently for class when anticipating the use of clickers and perceived clickers as useful to learning in a clinic-based course. Williams, Lewis, Boyle, Brown, and Holt (2008) found that 85% or more of occupational therapists and other health profession students viewed wireless keypads as a useful learning tool when answering critical thinking questions during an interprofessional lecture.

Simulation and Virtual Reality

Simulated clinical environments offer a valuable safety net for students to practice lifelike patient scenarios within an artificial environment. Simulation options range from low fidelity, such as paper or computer-based patient scenarios, to high fidelity, which include standardized patients or computerized mannequins. Benefits of simulation are well documented in the medical field and are more effective when combined with principles of distributed practice, repetitive practice, individualized learning, mastery learning, and feedback (Cook et al., 2013).

Table 18-1	
EDUCATIONAL TECHNOLOGY TOOLS	
COMMUNICATION TECHNOLOGY	e-mail, text message (Internet relay chat), Audience Response Systems (ARS; Poll Everywhere, clickers), synchronous audio/video conference (Skype, Cisco WebEx, Zoom, Adobe Connect, GoToMeeting), social media (Facebook, LinkedIn, Twitter, Instagram, Snapchat, blogs, wiki, social media stories), podcasts, bulletin and/or discussion boards, listservs, online scheduling tools (Doodle, Rally, NeedToMeet, YouCanBook.me)
COURSE MANAGEMENT SYSTEMS AND ASSESSMENT TOOLS	Open source and proprietary learning management systems (Moodle, Blackboard, Skillsoft, Desire2Learn, Canvas, Sakai, Jenzabar, Pearson LearningStudio), content management systems (SharePoint, WordPress), massive open online courses (edX, Khan Academy, Coursera), collaborative peer grading (Mobius SLIP), assessment tools (ExamSoft, Respondus Lockdown Browser, BioSig-ID), plagiarism checkers (TurnItIn, SafeAssign)
ORGANIZATION AND PRESENTATION TECHNOLOGY	Presentation software (PowerPoint, Keynote, Prezi), lecture capture tools (Panopto, Tegrity, Camtasia), animation and video software (Flash, iMovie, GoAnimate, CrazyTalk), webinars, interactive whiteboards (SMART board, Promethean), content engagement tools (Piazza, VoiceThread)
INFORMATION SEARCH AND MANAGEMENT TECHNOLOGY	Internet, electronic databases (PubMed, CINAHL, ProQuest, OvidSP, Eric), reference management software (Procite, EndNotes, Refworks, Covidence), data collection and analysis software (Excel, SPSS, REDCap, SurveyMonkey), file hosting services (OneDrive, Google Docs, Dropbox, Box)
SPECIALIZED SIMULATION EQUIPMENT	High-fidelity mannequin-based simulators (SimMan, VitalSim), task trainers (blood pressure training arm), virtual and augmented reality (Second Life, Active Worlds)
ELECTRONIC RESOURCES	e-books, e-journals, mobile applications (GONI: Goniometry for Clinicians, MOBI: Mobility Aids, OT Exam Prep, OT Kinesiology), asynchronous video platforms (International Clinical Educators [ICE] Video Library, YouTube, OccupationalTherapy.com)
Note: Examples listed in parentheses represent a sample of what is available and are not intended to be all inclusive. Any reference to a specific educational technology within this chapter does not constitute or imply the endorsement, recommendation, or favoring of that product.	

Based on survey responses from 245 occupational therapy assistant and occupational therapy entry-level programs, Bethea, Castillo, and Harvison (2014) found that 175 programs engage in some manner of simulation, most commonly human or video based. The use of simulation was more prevalent in clinical intervention courses and with acute care scenarios. Despite the inherent challenges, such as the time needed to develop scenarios, equipment costs, and scheduling difficulties, simulation offers far-reaching positive impacts in the areas of student clinical reasoning, fieldwork preparation, communication skills, and safety awareness.

Simulation-based assessments also provide an effective way of measuring clinical competency, particularly in preparation for fieldwork. Tomlin (2005) revealed that occupational therapy student simulation scores from an interactive client video scenario were more effective than academic grades at predicting Level II Fieldwork Performance Evaluation (American Occupational Therapy Association, 2002) scores because of their ability to measure efficient time management within a realistic clinical context.

Virtual world (VW) role-play simulations provide a less costly and less time-consuming alternative to high-fidelity methods while still preserving the benefits of a complex simulated environment. VW simulations engage the user in a multisensory, computer-generated environment using a helmet and/or gloves. Toth-Cohen and Mitchell (2010) described an interprofessional collaboration using an online VW training platform to provide health care to the homeless and recently homeless population. Preliminary results showed valuable lessons for patient-centered, interprofessional teamwork across multiple geographic locations.

The Accreditation Council for Occupational Therapy Education Standards recommends that simulated environments be considered as an alternative option for Level I fieldwork placement (Accreditation Council for Occupational Therapy Education, 2018). Occupational therapy students also perceive that the use of video simulations could potentially supplement fieldwork placement (Brown & Williams, 2009). Advances in technology have expanded the possibilities for simulation as a teaching tool, and it is expected that technology-enhanced simulation will continue to grow as a core component of occupational therapy education.

Social Media

Social media includes any easy-to-use form of online communication and collaboration (Junco, 2014). Academic institutions use social media to deepen connections with a myriad of stakeholders for the purposes of recruitment, networking, marketing, fundraising, crisis communication, and communication of special events, research, and innovation, among others. In addition, students and faculty use social media to communicate about course activities and to facilitate the learning process; for example, occupational therapy educators reported using blogs as an avenue for reflection and discussion of ethical issues (Hudon et al., 2016). Occupational therapy educators also use discussion forums, such as the American Occupational Therapy Association CommunOT (https://communot. aota.org) platform to exchange ideas and information. Twitter, an online news and networking site, can be used to create a community of learners within a classroom and across the globe (Maclean, Jones, Carin-Levy, & Hunter, 2013). However, data out of the United Kingdom suggest that the majority (89%) of occupational therapy students use Facebook, whereas only 30% use Twitter (Parks et al., 2017). In general, health profession students reported that they prefer to receive information online over other formats (Giordano & Giordano, 2011).

Video

Video serves as a multifunctional medium across a variety of educational technology tools and methods and can be used to improve student learning and satisfaction in both asynchronous and synchronous formats. Videos have been distributed within occupational therapy education via e-learning modules, mobile applications, learning management systems (LMSs), and DVD platforms. Occupational therapy faculty report that instructional videos are among the most useful educational resources, well beyond online resources more generally (Reynolds, Watling, Zapletal, & May-Benson, 2012).

Video Provides Meaningful Feedback

Occupational therapy students reported that reflective video analysis "was the best part [of a comprehensive practical exam] because I could see how I actually looked" (Giles, Carson, Breland,

Coker-Bolt, & Bowman, 2014). Furthermore, students who received annotated video feedback on transfer skills scored higher on the examination than students who received traditional feedback during labs (Truskowski & VanderMolen, 2017).

Video Is Useful for Introducing Foundational Clinical Skills

Occupational therapy students have used instructional videos to learn goniometry skills (Giles, Annan-Coultas, Gober, & Greene, 2018), manual muscle testing (McAlister, 2014), wheelchair transfers (Hayden, 2013), dependent hoist transfers (Gallagher, Gilligan, & McGrath, 2014), and kinesiology taping techniques (Rice, Amerih, & Brown, 2017). All of these studies used video as a lab supplement and found positive student responses, except for Gallagher et al. (2014), who found that confidence and preference was greater for face-to-face instruction over video instruction only; however, their small sample size warrants further investigation.

Case-Based Videos Connect Student Learning to Clinical Application

In Murphy and Stav (2018), occupational therapy students exhibited greater inductive reasoning skills when using video case studies vs text-based case studies. Bagatell and Broggi (2014) used pediatric video cases to improve communication between occupational therapy and physical therapy students. After analyzing dental student postures via video, occupational therapy students educated dental students in ergonomics and repetitive stress injury prevention during dental examinations (Bowman, Murphy, & Schaner, 2016).

Video Facilitates Global Collaborative Learning

Using Web conferencing software, students in the United States have interacted synchronously with students in Sweden, India, South Africa, and the Philippines (Aldrich & Grajo, 2017; Aldrich & Johansson, 2015; Asher, Estes, & Hill, 2014; Cabatan & Grajo, 2017). Global interactions occurred within the context of occupational therapy and occupational science courses, with topics ranging from culture and occupational justice to case-based intervention planning. Students in these studies perceived these cross-cultural interactions as positive learning experiences.

Learning Management Systems

An LMS, also known as a *virtual learning environment*, is a Web-based software platform commonly used to deliver course material via a single, consistent, organized, and intuitive user interface with special features, such as examinations, discussion boards, feedback, and tracking options. LMSs have often been used within occupational therapy education to support online, hybrid, and traditional brick-and-mortar educational programs. For example, LMS discussion boards have been used as a supplement to traditional classroom activities (Gallew, 2004) and for peer coaching and self-directed learning during fieldwork (Thomas & Storr, 2005) with positive reports of student satisfaction. Occupational therapy educators have pursued virtual learning environments to meet the needs of students in rural communities (Bracciano, Lohman, Coppard, Bradberry, & Easley, 2011) and have acknowledged the critical need for information technology support when integrating an online platform (Barnard-Ashton, Rothberg, & McInerney, 2017). As online learning continues to expand, educational programs are expected to become more reliant on LMS for course delivery.

LIMITATIONS OF EDUCATIONAL TECHNOLOGY

Educational technology is not a panacea. Barriers related to perceived usefulness and perceived ease of use can derail a learner's engagement with any educational technology, regardless of the intended educational value (Davis, 1985). Furthermore, inequitable and inconsistent access to educational technology can limit successful implementation at individual, institutional, and societal levels.

Individual Barriers

Although modern occupational therapy students are widely regarded as being confident with technology and preferring to use the Internet as their primary learning resource (Hills, Ryan, Smith, & Warren-Forward, 2012), this perception lacks empirical support (Bennett, Maton, & Kervin, 2008). If users are inherently anxious about their own technological savvy and do not perceive sufficient environmental support to ensure a successful experience, they are less likely to engage with a new technology.

However, initial acceptance of a new technology does not guarantee success. Students in a collaborative, international occupational therapy program identified additional barriers to using a virtual environment, including scheduling difficulty for synchronous conversations, poor fit of social interactions for self-described introverts, and poor Internet connections (Cabatan & Grajo, 2017). Reliability and speed of access influence perceptions of both ease of use and usefulness of technology. For example, students with slow or unreliable Internet access may find an LMS both difficult to use and not useful. Connectivity issues tend to disproportionately influence ratings of usefulness rather than ease of use of social media for higher education (Dumpit & Fernandez, 2017), suggesting that learners discount the utility of the platform and its associated content when Internet connections are unstable.

Institutional Barriers

Implementing a new educational technology requires institutional investments not just in the technology itself but also in setup, training, infrastructure, user support, and faculty time to develop new materials or adapt existing content. Lack of institutional support is a barrier to developing new educational approaches around the world, particularly in regions where new educational technologies have been rushed into practice without adequate faculty training and release time to maximize their value (Jacob, Xiong, & Ye, 2015). Institutions that do invest in educational technology must brace for rapid knowledge obsolescence; new technologies will eventually be outdated or discontinued, requiring educators to restart the entire technology adoption process at additional cost (Adams Becker et al., 2017).

Societal Barriers

Inequitable access to educational technologies disproportionately impacts students in financially disadvantaged populations and geographic regions (Adams Becker et al., 2017). Eighty percent of the population in developed countries has Internet access; only 41.3% in developing countries and 17.5% in less-developed countries have access (International Telecommunications Union, 2017). The relationship between connectivity and technology usefulness is amplified in areas where Internet access is less widespread and reliable. For example, university students in Turkey rated a virtual learning environment less useful than their classmates in the United Kingdom because of differences in accessibility and reliability (Kurt & Tingöy, 2017). Consistent with their peers across higher education, occupational therapy educators in South Africa report unstable power and Internet bandwidth as two of the largest barriers to blended occupational therapy education (Barnard-Ashton et al., 2017).

Implications for Occupational Therapy Education

Innovation is inherently linked to educational technology because of the ever-changing state of technology itself. Educators must stay current on advances and opportunities afforded by educational technology. Taking into account students' occupational profiles, educators should consider how technology can be used to transfer information in an efficient, effective, and personalized manner. Furthermore, educators should advocate for the development of new technologies and create evidence regarding their effectiveness (Bondoc, 2005). The following suggestions are supported by the literature reviewed in the preceding sections.

- Best practices for implementing educational technology within the occupational therapy curriculum
  - Reinforce active participation and a sense of classroom community via ARS.
  - Promote realistic, meaningful clinical applications with virtual reality and computerized simulation.
  - Consider the academic use of social media to enhance dialogue and share resources.
  - Use video as a means for immediate student feedback, clinical skill introduction and application, and observation of real patient-therapist interactions.
  - Collaborate globally using technology within existing coursework to enrich understanding of occupation and culture.
  - Provide adequate information technology support to reduce anxiety associated with new technologies.
  - Tightly integrate educational technology tools and established teaching methods within the prevailing pedagogical theory underlying the existing curriculum.
  - Collect data on student perceptions and technology effectiveness. Make adjustments as indicated.
- How to advocate for improvements in educational technology tools and methods
  - Create and/or support emerging technologies in education.
  - Advocate for continued awareness of the importance of education research.
  - Seek funding for up-to-date educational technology tools and research.
  - Engage in local and global research into the effective use of technology in occupational therapy education, preferably using adequately powered experimental designs.
  - Collaborate and share innovative ideas for incorporating technology into the curriculum via networking and publications.
  - Request institutional- and national-level support for educational technology and teaching effectiveness programs, particularly information technology support and faculty mentorship.

Educational technology has gained widespread momentum, even as it attempts to keep up with the popularity of everyday technology in society. Before investing in new educational technologies, it is important to carefully and thoughtfully select tools that effectively pair with the intended pedagogical approach. Educational technology serves as a modality for improving student learning; it does not replace the teacher. "The [education] product we need today must serve the 21st century and ensure preparation for that which is to come, some known and still much unknown, much that will need to be thought through carefully before significant change comes" (Mitcham, 2014, p. 637).

Key Reflection Questions

1. What role does technology play in the occupational profiles of your students?
2. How could you intentionally combine tool, method, and theory when integrating a new educational technology within your course?
3. What individual, institutional, and societal barriers must you consider when implementing new educational technologies for students in your program?
4. How can you advocate for improvements in educational technology within your own curriculum and within occupational therapy education globally?

What led you to become an occupational therapy educator?

Occupational therapists are natural teachers. We break down complex tasks into their component parts and grade the challenge to achieve the highest level of independence. Engaging in this process with students as they transform into independent clinicians brings great joy and satisfaction, particularly when confidence leads to compassionate, authentic therapeutic intervention.

Amanda K. Giles, OTD, OTR/L

I became an occupational therapy educator because I am passionate about nurturing client-centered, evidence-based practice in future occupational therapy practitioners. Our profession's goals of maximizing health, well-being, and quality of life can only be met with an appreciation for the evidence and that evidence is only valuable to the extent that it informs and is informed by practice.

William E. Janes, OTD, MSCI, OTR/L

REFERENCES

Accreditation Council for Occupational Therapy Education. (2018). 2018 Accreditation council for occupational therapy education (ACOTE) standards and interpretive guide. Retrieved from https://www.aota.org/~/media/Corporate/Files/EducationCareers/Accredit/StandardsReview/2018-ACOTE-Standards-Interpretive-Guide.pdf

Adams Becker, S., Cummins, M., Davis, A., Freeman, A., Hall Giesinger, C., & Ananthanarayanan, V. (2017). *NMC horizon report: 2017 higher education edition.* Austin, TX: The New Media Consortium.

Aldrich, R. M., & Grajo, L. C. (2017). International educational interactions and students' critical consciousness: A pilot study. *American Journal of Occupational Therapy, 71*(5), 7105230020. doi:10.5014/ajot.2017.026724

Aldrich, R. M., & Johansson, K. E. (2015). US and Swedish student learning through online synchronous international interactions. *American Journal of Occupational Therapy, 69*(Suppl. 2), 6912350010p1-5. doi:10.5014/ajot.2015.018424

American Occupational Therapy Association. (2002). *Fieldwork Performance Evaluation for the occupational therapy student.* Bethesda, MD: AOTA Press.

Asher, A., Estes, J., & Hill, V. (2014). International outreach from the comfort of your classroom! *Education Special Interest Section Quarterly, 24*(4), 1.

Bagatell, N., & Broggi, M. (2014). Occupational therapy and physical therapy students' perceptions of a short-term interprofessional education module. *Education Special Interest Section Quarterly, 24*(2), 1-4.

Barnard-Ashton, P., Rothberg, A., & McInerney, P. (2017). The integration of blended learning into an occupational therapy curriculum: A qualitative reflection. *BMC Medical Education, 17*(1), 135. doi:10.1186/s12909-017-0977-1

Bennett, S., Maton, K., & Kervin, L. (2008). The 'digital natives' debate: A critical review of the evidence. *British Journal of Educational Technology, 39*(5), 775-786. doi:10.1111/j.1467-8535.2007.00793.x

Bethea, D. P., Castillo, D. C., & Harvison, N. (2014). Use of simulation in occupational therapy education: Way of the future? *American Journal of Occupational Therapy, 68*(Suppl. 2), S32-S39. doi:10.5014/ajot.2014.012716

Bondoc, S. (2005). Occupational therapy and evidence-based education. *Education Special Interest Section Quarterly, 15*(4), 1-4.

Bowman, P., Murphy, C., & Schaner, M. (2016). Engaging dental students in ergonomics. *American Journal of Occupational Therapy, 70*(4 Suppl. 1), 7011515249p1. doi:10.5014/ajot.2016.70S1-PO1097

Bracciano, A., Lohman, H., Coppard, B. M., Bradberry, J. C., & Easley, C. (2011). Development of a hybrid distance occupational therapy program in Alaska. *Journal of Allied Health, 40*(2), 90-95.

Brown, T., & Williams, B. (2009). The use of DVD simulation as an interprofessional education tool with undergraduate occupational therapy students. *British Journal of Occupational Therapy, 72*(6), 266-274. doi:10.1177/030802260907200607

Cabatan, M. C. C., & Grajo, L. C. (2017). Internationalization in an occupational therapy curriculum: A Philippine–American pilot collaboration. *American Journal of Occupational Therapy, 71*(6), 7106165010p1-7106165010p9. doi:10.5014/ajot.2017.024653

Cook, D. A., Hamstra, S. J., Brydges, R., Zendejas, B., Szostek, J. H., Wang, A. T., ... Hatala, R. (2013). Comparative effectiveness of instructional design features in simulation-based education: Systematic review and meta-analysis. *Medical Teacher, 35*(1), e867-e898. doi:10.3109/0142159X.2012.714886

Davis, F. D. (1985). *A technology acceptance model for empirically testing new end-user information systems: Theory and results.* Cambridge, MA: Massachusetts Institute of Technology.

Dumpit, D. Z., & Fernandez, C. J. (2017). Analysis of the use of social media in higher education institutions (HEIs) using the technology acceptance model. *International Journal of Educational Technology in Higher Education, 14*(1), 5. doi:10.1186/s41239-017-0045-2

Gallagher, A. M., Gilligan, R., & McGrath, M. (2014). The effect of DVD training on the competence of occupational therapy students in manual handling: A pilot study. *International Journal of Therapy and Rehabilitation, 21*(12), 575-583. doi:10.12968/ijtr.2014.21.12.575

Gallew, H. A. (2004). Brief or new: The benefits of on-line learning in occupational therapy. *Occupational Therapy in Health Care, 18*(1-2), 117-125. doi:10.1080/J003v18n01_12

Gee, B., Porter, J., Clark, C., & Peterson, T. (2017). Overview of instructional technology used in the education of occupational therapy students: A survey study. *Open Journal of Occupational Therapy, 5*(4), 13. doi:10.15453/2168-6408.1352

Giles, A. K., Annan-Coultas, D., Gober, A., & Greene, L. (2018). E-Learning innovations: Implementation of video in an occupational therapy classroom. *Journal of Occupational Therapy Education, 2*(1). doi:10.26681/jote.2018.020103

Giles, A. K., Carson, N. E., Breland, H. L., Coker-Bolt, P., & Bowman, P. J. (2014). Use of simulated patients and reflective video analysis to assess occupational therapy students' preparedness for fieldwork. *American Journal of Occupational Therapy, 68*(Suppl. 2), S57-S66. doi:10.5014/ajot.2014.685S03

Giordano, C., & Giordano, C. (2011). Health professions students' use of social media. *Journal of Allied Health, 40*(2), 78-81.

Hayden, C. L. (2013). Online learning of safe patient transfers in occupational therapy education. *Open Journal of Occupational Therapy, 1*(2), 7. doi:10.15453/2168-6408.1021

Hills, C., Ryan, S., Smith, D. R., & Warren-Forward, H. (2012). The impact of 'Generation Y' occupational therapy students on practice education. *Australian Occupational Therapy Journal, 59*(2), 156-163. doi:10.1111/j.1440-1630.2011.00984.x

Hudon, A., Perreault, K., Laliberté, M., Desrochers, P., Williams-Jones, B., Ehrmann Feldman, D., ... Mazer, B. (2016). Ethics teaching in rehabilitation: Results of a pan-Canadian workshop with occupational and physical therapy educators. *Disability and Rehabilitation, 38*(22), 2244-2254. doi:10.3109/09638288.2015.1123308

International Telecommunications Union. (2017). Measuring the information society report (Vol. 1). Geneva, Switzerland. Retrieved from https://www.itu.int/en/ITU-D/Statistics/Documents/publications/misr2017/MISR2017_Volume1.pdf

Jacob, W. J., Xiong, W., & Ye, H. (2015). Professional development programmes at world-class universities. *Palgrave Communications, 1*, 15002. doi:10.1057/palcomms.2015.2

Junco, R. (2014). *Engaging students through social media: Evidence-based practices for use in student affairs.* San Francisco, CA: Jossey-Bass.

Kurt, Ö. E., & Tingöy, Ö. (2017). The acceptance and use of a virtual learning environment in higher education: An empirical study in Turkey, and the UK. *International Journal of Educational Technology in Higher Education, 14*(1), 26. doi:10.1186/s41239-017-0064-z

Maclean, F., Jones, D., Carin-Levy, G., & Hunter, H. (2013). Understanding Twitter. *British Journal of Occupational Therapy, 76*(6), 295-298. doi:10.4276/030802213X13706169933021

McAlister, R. B. (2014). Use of instructor-produced YouTube videos to supplement manual skills training in occupational therapy education. *American Journal of Occupational Therapy, 68*(Suppl. 2), S67-S72. doi:10.5014/ajot.2014.685S04

Mernar, T. (2015). Using clicker technology: Comparing student perceptions of learning and participation. *American Journal of Occupational Therapy, 69*(Suppl. 1), 6911520075p1. doi:10.5014/ajot.2015.69S1-PO1102

Mitcham, M. D. (2014). Education as engine. *American Journal of Occupational Therapy, 68*(6), 636-648. doi:10.5014/ajot.2014.686001

Murphy, L. F., & Stav, W. B. (2018). The impact of online video cases on clinical reasoning in occupational therapy education: A quantitative analysis. *Open Journal of Occupational Therapy, 6*(3), 4. doi:10.15453/2168-6408.1494

Parks, M., Sorby, K., Davis, B., McFarland, J., Wallbank, H., King, R., & Adams, D. (2017). Exploring the use of social media by occupational therapy students. *Research at the University of York St John.* Retrieved from http://ray.yorksj.ac.uk/id/eprint/2302/

Reynolds, S., Watling, R., Zapletal, A., & May-Benson, T. (2012). Sensory integration in entry-level occupational therapy education. *Sensory Integration Special Interest Section Quarterly Newsletter, 35*(4), 1-4.

Rice, T., Amerih, H., & Brown, D. (2017). The impact of instructional method on the application of Kinesio Taping techniques for occupational therapy students. *Journal of Occupational Therapy Education, 1*(3), 2. doi:10.26681/jote.2017.010302

Smith, R. O. (2017). Technology and occupation: Past, present, and the next 100 years of theory and practice. *American Journal of Occupational Therapy, 71*(6), 7106150010p1-7106150010p15. doi: 10.5014/ajot.2017.716003

Taylor, M., Benson, J. D., & Szucs, K. (2017). Student response system and learning: Perceptions of the student. *American Journal of Occupational Therapy, 71*(4 Suppl. 1). doi:10.5014/ajot.2017.71S1-PO2019

Thomas, A., & Storr, C. (2005). WebCT in occupational therapy clinical education: Implementing and evaluating a tool for peer learning and interaction. *Occupational Therapy International, 12*(3), 162-179. doi:10.1002/oti.3

Tomlin, G. (2005). The use of interactive video client simulation scores to predict clinical performance of occupational therapy students. *American Journal of Occupational Therapy, 59*(1), 50-56. doi:10.5014/ajot.59.1.50

Toth-Cohen, S., & Mitchell, P. R. (2010). Second Life project development as a venue for interdisciplinary collaboration. In R. Russell (Ed.), *Cases on collaboration in virtual learning environments: Processes and interactions* (pp. 239-248). Hershey, PA: IGI Global.

Truskowski, S., & VanderMolen, J. (2017). Outcomes and perceptions of annotated video feedback following psychomotor skill laboratories. *Journal of Computer Assisted Learning, 33*(2), 97-105. doi:10.1111/jcal.12167

Williams, B., Lewis, B., Boyle, M., Brown, T., & Holt, T. (2008). A survey of undergraduate health science students' views on interprofessional education and the use of educational technology: Preliminary analyses and findings. *Journal of Emergency Primary Health Care, 6*(4).

19

Fieldwork Education
New and Emerging Models to Support the Future of Practice

Susan Coppola, OTD, OT/L, FAOTA
and Susan M. Higgins, OTD, OTR/L

Chapter Objectives

By the end of this chapter, the reader will be able to:

1. Identify the shared origins and philosophies of occupational therapy and progressive education as they are evidenced in fieldwork.
2. Relate key principles of John Dewey's pedagogy to fieldwork in occupational therapy.
3. Describe the current and proposed structure of fieldwork in the United States and how progressive education principles are or could be emphasized in processes and structure of fieldwork.
4. Discuss ways that principles of progressive education can be used in fieldwork to advance the profession, using the concepts and pillars of the American Occupational Therapy Association's Vision 2025.

INTRODUCTION

This chapter addresses the history and evolution of occupational therapy pedagogy in fieldwork from the beginnings of the profession over 100 years ago to an imagined future. We build on Schwartz's (1992) discussion of the shared beginning of occupational therapy with the progressive education movement. Then, using principles of progressive education initially described by Dewey, we explore how those principles appear in occupational therapy fieldwork design. We also use Vision 2025 from the American Occupational Therapy Association (AOTA, 2017b) along with these principles to envision occupational therapy fieldwork for the future.

Taff, S. D., Grajo, L. C., & Hooper, B. R. (Eds.). *Perspectives on Occupational Therapy Education: Past, Present, and Future* (pp. 201-211). © 2020 Taylor & Francis Group.

SHARED HISTORY OF OCCUPATIONAL THERAPY
AND PROGRESSIVE EDUCATION INFORMING FIELDWORK

Schwartz (1992) argued that although the moral treatment movement spawned occupational therapy, the progressive education movement exerted a significant influence on essential principles of the profession. The progressive education movement, begun in the early 1900s, shared leaders with occupational therapy as a profession. Noted names from the field of education were John Dewey and Susan Cox Johnson. Social workers Jane Addams, Julia Lathrop, and Eleanor Clarke Slagle and Susan Tracy, a nurse, were pragmatists, humanists, and occupationalists. These were some of the social reformers associated with innovative programs, most notably the Lab School and Hull House in Chicago, who shared a worldview and philosophy of occupation as learning and of education as a doing process. That philosophy was infused with morality about the benefits of educative experiences for individuals as well as for generating a just and democratic society. These beliefs about the nature of learning and the ideals about the renewal of society exist in present-day occupational therapy fieldwork.

Fieldwork combined with academic coursework in occupational therapy aligns with Deweyan views that professional education should contain focused time for apprenticeship and for developing complex reasoning (Cohn, 1989). Fieldwork was a required learning and proving ground in the first occupational therapy education standards (Presseller, 1983). The initial 1923 standards required 2 months of fieldwork that increased to 9 months in 1935 and decreased to 6 months in 1973. Entry-level doctoral programs currently also require a 14-week experiential component distinct from fieldwork (Accreditation Council for Occupational Therapy Education [ACOTE], 2011; AOTA, 2018). Variation in the length of fieldwork occurred when wartime needs accelerated education programs in the military (Colman, 1990). The early standards required experience with specific types of diagnostic groups. These early prescriptive standards have been replaced by requirements for experiences in diversity of client age and settings, as well as innovative fieldwork placements to expand practice in emerging arenas (AOTA, 2016; Rodger et al., 2007). Fieldwork can now include practices beyond direct services to clients, such as clinically based research (e.g., clinical reasoning study of providers of prevention-based services for older adults), community-level practice (e.g., accessible tourism, adaptive sports, parks and gardens accessibility, and camp for children of immigrant farm workers), consultation (e.g., dementia care, soldiers with brain injury, and school-based inclusion in under-resourced countries), administration (e.g., private practice, career ladder projects, and developing a memory care unit), and policy (AOTA, 2016). Practices with underserved persons in prisons, homeless shelters, and refugee communities represent exciting places for students to learn and serve. In some regions, these examples are not novel, and in others they are innovative. Fieldwork coordinators and faculty can look to their local communities and networks to identify needs and opportunities for students to extend beyond traditional direct care such as those mentioned previously.

In this chapter, we consider these differing types of fieldwork (i.e., traditional and role-emerging settings considered innovative or pioneering) in light of their pedagogy and purposes. In particular, we will address how opportunities for innovation and engagement in communities can foster depth of learning in important areas such as leadership, advocacy, inquiry, collaboration, and creativity.

Intentional Use of Progressive Pedagogy to Deepen Learning and Innovation

The essence of progressive education is involvement in meaningful experiences to build habits of inquiry for solving problems of the future. This philosophy challenged traditional passive and decontextualized learning and instead engaged students with complexity in each situation. Fieldwork is the natural place to enact principles of progressive education centered on learning as transaction in real situations as described by Dewey and Small (1897).

This section explores progressive education principles described by Dewey, namely education as experience, reflection, learning as a social process, experience of learning, inquiry, role of teacher/supervisor, and outcomes of learning (Dewey, 1938; Dewey & Small, 1897). Deweyan learning principles inform and exist in occupational therapy practice and learning. Reexamining pedagogical origins enables fieldwork coordinators and educators to intentionally and explicitly optimize learning on traditional and innovative fieldwork.

The phrase "education as experience" captures the essence of Deweyan theory (i.e., we learn by doing things). Engaging in the world develops habits to be used for future situations. An accessible tourism project may prepare students to communicate about inclusion and disability with community businesses and the transportation industry. Fieldwork gives students authentic experiences to form habits of effective problem solving in context and habits of advocacy. It is a full-body experience that engages senses, movements, thinking, and feeling. It is no wonder that fieldwork can be both exhausting and exhilarating. As fieldwork challenges students toward more creative problem solving in unchartered territory, such as having responsibility for a new community program, a deeper level of engagement can foster transformative learning.

Reflection for Learning

Reflection, in Deweyan pedagogy, is essential for turning experience into learning. Schön (1983) extended Dewey by postulating that professional development is a process of learning through reflection in action and reflection on action. Ideally, fieldwork supervisors model and encourage students to reflect as an ongoing part of practice and create time for looking back over experiences in a way that turns those experiences into professional reasoning. The concept of reflexivity built upon Schön's work on reflection by adding dimensions of self-awareness and interpretation. Reflexivity involves critical reflection into situations in light of one's own perspectives and biases and also considers the influence of one's presence in the situation. Reflexivity underpins client-centered practice and enables students to act knowingly and ethically in complex situations. Innovative fieldwork experiences are inherently complex, given the uncertainty and diversity of interests, cultures, stakeholders, and other matters. For example, reflexivity would inform school-based fieldwork on inclusion for children in an underresourced country. In any fieldwork, reflexivity is valuable and sharpened in navigating interpersonal situations effectively.

Learning is a Social Process

Learning is a social process (Dewey, 1938). Fieldwork is a powerful social situation saturated with meanings, novelty, reasoning, and emotion. Students learn through engaging in socially constructed understandings in real-life situations. Peer learning models of fieldwork can offer richly coconstructed interprofessional and intraprofessional learning. What students learn on fieldwork is multifaceted and dominated by learning through interacting with others. Thus, the socialization process teaches personal conduct, subtle rules for team membership, and how to influence others. Wenger (1998) extended Dewey's social learning theories to the concept of "communities of practice." In this theory, high-performing teams comprise diverse individuals who share objectives and conduct their work as a negotiated learning process. Critically reflecting on social processes and power dynamics positions students to work toward fairness in exchanges in future situations (Freire, 1970). Fieldwork education is a place where students can enact and deepen their beliefs about occupational justice. According to Dewey, learning habits of ethical conduct and reasoning occur within real-life social experiences that form and reinforce those habits. Well-established institutional practices may offer students limited freedom to question or change boundaries and rules for practice and interaction. Novel fieldworks, such as an interprofessional student team project for clients with aphasia, may afford more opportunities to negotiate and advance collaboration than well-established settings.

Experience of Learning

The experience of learners is central in progressive education. Learner-centered education (Henson, 2003) further emphasizes the students' perspective. In fieldwork, educators typically consider students' prior experiences and the importance of continuity and coherence. However, as professional preparation, occupational therapy fieldwork must be more subject centered, therefore emphasizing the subjects of occupation and occupational therapy (Hooper, 2010). Ideally, educators address both learner and subject, gradually building challenges and expectations for standards of professional reasoning and performance. When fieldwork is in a long-standing practice setting, such as an inpatient rehabilitation unit, students learn valuable established content and practice applications through problem solving in circumscribed roles. In novel settings, for example with refugees adjusting to a new country, broader questions may arise for clients, and students may wonder if the work is real occupational therapy. Attention to these questions may guide their work toward highly creative responses to occupational needs and quite authentic occupational therapy. Role-emerging experiences may build more advanced habits of inquiry because of the challenge posed in uncertain situations.

Role of Educator

The role of the educator is to help students learn how to approach problematic situations through sound inquiry processes (Dewey, 1916, 1938; Dewey & Small, 1897). The fieldwork educator sequences and scaffolds learning so the student is engaged in the doing of practice as a problem-solving process. Didactic sessions may occur briefly during fieldwork, but the heart of learning is supporting the student's inquiry and action in real-life practice. Supervisors bring differing theories, skills, and expectations to the process. Their beliefs about learning may be "sink or swim," observe then do, or learn by active experimentation. Ideally, the supervisor uses the principles of the "just-right challenge" for learning while learning with the student. Novel situations may prompt strong collaboration between the fieldwork educator and the student because it is uncertain territory for both. The discourse may rely heavily on the student's knowledge and judgment (e.g., when the student visits homes of people with mental illness and therefore knows more about the clients' needs and situations). The educator must also consider that experiences can be miseducative (Dewey, 1938) if they stifle curiosity or promote overgeneralizing or hopelessness rather than inspiring inquisitiveness and future learning.

Outcomes of Learning

Outcomes of learning described by Dewey (1938) relate to contemporary views of education as building strong habits of inquiry and quest for more learning. It is essential for students to acquire knowledge and discrete skills in each fieldwork setting. Then by developing competent performance in multiple settings they hone their capacity to learn skills and problem solve. In novel areas, like developing a rural home-based consultant practice, this ability of inquiry and problem solving is taken to a higher level. The success and satisfaction they gain in fieldwork should inspire them to continue to learn and contribute.

In summary, fieldwork is the most contextualized and engaging component of the occupational therapy curriculum. It is not just apprenticeship but a process that integrates theory and practice. Theory guides problem-solving processes, but the situation is emotional because of the reality and urgency of human need. Fieldwork has waves of information and demands, not controlled sequence and timing like learning in the classroom. Fieldwork is a messy and authentic paradise for using the principles of progressive education to prepare students for the uncertainties of the future.

CURRENT STRUCTURES AND SITUATION OF FIELDWORK EDUCATION IN THE UNITED STATES

ACOTE identifies fieldwork education as a "crucial part of professional preparation" (ACOTE, 2018, p. 39) and sets the standards for implementation of both Level I and Level II fieldwork experiences. Level I fieldwork was designed to "introduce students to the fieldwork experience, apply knowledge to practice, and develop understanding of the need of clients" (ACOTE, 2018, p. 40), whereas Level II fieldwork aims to "develop competent, entry-level, generalist occupational" therapy practitioners (p. 41). There are 16 standards in the current ACOTE standards (ACOTE, 2018) that address Level I and Level II fieldwork. These standards address aspects such as psychosocial factors, client centeredness, and occupation-based services. Occupational therapy students are required to complete 24 weeks of Level II fieldwork, and occupational therapy assistant students are required to complete 16 weeks of Level II fieldwork in at least two different practice areas, with the ultimate goal of competent generalist entry-level practice.

A recent survey conducted by the AOTA Commission on Education (AOTA, 2017a) found that during the past 3 years, 2014 to 2016, over 50% of all Level II fieldwork placements for occupational therapy and occupational therapy assistant students were in traditional hospital-based placements. This includes placements in inpatient acute care, inpatient rehabilitation, skilled nursing facilities, subacute long-term care, general rehabilitation outpatient, outpatient hand clinics, pediatric hospital/units, pediatric hospital outpatient, and inpatient psychiatry (AOTA, 2017a). Level II placements in community-based programs, defined as pediatric community, behavioral health, older adult community living, older adult day program, outpatient/hand private practice, adult day program for developmental disabilities, home health, and pediatric outpatient clinic, accounted for 37% of total responses. Eleven percent of the Level II placements occurred in school-based practice areas, schools, and early intervention. Lastly, approximately 1% of placements did not fit into these categories, which included placements in low vision therapy, role-emerging settings, homeless shelters, hippotherapy, animal-assisted intervention programs, lymphedema, work hardening, jail/prison, mixed experience rural, and community mental health emergent areas.

In their national survey, Evenson, Roberts, Kaldenberg, Barnes, and Ozelie (2015) found similar results in that traditional practice areas were most frequently offered fieldwork placements for Level II fieldwork, with the highest number in physical medicine followed by pediatric settings. The report also found that the majority of fieldwork educators surveyed typically supervised two or fewer occupational therapy and/or occupational therapy assistant students per year. The preferred method of supervision for students remains the traditional one supervisor to one student (1:1) model. Although fieldwork educators were able to identify the benefits and supports to hosting Level II students, these did not appear to outweigh the perceived challenges to increase overall fieldwork availability.

Anecdotal evidence also suggests that the majority of Level I fieldwork placements also occur in traditional settings, although current standards allow for placements in a variety of traditional, community-based and nontraditional settings. Programs have started using innovative Level I fieldwork opportunities (Overton, Clark, & Thomas, 2009); however, because there is not a method to collect data related to Level I and Level II fieldwork usage, the exact numbers are not available.

There is limited published information on the status and effectiveness of fieldwork education. Empirical evidence for currently used fieldwork models is absent from the literature; instead, evidence comes from educational theory about learning and student reports of experiences of fieldwork. Although academic programs seek to place students in settings that align with their curriculum philosophies, a shortage of fieldwork sites in many regions makes for a pragmatic approach of placing students where there are available supervisors.

Doctoral Capstone Experience

The Doctoral Capstone Experience is a component of entry-level Clinical Doctorate programs that occurs after completion of course work and Fieldwork (AOTA, 2018). Unlike Fieldwork II designed to prepare students for entry-level practice, the Capstone offers an extended exposure in one or more areas: administration, education, leadership, advocacy, research, clinical practice skills, policy and program development, theory development (AOTA, 2018). This Doctoral Capstone Experience is built upon a Capstone Project for a planned, mentored and evaluated 'real-world' endeavor. Pedagogy for the experience ideally draws upon the progressive education conditions described in this chapter that emphasize learning through doing, reflection, social processes, and attention to the experience of the student. A Capstone Coordinator works with an identified mentor, possibly from another discipline, to support this active learning experience. Products of the Doctoral Capstone may include presentations, manuals, programs and manuscripts. Educational outcomes are ultimately to advance the student's inquiry skills, problem solving in new situations, and inspiration for future learning.

International Fieldwork

Over the past decade, there has been much activity and interest about international placements. Increasingly, students come to occupational therapy programs with global connections, an interest in cross-cultural learning, and a desire to enact/promote justice beyond their local area. We authors have been part of this globalization trend and inspired by student interests. Yet, there is a paucity of guidance for developing and evaluating these learning experiences (Kirke, Layton, & Sim, 2007; Simonelis, Njelesani, Novak, Kuzma, & Cameron, 2011). Many types and lengths of fieldworks have emerged (Cameron et al., 2013). Some are faculty-led trips to other countries. Other experiences are supervised by host country occupational therapists or other disciplines in the case of Level I fieldwork. Although students often find these experiences transformative and applicable to their future practice in country, there have been numerous pitfalls to these endeavors from the standpoint of the host country (Elliot, 2015; Mu, Coppard, Bracciano, Doll, & Matthews, 2010). In underresourced countries, students can inadvertently escalate the sense of inequity that locals face or may act culturally insensitive or insulting to the very people they hope to help. Bringing and removing short-term resources is proven to be damaging in underresourced areas for the long-term rather than the short-term goals (Thibeault, 2006, 2013). International fieldwork is ethical when guided by humble respect, genuine client centeredness, deep cultural responsiveness, and long-term sustainable relationships. In short, it is difficult and time-consuming to do well. However, there is great value in learning how to learn in new cultures and, given trends in international migration and human displacement, to build international connections.

PROPOSED FUTURE OF FIELDWORK EDUCATION IN THE UNITED STATES

The near future of fieldwork education includes several changes to newly adopted ACOTE standards. The first major significant change is the addition of the requirement that all experiences must include a psychosocial objective (AOTA, 2018). Another change is the expansion of options for Level I fieldwork to include a combination of simulation, standardized patients, faculty practice, faculty-led site visits, and traditional practice experiences (AOTA, 2018). Innovation in fieldwork, such as the examples cited in Table 19-1, will contribute to the profession's future.

Table 19-1

EXAMPLES OF INNOVATION IN FIELDWORK RELATING TO THE AMERICAN OCCUPATIONAL THERAPY ASSOCIATIONS VISION 2025

VISION 2025	INNOVATIVE EXAMPLES
Maximizes health, well-being, and quality of life	The Allegheny County Jail Project (ACJ Project; Provident & Joyce-Gaguzis, 2005) Project Based Fieldwork (Fortune & McKinstry, 2012) On-Campus Occupational Therapy Clinics (Erickson, 2018)
For all people, populations, and communities	University of Utah Division of Occupational Therapy Immigration and Refugee Resettlement Community Fieldwork Program (Smith, Cornella, & Williams, 2014) Adaptive Skiing Fieldwork Program (White et al., 2016) Level II Fieldwork at Community Based Mental Health Centers (Tippie, Bauer, & Dillon, 2016) Innovative Practice in Accessible and Inclusive Tourism (Coppola, Sakornsatian, Thongkuay, & Trevittaya, 2012)
Through effective solutions that facilitate participation in everyday living	Fieldwork in Disaster Relief and Recovery Program, (Santoso, 2013) The Promoting Environments that Measure Outcomes (PrEMO) Model, (Schaaf et al., 2017) Creating Community Collaboration with a Fieldwork Advisory Board, (Iliff et al., 2015) Collaborative Model of Clinical Education (Rindflesch et al., 2008) Specialty Level II in Low Vision Rehabilitation, (Nastasi, 2013)

ADVANCING THE PROFESSION THROUGH VISION AND PEDAGOGY

The year 2017 was significant in the history of the profession of occupational therapy; 2017 was the centennial year, 100 years as a profession. The first part of the year 2017 was spent celebrating the history, looking at the major events and people who have formed the profession as it is today, and proclaiming the accomplishments of the centennial vision. By the end of 2017, major changes were proposed to occupational therapy education while planning for the future with Vision 2025.

AOTA's Vision 2025 states that, "Occupational therapy maximizes health, well-being, and quality of life for all people, populations, and communities through effective solutions that facilitate participation in everyday living" (AOTA, 2017b). Hooper (2010) described how a centennial vision could guide occupational therapy education. Throughout history, fieldwork has been an integral part of occupational therapy education; it is the key to transitioning to professional practice. Quality fieldwork experiences will continue to be integral to the future of occupational therapy. In the next section, we explore how the plan and pillars of Vision 2025 (Phipps, 2017), along with Deweyan principles, might optimally guide the future of fieldwork.

Maximizes Health, Well-Being, and Quality of Life

Through the provision of quality and effective fieldwork opportunities for occupational therapy and occupational therapy assistant students, we can increase access to occupational therapy services in traditional and role-emerging practice areas. This might occur through highly collaborative programs that are centered on lifestyle, prevention, and psychosocial well-being rather than focusing on impairments and functional independence in activities of daily living.

For All People, Populations, and Communities

Fieldwork opportunities can address society's emerging needs, such as school mental health programs, domestic violence shelters, community mental health, caregiver support, and adaptive sports. Deweyan pedagogy teaches awareness of ethics in all actions and how people can work together for social equality and building a better society.

Through Effective Solutions That Facilitate Participation in Everyday Living

Deweyan tenets teach inquiry, creativity, and problem-solving processes so that students can negotiate the problems of the future. Using problem-based and solution-focused learning, students form habits that enable them to enter new situations and contribute an occupational lens on cross-sector issues.

The pillars of AOTA's plan to achieve Vision 2025 are effectiveness, leadership, collaboration, and accessibility. We can apply these pillars to the future of fieldwork education in the following ways.

Effectiveness

Fieldwork education needs to be evidence based and cost effective. Yet, there is limited evidence to support current fieldwork models, and newer models may hold promise for effectiveness. The 2:1 or 3:1 collaborative model of student placement has been described as an effective method for providing fieldwork education for occupational therapy students (Thomas, Penman, & Williamson, 2005). Although the collaborative model challenges traditional beliefs of 1:1 fieldwork, students involved in the collaborative model present as more confident, engage in peer support and peer learning, and appear more independent, with increased clinical reasoning and clinical competence. Fieldwork educators may prefer the traditional 1:1 model because this may be the model in which they themselves were trained; however, this traditional model does not appear to be a viable long-term option given the ratio of students to available fieldwork sites.

Leadership

Ways that fieldwork can contribute to leadership in the future include increasing experiences in community-based and nontraditional fieldwork settings and experiences in research, administrative roles, advocacy, and policy development.

Collaboration

Occupational therapy practice is a collaborative process involving clients (including caregivers, families, and others) and colleagues within and outside of the profession. Stressing collaboration in serving clients can be done in any setting. The increasing use of interprofessional and 2:1 supervision models in fieldwork prepares students in this important arena. Preparing fieldwork educators for these models can better ensure the success of learning.

Accessibility

Fieldwork can contribute to the quest to build diversity of practitioners in the profession. For example, fieldwork is an important place to endorse and promote accommodations and technologies for students with disabilities, provide opportunities for cross-cultural engagement, and embrace differing learning preferences.

This chapter offers guidance for occupational therapy fieldwork education by looking back on the pedagogies of John Dewey and learning theorists, with consideration for a vision for the future of the profession in the United States. Key elements of those pedagogies promote active learning situated in practice, reflection, ethics, and collaboration. We believe that thoughtful pedagogy is key to professional development and building the kind of practitioner and workforce needed for the future of the profession. We encourage awareness of the language and pedagogy of fieldwork and how these structures can support the AOTA's Vision 2025 to advance the profession to meet society's needs.

Implications for Occupational Therapy Education

- Intentional pedagogy in fieldwork can prepare students for uncertainty and innovation in future practice.
- Critical evaluation of fieldwork structures, power, and pragmatics can generate new possibilities about the benefits of nontraditional or role-emergent settings.
- A future vision of the profession serving occupational needs of all people, populations, and communities will require pioneering practices and fieldwork that create practitioners who embrace innovation, uncertainty, leadership, advocacy, and collaboration.

Key Reflection Questions

1. In your current (past or future) fieldwork situation, in what ways might students be supported to engage in socially constructed learning experiences (e.g., with peers and interprofessional learners)?
2. How might a creative inquiry and problem-solving process be part of ongoing supervisory processes with students?
3. In what ways might supervisors shift to facilitating learning rather than instructing students about practice, and how might students benefit from this approach?
4. How do you see your role in supporting AOTA's Vision 2025 through fieldwork education?

What led you to become an occupational therapy educator?

As a fieldwork educator, I realized how much I learned from students when I gave them support and freedom to be creative. Their fresh eyes and young hearts kept me thinking and in touch with my passion for our clients. I am drawn to the challenge of teaching students how to reason and to perform the art of therapy, in heart and mind, for truly client-centered practice.

Susan Coppola, OTD, OT/L, FAOTA

I became a fieldwork educator because I wanted to help students to develop and thrive as occupational therapy practitioners. I became an academic educator so that students could have the opportunity to share in my experiences and expertise in fieldwork and mental health practice. I continue to teach so that students can take the lessons learned and go out into the world and make their clients' lives a little better one encounter at a time.

Susan M. Higgins, OTD, OTR/L

REFERENCES

Accreditation Council for Occupational Therapy Education (2018). 2018 ACOTE standards and interpretive guide. Retrieved from https://www.aota.org/~/media/Corporate/Files/EducationCareers/Accredit/StandardsReview/2018-ACOTE-Standards-Interpretive-Guide.pdf

American Occupational Therapy Association. (2016). Occupational therapy fieldwork education: Value and purpose. *American Journal of Occupational Therapy, 70*(Suppl. 1-2), 7012410060. doi:10.5014/ajot.2016.706S06

American Occupational Therapy Association. (2017a). *Commission on education report to the AOTA Board*. Bethesda, MD: Higgins, Amin-Arsala, Jackson.

American Occupational Therapy Association. (2017b). Vision 2025. *American Journal of Occupational Therapy, 71*, 7103420010. doi:10.5014/ajot.2017.713002

American Occupational Therapy Association. (2018). Accreditation Council for Occupational Therapy Education (ACOTE) standards and interpretative guide. Retrieved from https://www.aota.org/~/media/Corporate/Files/EducationCareers/Accredit/StandardsReview/2018-ACOTE-Standards-Interpretive-Guide.pdf

Cameron, D., Cockburn, L., Nixon, S., Parnes, P., Garcia, L., Leotaud, J., ... Williams, T. (2013). Global partnerships for international fieldwork in occupational therapy: Reflection and innovation. *Occupational Therapy International, 20*(2), 88-96.

Cohn, E. S. (1989). Fieldwork education: Shaping a foundation for clinical reasoning. *American Journal of Occupational Therapy, 43*(4), 240-244.

Coppola, S., Sakornsatian, S., Thongkuay, S., & Trevittaya, P. (2012). Innovative practice in accessible and inclusive tourism. *World Federation of Occupational Therapists Bulletin, 66*(1), 43-46.

Colman, W. (1990). Evolving educational practices in occupational therapy: The war emergency courses, 1936–1954. *American Journal of Occupational Therapy, 44*(11), 1028-1036.

Dewey, J. (1916). *Democracy and education*. New York, NY: Macmillan.

Dewey, J. (1938). *Education and experience*. New York, NY: Macmillan.

Dewey, J., & Small, A. W. (1897). *My pedagogic creed*. New York, NY: EL Kellogg & Company.

Elliot, M. L. (2015). Critical ethnographic analysis of "doing good" on short-term international immersion experiences. *Occupational Therapy International, 22*(3), 121-130.

Erickson, K. (2018). On-campus occupational therapy clinic enhances student professional development and understanding. *Journal of Occupational Therapy Education, 2*(2). doi:10.26681/jote.2018.020202

Evenson, M. E., Roberts, M., Kaldenberg, J., Barnes, M. A., & Ozelie, R. (2015). Brief report–National Survey of Fieldwork Educators: Implications for occupational therapy education. *American Journal of Occupational Therapy, 69*(Suppl. 2), 6912350020p1-6912350020p5.

Fortune, T., & McKinstry, C. (2012). Project-based fieldwork: Perspectives of graduate entry students and project sponsors. *Australian Occupational Therapy Journal, 59*(4), 265-275.

Freire, P. (1970). *Pedagogy of the oppressed*. New York, NY: Bloomsbury.

Henson, K. T. (2003). Foundations for learner-centered education: A knowledge base. *Education, 124*(1), 5-17.

Hooper, B. (2010). On arriving at the destination of the centennial vision: Navigational landmarks to guide occupational therapy education. *Occupational Therapy in Health Care, 24*(1), 97-106. doi:10.3109/07380570903329636

Iliff, S., Allen, A., Alley, S. T., Burns, R., Lopez, L., Luke, B. J., ... & Rhee, V. I. (2015). Creating community collaboration with a fieldwork advisory board. *OT Practice, 19*(1), 16-19.

Kirke, P., Layton, N., & Sim, J. (2007). Informing fieldwork design: Key elements to quality in fieldwork education for undergraduate occupational therapy students. *Australian Occupational Therapy Journal, 54*(s1).

Mu, K., Coppard, B. M., Bracciano, A., Doll, J., & Matthews, A. (2010). Fostering cultural competency, clinical reasoning, and leadership through international outreach. *Occupational Therapy in Health Care, 24*(1), 74-85.

Nastasi, J. A. (2013). Specialty level II fieldwork in low vision rehabilitation. *Work, 44*(3), 361-378.

Overton, A., Clark, M., & Thomas, Y. (2009). A review of non-traditional occupational therapy practice placement education: a focus on role-emerging and project placements. *British Journal of Occupational Therapy, 72*(7), 294-301.

Phipps, S. (2017). *Bridging the centennial vision with Vision 2025*. Paper presented at the Massachusetts Occupational Therapy Association. Nordwood, MA.

Presseller, S. (1983). Fieldwork education: The proving ground of the profession. *American Journal of Occupational Therapy, 37*(3), 163-165.

Provident, I. M., & Joyce-Gaguzis, K. (2005). Brief report—Creating an occupational therapy Level II fieldwork experience in a county jail setting. *American Journal of Occupational Therapy, 59*, 101-106.

Rindflesch, A., Dunfee, H., Cieslak, K., Eischen, S., Trenary, T., Calley, D., & Heinle, D. (2008). Collaborative model of clinical education in physical and occupational therapy at the Mayo Clinic. *Journal of Allied Health, 38*, 132-142.

Rodger, S., Thomas, Y., Dickson, D., McBryde, C., Broadbridge, J., Hawkins, R., & Edwards, A. (2007). Putting students to work: Valuing fieldwork placements as a mechanism for recruitment and shaping the future occupational therapy workforce. *Australian Occupational Therapy Journal, 54*(s1), S94-S97.

Santoso, B. T. (2013). Occupational therapy fieldwork experience in disaster response and recovery. *World Federation of Occupational Therapists Bulletin, 68*(1), 31-43.

Schaaf, R. C., Carroll, A. P., Toth-Cohen, S., Burke, J. P., Johnson, C., & Herge, E. (2017). Promoting environments that measure outcomes: partnerships for change. *Journal of Occupational Therapy Education, 1*(2). Retrieved from http://encompass.eku.edu/jote/vol1/iss2/5

Schön, D. A. (1983). *The reflective practitioner: how professionals think in action.* New York, New York: Basic Books.

Schwartz, K. B. (1992). Occupational therapy and education: A shared vision. *American Journal of Occupational Therapy, 46*(1), 12-18.

Simonelis, J., Njelesani, J., Novak, L., Kuzma, C., & Cameron, D. (2011). International fieldwork placements and occupational therapy: Lived experiences of the major stakeholders. *Australian Occupational Therapy Journal, 58*(5), 370-377.

Smith, Y. J., Cornella, E., & Williams, N. (2014). Working with populations from a refugee background: An opportunity to enhance the occupational therapy educational experience. *Australian Occupational Therapy Journal, 61*(1), 20-27.

Thibeault, R. (2006). Globalisation, universities and the future of occupational therapy: Dispatches for the majority world. *Australian Occupational Therapy Journal, 53*(3), 159-165.

Thibeault, R. (2013). Occupational justice's intents and impacts: From personal choices to community consequences. In *Transactional perspectives on occupation* (pp. 245-256). Dordrecht, Netherlands: Springer Netherlands.

Thomas, Y., Penman, M., & Williamson, P. (2005). Australian and New Zealand fieldwork: Charting the territory for future practice. *Australian Occupational Therapy Journal, 52*, 78-81.

Tippie, M., Bauer, E., & Dillon, M. B. (2016). Level II fieldwork at community-based mental health centers. *OT Practice, 4*(6), 21-23.

Wenger, E. (1998). *Communities of practice: Learning, meaning, and identity.* Cambridge, UK: Cambridge University Press.

White, B. P., Drake, R. L., Merrill, S. C., Blodgett, A. M., Collins, K. V., Hubbard, C. B., … Smith, K. (2016), Adaptive skiing and OT: UNH fieldwork students help people with disabilities hit the slopes. *OT Practice, 18*(1), 17-19.

20

Interprofessional Education
Where to Next?

Nancy E. Carson, PhD, OTR/L, FAOTA

Chapter Objectives

By the end of this chapter, the reader will be able to:
1. Define interprofessional education.
2. Examine the interprofessional collaborative practice core competencies and subcompetencies.
3. Recognize the scope of the current evidence on the impact of interprofessional education on clinical practice, including patient/population health outcomes and health care delivery systems outcomes.
4. Discuss the factors necessary for interprofessional practice and team-based care to be consistently evident in health care.

INTRODUCTION

Current occupational therapy accreditation standards for educational programs require programs to prepare graduates who can effectively work with other professionals in the provision of care for individuals and/or populations (Accreditation Council for Occupational Therapy Education, 2012). Most other professional education associations, such as the Association of American Medical Colleges, the American Physical Therapy Association, and the American Academy of Physician Assistants, also require students to be prepared for interprofessional practice as stipulated in their profession's educational program accreditation standards (Accreditation Review Commission on Education for the Physician Assistant, Inc., 2016; Commission on Accreditation in Physical Therapy Education, 2015; Liaison Committee on Medical Education, 2017). The current focus on health professions education as an effective method for developing interprofessional competencies and collaborative practice developed out of an increasing concern for health care quality, safety, and cost disseminated in Institute of Medicine (IOM) reports (IOM, 2000, 2001). In 2009, the Interprofessional

Taff, S. D., Grajo, L. C., & Hooper, B. R. (Eds.). *Perspectives on Occupational Therapy Education: Past, Present, and Future* (pp. 213-220).
© 2020 Taylor & Francis Group.

Table 20-1	
INTERPROFESSIONAL EDUCATION COLLABORATIVE	
YEAR JOINED	**INSTITUTIONAL MEMBERS**
2011	American Association of Colleges of Nursing (AACN) American Association of Colleges of Osteopathic Medicine (AACOM) American Association of Colleges of Pharmacy (AACP) American Dental Education Association (ADEA) Association of Schools of Public Health (ASPH) Association of American Medical Colleges (AAMC)
2016	American Association of Colleges of Podiatric Medicine (AACPM) American Council of Academic Physical Therapy (ACAPT) American Occupational Therapy Association (AOTA) American Psychological Association (APA) Association of American Veterinary Medical Colleges (AAVMC) Association of Schools and Colleges of Optometry (ASCO) Association of Schools of Allied Health Professions (ASAHP) Council on Social Work Education (CSWE) Physician Assistant Education Association (PAEA)

Education Collaborative (IPEC) was formed when six national education associations came together to support efforts for developing and promoting interprofessional education (IPE) and learning experiences and instilling the skills needed for team-based care in future clinicians (IPEC Expert Panel, 2011). In 2016, nine additional professional organizations joined IPEC (Table 20-1).

WHAT IS INTERPROFESSIONAL EDUCATION?

IPE "occurs when two or more professions learn about, from, and with each other, to enable effective collaboration and improve health outcomes" (World Health Organization, 2010, p. 13). IPEC formed the IPEC Expert Panel, and in 2011 the panel's published report identified four interprofessional collaborative practice competency domains. Each domain included a general competency statement and 8 to 10 subcompetencies. In 2016, IPEC published an update that established interprofessional collaboration as the central domain encompassing the four original domains, the domains now being organized as core competencies within interprofessional collaboration. Establishing interprofessional collaboration as the central domain was based on an extensive review of health professions' competency frameworks that validated this approach (Englander et al., 2013). Additionally, the 2016 report puts an increased focus on achieving the Triple Aim, a framework of the Institute for Healthcare Improvement that focuses on simultaneously improving patient care, improving population health, and reducing health care cost (Berwick, Nolan, & Whittington, 2008). The report suggests expanding the interprofessional competencies to include a greater emphasis on population health approaches (IPEC, 2016). The competency statements and subcompetencies (now 8 to 11 per core competency) were updated to reflect these changes in health care and the current focus of IPE (Table 20-2).

As of 2016, the number of required interprofessional learning experiences has increased in health education programs, and the IPEC Faculty Development Institutes have trained over 300 teams to foster IPE initiatives in their respective institutions (IPEC, 2016). Research on the effectiveness of

Table 20-2

INTERPROFESSIONAL COLLABORATIVE PRACTICE CORE COMPETENCIES

CORE COMPETENCY	GENERAL COMPETENCY STATEMENT WITH SELECTED SUBCOMPETENCIES
Values/ethics for interprofessional practice	Work with individuals of other professions to maintain a climate of mutual respect and shared values. VE1. Place interests of patients and populations at center of interprofessional health care delivery and population health programs and policies, with the goal of promoting health and health equity across the life span. VE4. Respect the unique cultures, values, roles/responsibilities, and expertise of other health professions and the impact these factors can have on health outcomes. VE8. Manage ethical dilemmas specific to interprofessional patient/population-centered care situations.
Roles/ responsibilities	Use the knowledge of one's own role and those of other professions to appropriately assess and address the health care needs of patients and to promote and advance the health of populations. RR3. Engage diverse professionals who complement one's own professional expertise, as associated resources, to develop strategies to meet specific health and health care needs of patients and populations. RR5. Use the full scope of knowledge, skills, and abilities of professionals from health and other fields to provide care that is safe, timely, efficient, effective, and equitable. RR10. Describe how professionals in health and other fields can collaborate and integrate clinical care and public health interventions to optimize population health.
Interprofessional communication	Communicate with patients, families, communities, and professionals in health and other fields in a responsive and responsible manner that supports a team approach to the promotion and maintenance of health and the prevention and treatment of disease. CC3. Express one's knowledge and opinions to team members involved in patient care and population health improvement with confidence, clarity, and respect, working to ensure common understanding of information, treatment, care decisions, and population health programs and policies. CC4. Listen actively and encourage ideas and opinions of other team members. CC8. Communicate the importance of teamwork in patient-centered care and population health programs and policies.

continued

Table 20-2 (continued)	
INTERPROFESSIONAL COLLABORATIVE PRACTICE CORE COMPETENCIES	
CORE COMPETENCY	**GENERAL COMPETENCY STATEMENT WITH SELECTED SUBCOMPETENCIES**
Teams and teamwork	Apply relationship-building values and the principles of team dynamics to perform effectively in different team roles to plan, deliver, and evaluate patient/population-centered care and population health programs and policies that are safe, timely, efficient, effective, and equitable. TT3. Encourage health and other professional in shared patient-centered and population-focused problem solving. TT6. Engage self and others to constructively manage disagreements about values, roles, goals, and actions that arise among health and other professionals and with patients, families, and community members. TT9. Use process improvement to increase effectiveness of interprofessional teamwork and team-based services, programs, and policies.

IPE is also increasing. One recent example of an innovative IPE initiative focused on the impact of an interprofessional population health course that engaged students from five different health professions. Students participated in interprofessional teams in a clinical setting, and positive outcomes related to interprofessional learning, team-based communication, and clinical practice outcomes were found (Zomorodi et al., 2017). Another example of a clinical-based IPE initiative involved three different health profession students implementing an IPE fall prevention program for older adults in a community setting. Positive outcomes were found for teamwork and communication among the student participants, and applicability to future practice was acknowledged while community partners support it as an opportunity for increasing patient safety (Kurowski-Burt, Evans, Baugh, & Utzman, 2017).

Understanding the impact of IPE on clinical practice and health care delivery outcomes is ongoing. The IOM convened the Committee on Measuring the Impact of Interprofessional Education on Collaborative Practice and Patient Outcomes to provide recommendations to link IPE with patient, population, and system outcomes (IOM, 2015). The committee suggested four ways to create a foundation for evaluating the impact of IPE: "(1) more closely aligning the education and health care delivery systems, (2) developing a conceptual framework for measuring the impact of IPE, (3) strengthening the evidence base for IPE, and (4) linking IPE with changes in collaborative behavior" (IOM, 2015, p. 3). After examining the IPE literature, the committee concluded that targeted engagement between the education and health care delivery systems is needed along with a consistent taxonomy and framework for linking IPE with outcomes through purposeful and rigorous studies (IOM, 2015). Two recommendations emerged to address the findings:

- "Interprofessional stakeholders, funders, and policy makers should commit resources to a coordinated series of well-designed studies of the association between IPE and collaborative behavior, including teamwork and performance in practice. These studies should be focused on developing broad consensus on how to measure interprofessional collaboration effectively across a range of learning environment, patient populations, and practice settings" (IOM, 2015, pp. 5-6).
- "Health professions educators and academic and health system leaders should adopt a mixed methods research approach for evaluating the impact of IPE on health and system outcomes.

Table 20-3	
STRATEGIES AND ACTIVITIES	
RECOMMENDATIONS FOR EVALUATING THE IMPACT OF INTERPROFESSIONAL EDUCATION	**IMPLEMENTATION STRATEGIES AND TEACHING/LEARNING ACTIVITIES BASED ON INTERPROFESSIONAL CORE COMPETENCIES**
More closely align the education and health care delivery systems Develop a conceptual framework for measuring the impact of IPE Strengthen the evidence base for IPE Link IPE with changes in collaborative behavior	1. Train students in TeamSTEPPS and partner with health care delivery systems to have students evaluate interprofessional communication and teamwork skills. 2. Evaluate the impact of IPE by comparing the effectiveness of interprofessional communication and teamwork skills to better patient outcomes. 3. Evaluate the impact of IPE by measuring the knowledge of the role/responsibilities of the health care team on patient satisfaction. 4. Evaluate the impact of IPE by measuring the level of respect for the values/ethics of the health care team on employee satisfaction. 5. Develop innovative interprofessional Level I fieldwork rotations such as in a bariatric or chronic pain clinic to allow students to practice interprofessional communication and teamwork skills with other health professionals and develop an understanding of the role/responsibilities and values/ethics of other professionals. 6. Participate in community programs for underserved populations to understand roles/responsibilities and core values/ethics of team members for promoting health and health equity for individuals at higher risk for health disparities.
Developed for the Department of Defense Patient Safety Program in collaboration with the Agency for Healthcare Research and Quality. Adapted from United States., United States., & United States. (2010). *TeamSTEPPS: Strategies & tools to enhance performance and patient safety.* Falls Church, VA: TRICARE.	

When possible, such studies should include an economic analysis and be carried out by teams of experts that include educational evaluators, health services researchers, and economists, along with educators and others engaged in IPE" (IOM, 2015, p. 7).

Although all occupational therapy educational programs must address IPE, the method and approach vary greatly from institution to institution. Some institutions have comprehensive IPE approaches with administrative support and resources for implementation, whereas others bear the primary responsibility for developing IPE initiatives with limited resources. Logistical issues are one of the biggest barriers to IPE implementation. Scheduling common times for students to learn together can be challenging, and integrating consistent experiences for all health care team members continues to be a challenge. Finding classroom time for face-to-face interaction can be accomplished

Table 20-4

SELECTED ASSESSMENT TOOLS FOR PATIENT, POPULATION, AND HEALTH SYSTEM OUTCOMES

- TeamSTEPPS Perception Scale
  https://nexusipe.org/informing/resource-center/t-tpq-teamstepps%C2%AE-teamwork-perceptions-questionnaire-and-t-taq-teamwork
- Relational Coordination Survey
  https://nexusipe.org/informing/resource-center/rcs-relational-coordination-scale
- Practice Environment Checklist—Short Form
  https://nexusipe.org/informing/resource-center/assessing-teamwork-reliable-five-question-survey
- Interprofessional Collaboration Scale
  https://nexusipe.org/informing/resource-center/interprofessional-collaboration-scale
- Collaborative Practice Assessment Tool (https://nexusipe.org/informing/resource-center/cpat-collaborative-practice-assessment-tool)

easier than finding times for IPE embedded in community or clinical sites. In the future, requiring interprofessional clinical experiences to better train students for clinical practice should be the norm and should be supported and embraced by all health care professions and the institutions that support them. Some implementation strategies and teaching/learning activities based on interprofessional core competencies and supportive of evaluating the impact of IPE are provided in Table 20-3.

In order to design effective IPE activities that are linked to positive patient and population health outcomes, it is essential to identify the evidence for these initiatives and to disseminate them to all stakeholders. In 2012, the National Center for Interprofessional Practice and Education was created, and strategies were developed to achieve these aims. The strategies included the formation of a Nexus Incubator network for researching and assessing the impact of selected IPEC practice interventions, comparative effectiveness research to build the evidence for IEP, and the creation of a National Center Data Repository that will facilitate the generation of big data for observational studies as well as serve as an interactive repository for assessment tools being developed, validated, and improved (Pechacek, Cerra, Brandt, Lutfiyya, & Delaney, 2015). Selected assessment tools are provided in Table 20-4.

For interprofessional practice and team-based care to firmly take hold as the norm in health care, the recommendations of the IOM (2015) report need to be implemented. An analysis of the IOM report along with current IPE literature is suggested to support a new conceptual framework for thinking about IPE from early in professional curriculums through professional development offerings in health care settings (Cox, Cuff, Brandt, Reeves, & Zeirler, 2016). Consistent training across the professions and throughout the learning continuum is needed along with rigorous research to provide evidence on best practices. Occupational therapy educators are responsible for facilitating IPE with their students and need to be diligent in researching best practices and providing innovative approaches.

In order to achieve the IOM recommendations and move IPE into the future, occupational therapy educators must take a leadership role in designing innovative interprofessional experiences for students in a variety of clinical settings. As more graduate programs transition to the clinical doctorate, there is increased opportunity to expand on leadership skills and knowledge of population health. New graduates need to be prepared to take on leadership roles in interprofessional practice in a variety of clinical settings using outcome data to inform best practices.

Implications for Occupational Therapy Education

- Occupational therapy educators are responsible for facilitating IPE in the curriculum using best practices supported by the literature.
- Occupational therapy educators can use their skills in adaptation and creativity to be leaders in moving the evidence and innovation in IPE forward.
- Educating others about the role of the occupational therapist on the health care team is a core interprofessional competency that provides an opportunity for advocating broadly for occupational therapy services for those patients and populations who can benefit, thus expanding the impact of occupational therapy.

Key Reflection Questions

1. Discuss the importance of IPE for all health care students.
2. Describe an IPE experience you participated in and reflect on how the core competencies were used effectively, or, if they were not, explain why.
3. How can we best support IPE carryover into clinical practice?

What led you to become an occupational therapy educator?

My first job as an occupational therapist was on a psychiatric unit. I led many groups, with some being psychoeducational groups on topics such as stress management and communication skills. I enjoyed my role as a teacher in these groups, and I also enjoyed mentoring students in the clinical setting and helping them to develop their skills by collaborating and identifying their individual needs. I decided to become an occupational therapy educator after recognizing how much I enjoyed the role of teacher in multiple settings.

Nancy E. Carson, PhD, OTR/L, FAOTA

REFERENCES

Accreditation Council for Occupational Therapy Education. (2012). 2011 Accreditation council for occupational therapy education (ACOTE) standards. *American Journal of Occupational Therapy, 66*, S6-S74. doi:10.5014/ajot.2012.66S6

Accreditation Review Commission on Education for the Physician Assistant, Inc. (2016). *Accreditation standards for physician assistant education* (4th ed.). Retrieved from http://www.arc-pa.org/wp-content/uploads/2016/10/Standards-4th-Ed-March-2016.pdf

Berwick, D. M., Nolan, T. W., & Whittington, J. (2008). The triple aim: care, health, and cost. *Health Affairs, 27*(3). Retrieved from https://www.healthaffairs.org/doi/full/10.1377/hlthaff.27.3.759

Commission on Accreditation in Physical Therapy Education. (2015). Standards and required elements for accreditation of physical therapist education programs, revised 11/11/15. Retrieved from http://www.capteonline.org/uploaded-Files/CAPTEorg/About_CAPTE/Resources/Accreditation_Handbook/CAPTE_PTStandardsEvidence.pdf

Cox, M., Cuff, P., Brandt, B. F., Reeves, S., & Zeirler, B. (2016). Measuring the impact of interprofessional education on collaborative practice and patient outcomes. *Journal of Interprofessional Care, 30*(1), 1-3.

Englander, R., Cameron, T., Ballard, A. J., Dodge, J., Bull, J., & Aschenbrener, C. A. (2013). Toward a common taxonomy of competency domains for the health professions and competencies for physicians. *Academic Medicine, 88*, 1088-1094.

Institute of Medicine. (2000). *To err is human: Building a safer health system.* Committee on Quality of Health Care in America. Washington, DC: National Academy of Sciences.

Institute of Medicine. (2001). *Crossing the quality chasm: A new health system for the 21st century.* Committee on Quality of Health Care in America. Washington, DC: National Academy of Sciences.

Institute of Medicine. (2015). *Measuring the impact of interprofessional education on collaborative practice and patient outcomes.* Washington, DC: The National Academies Press.

Interprofessional Education Collaborative. (2016). *Core competencies for interprofessional collaborative practice: 2016 update.* Washington, DC: Author.

Interprofessional Education Collaborative Expert Panel. (2011). *Core competencies for interprofessional collaborative practice: Report of an expert panel.* Washington, DC: Interprofessional Education Collaborative.

Kurowski-Burt, A. L., Evans, K. W., Baugh, G. M., & Utzman, A. R. (2017). A community-based interprofessional education fall prevention project. *Journal of Interprofessional Education and Practice, 8,* 1-5. doi:10.1016/j.xjep.2017.04.001

Liaison Committee on Medical Education. (2017). *Functions and structures of a medical school: Standards for accreditation of medical education programs leading to the MD degree.* Washington, DC: Association of American Medical Colleges and the American Medical Association.

Pechacek, J., Cerra, F., Brandt, B., Lutfiyya, M. N., & Delaney, C. (2015). Creating the summary of evidence through comparative effectiveness research for interprofessional education and collaborative practice by deploying a national intervention network and a national data repository. *Healthcare, 3,* 146-161.

World Health Organization. (2010). *Framework for action on interprofessional education and collaborative practice.* Geneva, Switzerland: Author. Retrieved from http://www.who.int/hrh/resources/framework_action/en/

Zomorodi, M., de Saxe Zerden, L., Nance-Floyd, B., Alexander, L., Wilfert, R., & Byerley, J. (2017). Impact of an interprofessional population health course and clinical immersion experience: Students and practice outcomes. *Journal of Interprofessional Education and Practice, 9,* 91-94.

21

Imagining the Occupational Therapy Educational Landscape in 2050

Neil Harvison, PhD, OTR, FNAP, FAOTA;
Steven D. Taff, PhD, OTR/L, FNAP, FAOTA; Lenin C. Grajo, PhD, EdM, OTR/L;
and Barbara R. Hooper, PhD, OTR/L, FAOTA

Chapter Objectives

By the end of this chapter, the reader will be able to:

1. Recognize the key factors that have impacted the unprecedented growth of occupational therapy education in the past decade (2009-2019).
2. Describe how changes in health care and higher education policy influence changes in the occupational therapy curriculum.
3. Describe opportunities for occupational therapy education programs to prepare graduates and the profession to deal positively with impending changes.

OCCUPATIONAL THERAPY EDUCATION OVER THE PAST DECADE: 2009 TO 2019

Unprecedented Occupational Therapy Program Growth

The past decade has seen unprecedented growth in entry-level educational programs. During the 10-year period, the number of applicant, candidate, and accredited entry-level programs for the occupational therapist grew from 147 to 259, representing a 76% growth (Accreditation Council for Occupational Therapy Education, 2019). At the same time, the number of entry-level programs for the occupational therapy assistant grew from 130 to 253, representing a 95% growth (Accreditation Council for Occupational Therapy, 2019). This rapid proliferation in programs was in response to a number of factors. All health professions, including occupational therapy, have seen increased demand for skilled health care practitioners in response to changing societal needs. As reported by the U.S. Bureau of Labor Statistics, the projected growth of occupational therapists (24%) and

Taff, S. D., Grajo, L. C., & Hooper, B. R. (Eds.). *Perspectives on Occupational Therapy Education: Past, Present, and Future* (pp. 221-227).
© 2020 Taylor & Francis Group.

occupational therapy assistants (29%) is expected to outgrow that of other treating practitioners (16%) and all jobs in the U.S. economy (7%). The U.S. Bureau of Labor Statistics' report states that more occupational therapy practitioners will be needed to address the changing health needs of the U.S. population. Leading this demand will be the needs of an aging population, an increased incidence of autism spectrum disorders, and an increase in the prevalence of chronic conditions (U.S. Bureau of Labor Statistics, 2019). This strong demand for graduates has attracted applicants searching for career-oriented programs with strong employment and income potential.

At the same time, higher education institutions have been facing an increasing number of challenges. As costs of higher education have grown (Snyder, de Brey, & Dillow, 2018) and public funding has decreased (Mitchell, Leachman, Masterson, & Waxman, 2018), institutions have become more dependent on professional-focused programs that can attract strong applicant pools and tuition-driven revenues. More recently, the national applicant pool to undergraduate programs has begun to decline, and a number of smaller institutions have closed because of declining enrollments in the liberal arts (NSC Research Center, 2018). In response to these changes, new providers have entered the occupational therapy education market with the biggest growth among for-profit, faith-based, and smaller liberal arts–focused institutions (American Occupational Therapy Association [AOTA], 2018).

Profile of Students

Over the past 10 years, occupational therapy has been featured in widely disseminated publications as a "best job" for the future ("100 Best Jobs," 2019). This recognition drove record numbers of competitive applicants, higher admission criteria, and grade point averages of admitted students (AOTA, 2018); yet, despite the high number of applications, the community has had little success in diversifying the student population. Occupational therapy students overwhelmingly identify as non-Hispanic (93%), White (82%), and female (89%) (AOTA, 2019). Occupational therapy assistant students overwhelmingly identify as non-Hispanic (87%), White (74%), and female (86%) (AOTA, 2019).

Changes in Health Care and Higher Education Policy

In addition to growth in academic programs, health care and higher education policy debates revolve around rising costs and poor outcomes. Despite the reforms proposed in the Affordable Care Act (Patient Protection and Affordable Care Act, 2010), the health care system has remained largely focused on disease management with volume-based reimbursement. The majority of occupational therapy graduates enter the workforce employed in traditional health care facilities (AOTA, 2015). Health care costs continue to rise with unsatisfactory outcomes, leading policy makers to question the costs and benefits of both health care education and delivery systems to society. How these debates will impact future health delivery and reimbursement models remains uncertain (Wamble, Ciarametaro, Houghton, Ajmera, & Dubois, 2019).

At the same time, higher education has come under increased scrutiny for cost, student debt, and graduate default rates (Reauthorizing the Higher Education Act, 2018). Higher education institutions face pressure to address costs, accessibility, and innovative ways to deliver degrees outside of the costly brick-and-mortar institutions. Policy makers have introduced proposals linking access to federal student aid to institutional and programmatic outcomes. These outcomes include measures such as degree completion rates, graduate debt-to-earnings ratios, certification pass rates, and gainful employment in the field for which the degree program is designed (GovTrack.us., 2019).

The Occupational Therapy Curriculum

Since the publication of the occupational therapist and occupational therapy assistant model curriculum guides in 2008 (AOTA, 2008), there has been an increased recognition of the complexities and importance of well-designed curricula in delivering occupational therapy educational programs. However, in response to the demands of the health care market, the majority of the didactic components of occupational therapy curricula have continued to focus primarily on preparing graduates in addressing disease management. A recent survey of practitioners providing supervision to students on Level II fieldwork found that the most frequently represented practice setting was physical medicine (outpatient and inpatient acute care, skilled nursing, and inpatient rehabilitation; Evenson, Roberts, Kaldenberg, Barnes, & Ozelie, 2015).

Despite the continued focus on disease management, there have been some changes in curricula in response to national initiatives and proposals in the Affordable Care Act. Occupational therapy programs have acknowledged the growing emphasis on interprofessional and intraprofessional education and collaborative practice (Hughes et al., 2019). In the United States, this movement grew in response to the Institute of Medicine's report on the impact of health care errors and the importance of collaborative practice between health care providers (Kohn, Corrigan, & Donaldson, 2000). In addition, occupational therapy programs have begun to explore community-based delivery systems and the distinct contributions of the profession to health outcomes among individuals and populations (AOTA, 2018).

WHERE DO WE GO IN THE NEXT 30 YEARS?

Will Program Growth Continue?

The U.S. Bureau of Labor Statistics (2019) is projecting an increased demand for new graduate occupational therapy practitioners to address population changes. Strong job markets have traditionally resulted in program growth. However, the demand will be highly dependent on the impact of health reimbursement and delivery system changes. For example, the Centers for Medicaid and Medicare Services, other payers, and health systems are shifting reimbursement to emphasize the value of services provided rather than payments based on the volume or minutes of services. Practitioners will be financially rewarded for demonstrating value through outcome measures and potentially penalized for not meeting the value criteria or desired outcomes (Sandhu, Furniss, & Metzler, 2018). In another reimbursement change, Medicare will be changing the rate reimbursed for services provided by occupational therapy assistants in Part B settings from 100% of the rate paid for services by an occupational therapist to 85% of the occupational therapist rate by 2022 (CMS.gov, 2019). Although it is not clear what direct impact these and other potential reimbursement changes will have on skill mix and hiring patterns, there will likely be an impact on the job market in traditional settings.

In addition to changes in reimbursement policy, there is a continued desire by policy makers to shift delivery systems away from the traditional focus on disease management to community-based, primary care, and preventive services addressing health and wellness (Institute of Medicine, 2015). Although there is sufficient evidence to support the cost benefits of this proposal (Institute of Medicine, 2015), reimbursement systems do not currently support this practice. The expansion of practice in this area will be dependent to a large extent on the ability of occupational therapy practitioners to identify and measure outcomes demonstrating the value of their service.

Changes in Student Profiles

The decreasing number of high school graduates applying for college combined with the changing demographics of the applicant pool will offer particular challenges for occupational therapy educational programs (Grawe, 2018). There will be greater competition across all health professions for the decreasing number of qualified applicants. In addition, the applicant pool will become more diverse in respect to factors including socioeconomic status, race, sex, and ethnicity. It is projected that by 2025, White students will make up 11.5 million of the total 23.3 million, with the number of Latino (32%), Black (22%), Asian-Pacific Islander (16%), and multiracial (37%) students all growing more rapidly (Hussar & Bailey, 2017). Because occupational therapy has relied almost exclusively on applicant and student populations composed of predominantly White women from middle class backgrounds, this is going to be particularly challenging. This demographic group will no longer dominate an already shrinking applicant pool.

A number of health professions started major campaigns over the last decade addressing this issue. The campaigns have focused on a number of elements, including (a) student leader diversity programs, (b) summer preparation programs, (c) holistic admissions criteria, and (d) student retention initiatives (Association of American Medical Colleges, n.d.; American Dental Education Association, 2018). As a result, the profiles of the freshman class of these professions has changed significantly (Association of American Medical Colleges, n.d.). Occupational therapy programs will need to identify and implement strategies to address diversifying the applicant pool if the programs are to compete with the other health professions.

Health Care and Higher Education Policy

The shift in health care reimbursement from rewarding quantity (or minutes) of service to rewarding quality of services based on outcomes is likely to continue for the foreseeable future. For example, starting in 2019, the Centers for Medicaid and Medicare Services will implement the Patient-Driven Payment Model and will roll out similar systems in other payer settings over the next 10 years (CMS.gov, 2018; Sandhu et al., 2018). Although this change could negatively impact reimbursement of occupational therapy, it does provide opportunities for practitioners who can demonstrate the distinct value of occupational therapy by identifying and applying quality measures to everyday practice. These practitioners have the potential to prosper in the new system.

Health delivery systems will likely undergo significant change with a greater focus on promoting health as opposed to disease (HHS.gov, n.d.). This shift offers tremendous potential to the field of occupational therapy in addressing social determinants, adaptive performance patterns, habits, and routines to promote the health of individuals, groups, and populations, but this transition in practice settings is not without its challenges. Occupational therapy practitioners will need to be prepared to deal with change and to advocate for the role of occupation in promoting health and wellness in changing practice settings.

Higher education policy will continue to focus on the issues of access to higher education through affordability and innovation. Programs will be challenged to deliver occupational therapy curriculum through less expensive online and blended delivery models. Outcomes for professional programs, such as occupational therapy, will focus on the employability and earning potential of graduates irrespective of the changing practice settings.

The Occupational Therapy Curriculum

To succeed in this changing environment, occupational therapy educational programs will need to develop curricula that prepare entry-level practitioners with the competencies to thrive in existing practice settings while being prepared to adapt and change as the needs of society change.

In existing practice settings, occupational therapy practitioners will need to:

- Access, use, and help produce research, evidence, and knowledge translation
- Provide evidence-informed, occupation-based interventions
- Demonstrate resilience (avoid burnout)
- Identify and measure "value"
- Advocate for occupational therapy's distinct value; and practice at top of their license

In addition, occupational therapy practitioners will need to:

- Lead in health management, maintenance, and promotion (distinct from disease management model)
- Address social determinants and adaptive performance patterns (drivers of health and life expectancy)
- Identify and advocate for the role of occupations in achieving health and self-management (individuals, groups, and populations)
- Overcome the challenges of community-based practice while navigating new opportunities in community-based practices
- Articulate the distinct value of occupational therapy in new and emerging areas of practice

THE CHALLENGE FOR EDUCATORS: WEAVING THE PAST, PRESENT, AND FUTURE

As the landscape of occupational therapy education changes, occupational therapy educators need to continuously adapt to become innovators in this era of hyperchange (Hinojosa, 2007). In response to the trends and projections discussed in this chapter, this text has presented an overview of historical and philosophical perspectives that have shaped the current landscape of occupational therapy education. Drawing on the most salient lessons from the past and present, occupational therapy education must now continue to respond and evolve in a myriad of ways. Occupational therapy educators need to reframe and adapt signature pedagogies to optimize teaching and learning opportunities with the changing demographic of students in professional programs. Occupational therapy educators also must use and measure the value of new instructional technologies, use high- and low-technology simulation experiences to facilitate clinical reasoning and critical thinking, modify fieldwork experiences and expose students to new and emerging areas of practice, explore untapped areas of practice, and deliver occupational therapy education with inter- and intraprofessional perspectives. As health care changes constantly influence ways of measuring the effectiveness of therapy service provision, educators also need to modify ways they measure outcomes of education and engage in educational research to determine the effectiveness of teaching and learning strategies and curricular changes. Lastly, occupational therapy educators must also look at education and educational outcomes to not only be responsive to the American health care system and higher education system changes. The students of the new generation are becoming more globally and internationally connected than ever. While remaining faithful to the core principles of occupation-centered education, educators must also adapt curricula and instruction with the changing international landscape and foster collaborations with educators and scholars from other parts of the world. All of these dynamic changes are fundamental to the ongoing growth of not only occupational therapy education but also the profession itself. This never-ending process of becoming requires an education that is innovative, engaged, and transformative—one that is not simply explanatory but also emancipatory (Bingham & Biesta, 2010).

Implications for Occupational Therapy Education

- Health care and higher education policy debate is dominated by rising costs, changing societal demands, and limited outcomes.
- Policy will drive changes in health reimbursement and practice delivery models.
- Occupational therapy educational curricula must prepare entry-level practitioners with the competencies to thrive in existing practice settings while being prepared to adapt and change as the needs of society change.

Key Reflection Questions

1. How ready is the profession to identify and implement strategies to address diversifying the applicant pool if the programs are to compete with the other health professions?
2. How prepared are graduates from your program not only to practice in existing delivery models but to adapt and thrive in alternative practice settings addressing health of their clients?

What led you to become an occupational therapy educator?

My interest in education started in practice as I worked with new graduates and fieldwork students making the challenging transition from the primary role of student to the role of practitioner. Striving to understand how to mentor and support these new practitioners led to my exploration and questioning of the diversity of learning philosophies, instructional designs and pedagogy employed in our academic programs. I soon decided that I wanted to play a role in this process.

Neil Harvison, PhD, OTR, FNAP, FAOTA

REFERENCES

100 best jobs. (2019). *U.S. News & World Report.* Retrieved from https://money.usnews.com/careers/best-jobs/rankings/the-100-best-jobs

Accreditation Council for Occupational Therapy Education. (2019, January). Program director newsletter. Retrieved from https://www.aota.org/~/media/Corporate/Files/EducationCareers/Accredit/Announcements/PDenews/PDNewsletterWinter2019.pdf

American Dental Education Association. (2018). ADEA access, diversity and inclusion (ADI) strategic framework. Retrieved from https://www.adea.org/uploadedFiles/ADEA/Content_Conversion_Final/policy_advocacy/diversity_equity/ADEA_ADI_StrategyFrameworkGraphic_June15Revision.pdf

American Occupational Therapy Association. (2008). OT model curriculum. Retrieved from https://www.aota.org/Education-Careers/Educators/model-curriculum.aspx

American Occupational Therapy Association. (2015). *AOTA salary & workforce survey.* Bethesda, MD: AOTA Press.

American Occupational Therapy Association. (2018). Importance of primary care education in occupational therapy curricula. *American Journal of Occupational Therapy, 72*(Suppl. 2), 7212410040p1-7212410040p14. doi:10.5014/ajot.2018.72S202

American Occupational Therapy Association. (2019). *Academic programs annual data report.* Bethesda, MD: AOTA Press.

Association of American Medical Colleges. (n.d.). *Diversity in medical education: Facts & figures 2016.* Retrieved from http://www.aamcdiversityfactsandfigures2016.org/

Bingham, C., & Biesta, G. (2010). *Jacques Ranciere: Education, truth, emancipation.* London, England: Continuum International Publishing Group.

CMS.gov. (2018). *Patient driven payment model.* Retrieved from https://www.cms.gov/Medicare/Medicare-Fee-for-Service-Payment/SNFPPS/PDPM.html

CMS.gov. (2019). *CY 2019 therapy services update.* Retrieved from https://www.cms.gov/Medicare/Billing/TherapyServices/index.html

Evenson, M. E., Roberts, M., Kaldenberg, J., Barnes, M. A., & Ozelie, R. (2015). Brief report—National survey of fieldwork educators: Implications for occupational therapy education. *American Journal of Occupational Therapy, 69*(Suppl. 2), 6912350020. doi:10.5014/ajot.2015.019265

GovTrack.us. (2019). H.R. 4508—115th Congress: PROSPER Act. Retrieved from https://www.govtrack.us/congress/bills/115/hr4508

Grawe, N. (2018). *Demographics and the demand for higher education*. Baltimore, MD: Johns Hopkins University Press.

HHS.gov. (n.d.). *Strategic goal 1: Reform, strengthen, and modernize the nation's healthcare system*. Retrieved from https://www.hhs.gov/about/strategic-plan/strategic-goal-1/index.html#top

Hinojosa, J. (2007). Becoming innovators in an era of hyperchange [Eleanor Clarke Slagle lecture]. *American Journal of Occupational Therapy, 61*, 629-637.

Hughes, J., Allen, A., McLane, T., Stewart, J., Heboyan, V., & De Leo, G. (2019). Interprofessional education among occupational therapy programs: Faculty perceptions of challenges and opportunities. *American Journal of Occupational Therapy, 73*(1), 7301345010p1-7301345010p6. doi:10.5014/ajot.2019.030304

Hussar, W., & Bailey, T. (2017). Projections of education statistics to 2025 (NCES 2017-019). Retrieved from https://nces.ed.gov/pubs2017/2017019.pdf

Institute of Medicine. (2015). *Building health workforce capacity through community-based health professional education: Workshop summary*. Washington, DC: The National Academies Press. doi:10.17226/18973

Kohn, L. T., Corrigan, J., & Donaldson, M. S. (2000). *To err is human: Building a safer health system*. Washington, DC: National Academy Press.

Mitchell, M., Leachman, M., Masterson, K., & Waxman, S. (2018). *Unkept promises: State cuts to higher education threaten access and equity*. Retrieved from https://www.cbpp.org/research/state-budget-and-tax/unkept-promises-state-cuts-to-higher-education-threaten-access-and

NSC Research Center. (2018). *Current term enrollment-Fall, 2018*. Retrieved from https://nscresearchcenter.org/current-term-enrollment-estimates-fall-2018/

Patient Protection and Affordable Care Act, 42 U.S.C. § 18001 (2010).

Reauthorizing the Higher Education Act: Improving College Affordability: Hearing before the Committee on Health, Education, Labor and Pensions, Senate, 115th Cong. (2018).

Sandhu, S., Furniss, J., & Metzler, C. (2018). Using the new postacute care quality measures to demonstrate the value of occupational therapy. *American Journal of Occupational Therapy, 72*(2), 7202090010p1-7202090010p6. doi:10.5014/ajot.2018.722002

Snyder, T., de Brey, C., & Dillow, S. (2018). *Digest of Education Statistics, 2016* (NCES 2017-094). National Center for Education Statistics, Institute of Education Sciences, U.S. Department of Education. Retrieved from https://nces.ed.gov/programs/digest/d16/ch_3.asp

U.S. Bureau of Labor Statistics. (2019). *United States Department of Labor: Employment projections program*. Retrieved from https://www.bls.gov/ooh/healthcare/occupational-therapists.htm#tab-6

Wamble, D., Ciarametaro, M., Houghton, K., Ajmera, M., & Dubois, R. (2019). What's been the bang for the buck? Cost-effectiveness of health care spending across selected conditions in the US. *Health Affairs, 38*(1). doi:10.1377/hlthaff.2018.05158

Financial Disclosures

Dr. Rebecca M. Aldrich has not disclosed any relevant financial relationships.

Dr. Sue Baptiste has no financial or proprietary interest in the materials presented herein.

Dr. Andrea R. Bilics has no financial or proprietary interest in the materials presented herein.

Maria Concepcion Cabatan has no financial or proprietary interest in the materials presented herein.

Dr. Catherine Candler has not disclosed any relevant financial relationships.

Dr. Nancy E. Carson has no financial or proprietary interest in the materials presented herein.

Dr. Susan M. Cleghorn has no financial or proprietary interest in the materials presented herein.

Dr. Susan Coppola has no financial or proprietary interest in the materials presented herein.

Dr. Tina DeAngelis has no financial or proprietary interest in the materials presented herein.

R. Lyle Duque has no financial or proprietary interest in the materials presented herein.

Dr. Amy R. Early has no financial or proprietary interest in the materials presented herein.

Dr. Maria Luísa Guillaumon Emmel has not disclosed any relevant financial relationships.

Dr. Mirela de Oliveira Figueiredo has no financial or proprietary interest in the materials presented herein.

Dr. Roshan Galvaan has no financial or proprietary interest in the materials presented herein.

Dr. Amanda K. Giles has no financial or proprietary interest in the materials presented herein.

Dr. Lenin C. Grajo has no financial or proprietary interest in the materials presented herein.

Dr. Sharon A. Gutman has no financial or proprietary interest in the materials presented herein.

Dr. Neil Harvison has no financial or proprietary interest in the materials presented herein.

Dr. Susan M. Higgins has no financial or proprietary interest in the materials presented herein.

Dr. Barbara R. Hooper has no financial or proprietary interest in the materials presented herein.

Dr. William E. Janes has no financial or proprietary interest in the materials presented herein.

Dr. Sheama Krishnagiri has no financial or proprietary interest in the materials presented herein.

Dr. Giulianne Krug has no financial or proprietary interest in the materials presented herein.

Dr. Wanda J. Mahoney has no financial or proprietary interest in the materials presented herein.

Dr. Daniel Marinho Cezar da Cruz has no financial or proprietary interest in the materials presented herein.

Dr. Lauren E. Milton has no financial or proprietary interest in the materials presented herein.

Dr. Matthew Molineux has no financial or proprietary interest in the materials presented herein.

Dr. Jaime P. Muñoz has no financial or proprietary interest in the materials presented herein.

Dr. Monica S. Perlmutter has no financial or proprietary interest in the materials presented herein.

Liesl Peters has no financial or proprietary interest in the materials presented herein.

Dr. Bridgett Piernik-Yoder has no financial or proprietary interest in the materials presented herein.

Dr. Pollie Price has no financial or proprietary interest in the materials presented herein.

Melanie Roberts has no financial or proprietary interest in the materials presented herein.

Dr. Patricia Schaber has no financial or proprietary interest in the materials presented herein.

Dr. Stacy Smallfield has no financial or proprietary interest in the materials presented herein.

Dr. Yolanda Suarez-Balcazar has not disclosed any relevant financial relationships.

Dr. Steven D. Taff has no financial or proprietary interest in the materials presented herein.

Hanneke van Bruggen has no financial or proprietary interest in the materials presented herein.

Lyn Westcott has no financial or proprietary interest in the materials presented herein.

Dr. Hirokazu Yoshikawa has not disclosed any relevant financial relationships.

Index

and context, 121
intentional transfer of, 121
philosophical conceptualization of, 20
knowledge translation delays, 57
Knowles, Malcolm, 47

Lathrop, Julia, 202
Laval University, 166
leadership
fieldwork and, 208
need for, 148
learning
assessment of, 123–124
developing techniques for, 81–83
emotion and motivation sparking, 120
identifying objectives of, 65
lifelong, 59
linked to big ideas, 118–119
maximizing, 122
occupation-centered education mapped to
principles of, 118–124
reflection for, 203
requiring intentional knowledge transfer, 121
requiring practice, 121
as social process, 203
learning capacity, 47
learning environments, flexibility and choice in,
109
learning experience, 204
learning goals, of internationalization, 132
learning management systems, 195
learning outcomes, 204
categories of, 75–76
measurement rubrics for, 87–92
simulation impact on, 66–67
learning paradigms, 49
learning-shaping context, 122–123
learning situations, authenticity of, 121
Lisbon Treaty, Article 45, 172
local service learning, 132
Luther, Jessie, 160

Madagascar, 184–185
MAKER acronym, 178–180
Malaysia
bachelor's program in, 145
profile of occupational therapy education in,
146
managed care, 33
Manitoba University, 164
master's-level programs
in Africa, 184
in Brazil, 155–156
Maturing of the Profession Task Group, 41
McGill University, 165
McMaster University, 165
meaning making activities, 47
medical model, 33
in Canadian OT education, 161–162
medicine, OT relationship with, 23–24
mentorship, 58
metacognitive learning strategies, 47, 48

microlearning, 118
Middle East, employment opportunities in, 147
migration, of Southeast Asian occupational
therapists, 145–147
Minimum Standards for the Education of
Occupational Therapists
2002 version of, 144
2016 version of, 145
minority children, working with, 109
Model of Human Occupation, 185
Montreal University, 165
moral treatment movement, 202
Morocco, 184
motivation, sparking learning, 120
Mpokela, Awonke, 185
Multicultural, Diversity, and Inclusion Network
(MDI), 115
multicultural desires, assessment of, 138
Multicultural Experiences Questionnaire, 138
multidiscipline collaboration
in Brazil, 154
in Canada, 163
mutual accommodations model, 105

National Center for Interprofessional Practice
and Education, 218
National Society for the Promotion of
Occupational Therapy (NSPOT), founding
of, 13
Netherlands, nonrestraint approach in, 170
nonrestraint approach, 170
North Battleford, Saskatchewan, OT
department, 160

occupation
central concept of, 163
as concept unto itself, 119–120
learning as tool for practice, 120–121
learning through one's experiences, 119–120
as medium of change, 117
nature of, 117
occupational science and interdisciplinary
sciences illuminating, 121–122
subconcepts of, 117–118
occupation-based practice, 56, 120–121
occupation-centered education, 117–118
definition of, 117
measuring outcomes of, 76–80, 77
principles of, 118–124
occupational being, 117
occupational revolution, in Southeast Asia, 144
occupational science, 121–122, 163
occupational science partnership, 163
occupational therapist thinking, 117–118
occupational therapy
origins of, 3–4
professional status of, 14, 19–20
occupational therapy books, influencing African
OT education, 188
occupational therapy education
academic preparation in, 15–18
additional requirements for entry into

Printed in the United States
by Baker & Taylor Publisher Services